T0191799

# Bone Health Assessment in Pediatrics

Ellen B. Fung • Laura K. Bachrach
Aenor J. Sawyer
Editors

# Bone Health Assessment in Pediatrics

Guidelines for Clinical Practice

Second Edition

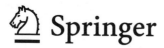 Springer

*Editors*
Ellen B. Fung
UCSF Benioff Children's Hospital Oakland
Children's Hospital Oakland Research
  Institute
Oakland, CA, USA

Laura K. Bachrach
Department of Pediatrics
Stanford University School of Medicine
Stanford, CA, USA

Aenor J. Sawyer
Director, UCSF Skeletal Health Service
Assistant Clinical Professor
Department of Orthopaedic Surgery
University of California
San Francisco

ISBN 978-3-319-80802-4          ISBN 978-3-319-30412-0   (eBook)
DOI 10.1007/978-3-319-30412-0

© Springer International Publishing Switzerland 2007, 2016
Softcover reprint of the hardcover 2nd edition 2016
This work is subject to copyright. All rights are reserved by the Publisher, whether the whole or part of the material is concerned, specifically the rights of translation, reprinting, reuse of illustrations, recitation, broadcasting, reproduction on microfilms or in any other physical way, and transmission or information storage and retrieval, electronic adaptation, computer software, or by similar or dissimilar methodology now known or hereafter developed.
The use of general descriptive names, registered names, trademarks, service marks, etc. in this publication does not imply, even in the absence of a specific statement, that such names are exempt from the relevant protective laws and regulations and therefore free for general use.
The publisher, the authors and the editors are safe to assume that the advice and information in this book are believed to be true and accurate at the date of publication. Neither the publisher nor the authors or the editors give a warranty, express or implied, with respect to the material contained herein or for any errors or omissions that may have been made.

Printed on acid-free paper

This Springer imprint is published by Springer Nature
The registered company is Springer International Publishing AG Switzerland

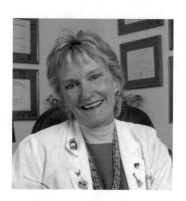

This second edition of Bone Health Assessment in
Pediatrics: Guidelines for Clinical Practice is dedicated to
Dr. Elizabeth Szalay, one of our coauthors and most
respected colleagues who passed away in December 2014.
She was a skilled surgeon, clinician, researcher, and
educator in the field of pediatric orthopedic surgery. She not
only transformed the lives of many children but her warmth,
enthusiasm, and generous mentorship inspired numerous
trainees under her leadership. Dr. Szalay was a devoted
advocate for underserved youth—Native American children,
children with physical disabilities, and those living in
extreme poverty. She worked tirelessly to optimize the
quality of life for her patients and their families. It is with
tremendous respect that her writing is memorialized in this
text. We, among many, are very grateful for her unparalleled
contributions to healthcare.

Ellen B. Fung, Ph.D., R.D., C.C.D.
Laura K. Bachrach, M.D.
Aenor J. Sawyer, M.D.

# Foreword

Over the past 20 years, the high interest in pediatric bone disease and the growing body of knowledge on skeletal development have led to the delineation of a new field where clinicians and investigators devote their efforts to the understanding, evaluation and treatment of bone diseases in children. Great momentum was obtained by the development of new non-invasive technologies, and among them densitometry. Such measurements in adult subjects have for a long time brought about unique information with high precision and reproducibility. Their major limitation however is that density results are expressed in two dimensions and extrapolated to represent volumetric density in a 3D bone structure. This is adequate if the size and shape of the studied bone are stable over time. It clearly does not apply to the bones of a growing child wheresize and shape change continuously until growth plates are fused. Thus two-dimensional DXA results had to be adapted to reflect this reality. This challenge has been met as described in details in the first chapters of this book. Interpretation of DXA data using correction parameters to take into account age, sex and body size have generated graphs and tables that are now integral parts of the evaluation of various conditions where bone development and structure are affected. As progress was made, new techniques have emerged that allow for three-dimensional imaging such as QCT, pQCT and HR-pQCT. Now trabecular and cortical bone compartments can be analyzed separately and bone formation evaluated with precision. It may become the equivalent of a non-invasive bone biopsy. Changes in cortical porosity, not captured by DXA will become an important end point in several studies. The only limitation of HR-pQCT is that it can only evaluate appendicular sites due to the amount of irradiation it generates and the design of the equipment. But this also may change in the future. All these considerations and more are covered in details in this Second Edition of *Bone Health Assessment in Pediatrics: Guidelines for Clinical Practice*. As such it represents an indispensable source of information and guidance for any clinician dealing with pediatric bone diseases.

Montreal, QC, Canada                                      Francis H. Glorieux, OC, MD, PhD

# Preface

Eight years ago, we published the textbook *Bone Densitometry in Growing Patients* to assist clinicians in evaluating bone health in children and adolescents. Since 2007, the field of pediatric bone densitometry has changed dramatically. Despite the emergence of alternative imaging devices, dual energy x-ray absorptiometry (DXA) remains the gold standard method for skeletal assessments in clinical practice. As such, we felt it was important to address some of the changes and new directions in the field with the second edition of the text, slightly modified in title to: *Bone Health Assessment in Pediatrics: Guidelines for Clinical Practice.*

Skeletal health determined in childhood and adolescence influences an individual's lifetime risk of bone fragility. Peak bone mass reached by early adulthood represents the "bone bank" for life. For this reason, optimizing bone acquisition in the first two decades can help prevent osteoporosis. As this awareness of the importance of early bone health has grown over the past decade, so has the concern for young patients facing threats to bone acquisition. These observations have led to greater demands for diagnostic and therapeutic tools to address bone fragility in children and adolescents.

Many of the chapter authors in this text have spent the past decade improving the ability to accurately assess pediatric bone health by DXA through the collection of, large and robust, ethnic-specific reference data sets. Moreover in October, 2013, many of these same individuals came together for the 2nd Pediatric Position Development Conference to draft what are now the 2013 International Society for Clinical Densitometry (ISCD) Guidelines for Pediatric DXA assessment, interpretation, and reporting. As part of these guidelines, a new definition of osteoporosis in pediatrics was adopted, and the relationship between DXA and fracture prediction clarified.

With all marked changes in the field since the last edition of this text, it was difficult to limit the discussion to 13 short chapters. Those that are included were considered to be the most relevant to the practicing pediatrician. Some of the highlights of this edition include an entire chapter on the assessment of infants and toddlers, a chapter devoted to the assessment of children with disabling conditions, an in-depth discussion of vertebral fracture and its etiologies, and a thorough review of the advantages and limitations of densitometry techniques including DXA, pQCT, HRpQCT, and MRI. New fracture prediction software including Trabecular Bone Score and Finite Element Analysis are described. In this edition, the limitations of DXA are addressed as are the most recent strategies for handling them including proposed DXA adjustments such as height Z-score. Our overarching goal is to provide the basic analysis and evaluation tools necessary for clinicians to optimize bone health for all children especially those with skeletal fragility.

This second edition is designed to provide distilled but multidimensional perspectives needed by clinicians interested in bone health. It is anticipated that those who work with the most challenging patients need practical guidance on how to measure and report on their bone health. Given that DXA will likely remain the recommended clinical method to clinically monitor bone health for the foreseeable future, this text can provide useful tools, images, and calculations necessary to be successful.

Oakland, CA, USA                                                                Ellen B. Fung
Palo Alto, CA, USA                                                            Laura K. Bachrach
San Francisco, CA, USA                                                        Aenor J. Sawyer

# Acknowledgments

This book is the culmination of work from dedicated experts in the field of pediatric densitometry. First and foremost we owe our deepest gratitude to the chapter authors who took time out of their busy schedules to share their knowledge and expertise in this second edition of *Bone Health Assessment in Pediatrics: Guidelines for Clinical Practice*.

It has been an honor and pleasure to work with many of these authors for a second time. It has also been truly inspiring to engage with the rising stars in this field who are new contributors to this text. The authors' commitment to this work over the past 18 months, despite many professional and personal demands, reflects their deep dedication to improving the skeletal health of all children and adults.

We are grateful for the enduring support and invaluable input from our mentors: Mary Bouxsein, Roland Fischer, Francis Glorieux, Paul Harmatz, James Kasser, Janet King, Mary Leonard, Bertram Lubin, Robert Marcus, Dolores Shoback, Virginia Stallings, Thomas P. Vail, Elliott Vichinsky, Babette Zemel, and our tireless colleagues Richard Capra, Lisa Calvelli, and Marcela Weyhmiller.

In the publishing arena, we thank Michael Griffin, our copy editor, for his patience and endurance with this text, as well as Richard Lansing from Springer Publishing Group for his foresight to consider a second edition of this unique text.

Despite all of the resources, talent, and commitment, we would not have been able to make this second edition a reality without generous support and sponsorship. We would like to thank the S.D. Bechtel Jr. Foundation, the major sponsor of this project and a decade of research and education in the Pediatric Bone Health Consortium. Last, but certainly not least, we are deeply indebted to our families for their patience, support, and unconditional love. We ask for their forgiveness for the many distracted evenings in front of the computer when we could have spent more focused time with them. They provide each of us the creativity, strength, and encouragement on a daily basis, without which we would not have had the inspiration or energy needed to accomplish this work.

Ellen B. Fung, Ph.D., R.D., C.C.D.
Laura K. Bachrach, M.D.
Aenor J. Sawyer, M.D.

# Contents

# Contributors

**Judith E. Adams, M.B.B.S., F.R.C.R., F.R.C.P.** Radiology & Manchester Academic Health Science Centre, Central Manchester University Hospitals NHS Foundation Trust, University of Manchester, Manchester, Lancashire, UK

**Laura K. Bachrach, M.D.** Department of Pediatrics, Stanford University School of Medicine, Stanford, CA, USA

**Maria Luisa Bianchi, M.D.** Experimental Laboratory for Children's Bone Metabolism Research, Bone Metabolism Unit, Istituto Auxologico Italiano IRCCS, Milan, Italy

**Teresa L. Binkley, Ph.D.** EA Martin Program, South Dakota State University, North Brookings, SD, USA

**Nicola J. Crabtree, Ph.D.** Department of Endocrinology, Birmingham Children's Hospital, Birmingham, West Midlands, UK

**Ellen B. Fung, Ph.D., R.D., C.C.D.** UCSF Benioff Children's Hospital, Oakland, CA, USA

**Catherine M. Gordon, M.D., M.Sc.** Division of Adolescent and Transition Medicine, Cincinnati Children's Hospital Medical Center, University of Cincinnati College of Medicine, Cincinnati, OH, USA

**H. Theodore Harcke, M.D., F.A.C.R., F.A.I.U.M.** Department of Medical Imaging, Nemours/A.I. duPont Hospital for Children, Wilmington, DE, USA

**Heidi J. Kalkwarf, Ph.D.** Gastroenterology, Hepatology and Nutrition, Cincinnati Children's Hospital, Cincinnati, OH, USA

**Tony M. Keavney, Ph.D.** Mechanical Engineering and Bioengineering, University of California, Berkeley, CA, USA

**Heidi H. Kecskemethy, M.S.Ed., R.D.N., C.S.P., C.B.D.T.** Departments of Biomedical Research and Medical Imaging, Nemours/A.I. duPont Hospital for Children, Wilmington, DE, USA

**Kyla Kent, B.A., C.B.D.T.** Stanford School of Medicine, Palo Alto, CA, USA

**Mary B. Leonard, M.D., M.S.C.E.** Department of Pediatrics, Stanford University School of Medicine, Stanford, CA, USA

**Thomas M. Link, M.D., Ph.D.** Department of Radiology and Biomedical Imaging, UCSF, San Francisco, CA, USA

**Jinhui Ma, Ph.D.** School of Epidemiology, Public Health and Preventive Medicine, University of Ottawa, Children's Hospital of Eastern Ontario Research Institute, Ottawa, ON, Canada

**Heather M. Macdonald, Ph.D.** Department of Family Practice and Centre for Hip Health and Mobility, University of British Columbia, Vancouver, BC, Canada

**Sharmila Majumdar, Ph.D.** University of California, San Francisco, CA, USA

**Heather A. McKay, Ph.D.** Departments of Orthopaedics and Family Practice, Centre for Hip Health and Mobility, Vancouver, BC, Canada

**M. Zulf Mughal, M.B., Ch.B., F.R.C.P.** Department of Paediatric Endocrinology, Royal Manchester Children's Hospital, Manchester, UK

**Sarah Pitts, M.D.** Divisions of Adolescent Medicine and Endocrinology, Harvard Medical School, Boston Children's Hospital, Boston, MA, USA

**Luis Del Rio, M.D., C.C.D.** Department of Bone Densitometry, Hospital Sant Joan De Deu, Barcelona, Spain

**Aenor J. Sawyer, M.D., M.S.** Director, UCSF Skeletal Health Service, Assistant Clinical Professor, Department of Orthopaedic Surgery, University of California, San Francisco

**Oliver Semler, M.D.** Department of Rare Skeletal Disease, Children's Hospital, University of Cologne, Cologne, Germany

**John Shepherd, Ph.D.** Department of Radiology and Biomedical Imaging, University of California, San Francisco, CA, USA

**Bonny L. Specker, Ph.D.** EA Martin Program, South Dakota State University, North Brookings, SD, USA

**Elizabeth Szalay, M.D.** (Deceased) Pediatric Orthopedic Surgery, Carrie Tingley Hospital, University of New Mexico, Albuquerque, NM, USA

**Kate A. Ward, Ph.D.** MRC Human Nutrition Research, Cambridge, Cambridge CB1 9NL and MRC Lifecourse Epidemiology Unit, University of Southampton, Southampton, UK

**Leanne M. Ward, M.D., F.A.A.P., F.R.C.P.C.** Division of Endocrinology and Metabolism, Department of Pediatrics, Children's Hospital of Eastern Ontario, University of Ottawa, Ottawa, ON, Canada

**Amanda T. Whitaker, M.D.** Department of Orthopaedic Surgery, Boston Children's Hospital, Boston, MA, USA

**Renaud Winzenrieth, Ph.D.** Research and Development Department, Medimaps SASU, Merignac, France

**Babette S. Zemel, Ph.D.** Department of Pediatrics, The Children's Hospital of Philadelphia, Philadelphia, PA, USA

# Chapter 1
# Rationale for Bone Health Assessment in Childhood and Adolescence

Maria Luisa Bianchi, Aenor J. Sawyer, and Laura K. Bachrach

## Introduction

Skeletal health in childhood and adolescence influences the lifetime risk of bone fragility. Peak bone mass (PBM) reached by early adulthood serves at the "bone bank" for life. For this reason, optimizing bone acquisition in the first two decades can help prevent osteoporosis. As awareness of the importance of early bone health has grown, so has concern for young patients facing threats to bone acquisition. This concern has led to increased use of bone densitometry in children and adolescents. Dual energy x-ray absorptiometry (DXA) is the recommended method for clinical use because of its speed, safety, precision, availability, and robust normative pediatric data. Although a valuable tool, DXA can be challenging to interpret in growing patients who represent a moving target for study. Variability in patterns of growth and maturity, particularly in children with chronic disease, must be considered when interpreting DXA findings. The goal of this book is to serve as a resource

M.L. Bianchi, M.D. (✉)
Experimental Laboratory for Children's Bone Metabolism Research, Bone Metabolism Unit, Istituto Auxologico Italiano IRCCS, via L. Ariosto 13, 20145 Milan, Italy
e-mail: ml.bianchi@auxologico.it

A.J. Sawyer, M.D., M.S.
Director, UCSF Skeletal Health Service, Assistant Clinical Professor,
Department of Orthopaedic Surgery, University of California, San Francisco

L.K. Bachrach, M.D.
Department of Pediatrics, Stanford University School of Medicine,
300 Pasteur Drive, Stanford, CA 94305-5208, USA
e-mail: lkbach@stanford.edu

© Springer International Publishing Switzerland 2016
E.B. Fung et al. (eds.), *Bone Health Assessment in Pediatrics*,
DOI 10.1007/978-3-319-30412-0_1

for those acquiring, interpreting, reporting, and utilizing densitometry in pediatric patients. DXA and newer 3-dimensional densitometry techniques (quantitative computed tomography, peripheral QCT, and high-resolution pQCT) are discussed in detail.

This chapter underscores the importance of optimizing PBM to reduce the risk of osteoporosis. The positive and negative factors influencing early bone health are reviewed. Finally, the strengths and limitations of DXA in the clinical management of children at risk for bone fragility are outlined.

## Bone Mineral Accrual

Childhood and adolescence are critical periods for establishing lifetime bone health. During the growing years, bones increase in length, width, and cortical thickness. Increases in bone mass (bone mineral content, BMC) and areal bone mineral density (aBMD) accompany these geometric changes. Gains in bone size and mass are most dramatic during adolescence and slow at the end of the second decade as bones reach their adult size and shape. Final consolidation of bone mineral occurs later and PBM is reached early in the third decade. From birth to adulthood, there is about a 40-fold increase in bone mass [1–4].

Two biologically similar but separate cellular processes direct skeletal development mediated by the bone-building osteoblasts and the bone-resorbing osteoclasts [5]. Bone modeling occurs only during the growing years prior to closure of the epiphyseal plates. Bone resorption and formation occur simultaneously or sequentially at different locations, in response to the various stimuli inducing and controlling bone growth and maturation. Bone modeling results in changes in bone size, shape, and mass. Bone remodeling, by contrast, is the process of bone turnover and maintenance which continues throughout life. With bone remodeling, bone resorption and formation occur at the same location without altering bone shape. Bone remodeling serves to replace old or damaged bone with new, healthy bone, thus repairing microfractures and preserving the tissue's mechanical properties. Remodeling also has a major role in the maintenance of the body's calcium homeostasis [5, 6].

Both cross-sectional and longitudinal studies have examined the tempo and patterns of skeletal growth and development [7–11]. Gender-related differences become manifest during puberty. The onset of puberty and peak height velocity occurs at an earlier age in girls, while the duration and magnitude of the pubertal growth spurt are greater in boys. Males eventually achieve a higher bone mass and density than females at both lumbar spine and femoral neck, but their peak values are reached at an older age [9, 11, 12]. In a longitudinal study of over 220 Canadian children aged 8–14 years, peak BMC velocity was reached at 12.5±0.9 years in females and 14±1 years in males; peak height velocity preceded peak BMC velocity by approximately 6 months [13]. The dissociation between linear growth and bone mass accrual may partially explain the increased rate of forearm fractures that is observed in girls aged 8–12 years and in boys aged 10–14 years [14, 15].

Kirmani et al. studied the changes in micro-architecture and strength at the ultra-distal radius through adolescence with pQCT [16]. Cortical thickness and density decreased from pre- to mid-puberty in girls (but not in boys), then rose to higher levels at the end of puberty in both sexes. Total bone strength increased linearly in both sexes, and after mid-puberty was higher in boys than in girls. The ratio of cortical to trabecular bone volume decreased transiently during mid- to late puberty in both sexes, with cortical porosity at its greatest. These changes would result in a transient reduction in cortical bone strength during mid-puberty which might explain the peak incidence of forearm fractures occurring at this age [16].

An estimated 40–60 % of adult bone mass is accrued during adolescence, with over 25 % of these gains accrued during the 2 years of peak skeletal growth. In both genders, about 90 % of PBM is accrued by 18 years of age with the remaining 10 % in the skeletal consolidation phase during the third decade [11, 17, 18]. About 85 % of the adult bone mass is cortical bone and 15 % is trabecular bone. Changes in these two bone compartments differ during periods of bone accrual and subsequent bone loss with aging [19]. PBM appears to be complete by the end of the second decade in the axial skeleton, which consists of mostly trabecular bone; PBM is achieved some time later in the appendicular skeleton, comprised primarily of cortical bone [20]. The peak density of trabecular bone is strongly influenced by the hormonal and metabolic factors associated with sexual maturation while mineral acquisition of cortical bone is slower [21]. Although the pattern of skeletal development follows these general timelines, the evolution of bone mass/density is subject to great individual variability.

## Determinants of Bone Acquisition and Peak Bone Mass

Bone mineral accrual and PBM are influenced by both heritable and modifiable factors as detailed below. Reaching one's genetic potential requires adequate nutrition, activity, and hormone production. Illness, prescribed medications (corticosteroids, anticonvulsants, etc.), and life habits (alcohol, tobacco, etc.) constitute additional influences [22, 23].

### Heritability

Genetic factors account for an estimated 60–80 % of the PBM variance as shown in studies of twins and parent/child pairs [24–26]. For example, one observational study of over 400 family participants reported a 3.8-fold increase in a son's likelihood of low bone density if his father had low bone density. The daughter's risk was increased 5.1-fold if her mother had low bone density [27].

The specific genes responsible for determining bone size and mass and the risk of osteoporosis have not yet been identified with certainty [28–31]. Polymorphisms in the vitamin D receptor (VDR) gene, estrogen receptor alpha (ESR1) gene, type I collagen A1 chain (*COL1A1*) genes have been associated with BMD, BMC, and fracture risk but each explains only 1–3 % of the variability in PBM. Genes encoding transforming growth factor-1 (TGF-1), apolipoprotein E, and low-density lipoprotein receptor-related protein-5 (*LRP5*) have also been investigated [32–35]. A large-scale meta-analysis of the genome-wide association studies (GWAS) found that 20 gene loci were associated with BMD but these genes contributed for only 2–3 % of the inter-individual variability of BMD [36].

## Modifiable Factors

An estimated 20–40 % of variability in PBM can be explained by modifiable factors such as nutrition and activity. Consequently, the achievement of an individual's full genetic potential of PBM can be influenced by these factors [37, 38]. The fact that the PBM is established in the first two decades of life underscores the importance of early lifestyle on bone health. Osteoporosis can be viewed as a disease of older adults with its roots early in life [39–41]. Bone health appears to begin in utero with calcium transport across the placenta to the fetus. Maternal serum concentration of 25(OH)-D is positively associated with the infant's bone mass at birth [42]. Birth weight, an indicator of healthy fetal development, is associated with bone mass in both early and late adulthood [43]. Conversely, poor early growth has been related to a higher risk of hip fracture in later life [44]. The Southampton Women's Survey [45], a prospective study of over 12,500 initially nonpregnant women aged 20–34 years and their children, has confirmed the importance of early bone health. To date, about 1000 children have been studied by DXA at birth, 4, and 6 years. The results confirm the hypothesis that "there may be critical periods where growth velocity relates very strongly to longer-term measures of bone development, thus offering potential opportunities for early intervention to optimize skeletal strength" [41]. Another mother-offspring cohort study found that fetal weight gain and post-natal catch-up in weight were associated with total-body BMD measured at 6 months of age. Children who remained in the lowest weight tertile after birth were much more likely to have low total-body BMD at 6 months of age [46].

### Nutrition

Calcium

Calcium is a key nutrient for skeletal health throughout life, allowing for optimal gains in bone mass during the growing years and reducing bone loss in later life [10, 47]. Calcium appears to be a threshold nutrient with skeletal mass increasing as calcium intake increases until a plateau is reached at which gains are constant. Defining the calcium "threshold" for children of varying ages remains controversial [48]. Estimates of the requirement for calcium come from studies of calcium balance, mineral accrual, and

**Table 1.1** Calcium and Vitamin D—dietary reference intakes

| Age | Calcium RDA[b] (mg/d) | UL[c] (mg/d) | Vitamin D[a] RDA[b] (IU/d) | UL[c] (IU/d) |
|---|---|---|---|---|
| 0–6 months | (200)[d] | 1000 | (400)[d] | 1000 |
| 6–12 months | (260)[d] | 1500 | (400)[d] | 1500 |
| 1–3 years | 700 | 2500 | 600 | 2500 |
| 4–8 years | 1000 | 2500 | 600 | 3000 |
| 9–13 years | 1300 | 3000 | 600 | 4000 |
| 14–18 years | 1300 | 3000 | 600 | 4000 |
| 19–30 years | 1000 | 2500 | 600 | 4000 |
| Females—Pregnancy and Lactation | | | | |
| 14–18 years | 1300 | 3000 | 600 | 4000 |
| 19–30 years | 1000 | 2500 | 600 | 4000 |

*Table adapted from*: A. C. Ross, C. L. Taylor, A. L. Yaktine, and H. B. Del Valle, *Editors;* Committee to Review Dietary Reference Intakes for Vitamin D and Calcium Food and Nutrition Board; Institute of Medicine. *Dietary Reference Intakes for Calcium and Vitamin D.* Washington, DC: The National Academies Press 2011 (ISBN 978-0-309-16394-1 available in PDF from The National Academies Press at *http://www.nap.edu/catalog.php?record_id=13050*) (page 7 and 9)
[a]Vitamin D: 40 International Units (IU)=1 μg
[b]RDA=Recommended Dietary Allowance: daily intake meeting or exceeding the requirements for 97.5 % of population
[c]UL=Tolerable Upper Intake Level: the highest average daily intake that is likely to pose no risk of adverse effects to almost all individuals in the general population
[d]RDAs have not been established for infants: this value is an adequate average intake (AI) based on observed or experimental intakes

fractures. In 2011, the Institute of Medicine published updated dietary reference intakes for calcium and vitamin D (see Table 1.1) [49], which were subsequently endorsed by the American Academy of Pediatrics [47]. During the critical period for bone acquisition from age 9 to 18, the recommended daily calcium intake is 1300 mg.

Despite persistent controversies about the optimal calcium intake, it is evident that calcium intake before and during puberty can contribute to the maximization of PBM within an individual's genetically determined potential. Several observational studies of children and adolescents in different countries have demonstrated an association between habitual calcium intake and BMC and/or BMD [48, 50–53]. A large, retrospective study of older, white American women also found that a higher milk intake during childhood and adolescence was associated with higher BMC and reduced fracture risk in adulthood [54]. Contrary to previous concerns, a calcium-rich diet in childhood has been linked to a reduced rather than increased mortality in adulthood from stroke [55].

The positive effects of calcium on height and BMC/BMD have also been supported by findings from several prospective randomized placebo-controlled trials [9, 56–58]. The skeletal effects have varied with the amount and source of calcium supplement, the skeletal region, and the age and maturity of the child [48, 57, 58]. Gains are greater at sites rich in cortical (appendicular skeleton) rather than trabecular bone (spine) [48].

Two meta-analyses have similarly confirmed the benefits of calcium supplementation and dairy products on bone mass during growth [59, 60]. The first one summarized 21 randomized controlled trials including 3821 subjects (aged 4–17.3 years) and found that greater calcium intake, with or without vitamin D, significantly increased total body and lumbar spine BMC in children with low intake at baseline [59]. The second one analyzed 19 randomized controlled trials including 2859 subjects (aged 3–18 years) and reported a small, positive effect of calcium supplementation (300–1200 mg/day) for total body BMC and upper limb BMD [60].

Whether the benefits from calcium supplementation are sustained after discontinuation is also controversial. Some studies have detected benefits for one or more years [9, 61] while other data suggest that the effects are lost soon after discontinuation [48]. A meta-analysis of several studies found that benefits of calcium supplementation persisted only at the upper limb [60].


Phosphorus

Despite the fact that phosphate makes up at least half of bone mineral mass, there is less concern about this nutrient in pediatrics. Phosphorus deficiency is rare because the element is abundant in common foods. In fact, concerns have been raised about overconsumption of phosphorus especially from soft drink consumption. Wyshak et al. found that the incidence of fractures in adolescent girls was correlated with the amount of carbonated beverages consumed [62]. The association between soft drinks and poor bone health is perhaps more likely explained by displacement of milk from diet than by high phosphorus intake [63]. A meta-analysis of 88 studies found an inverse relationship between soda consumption and intake of milk [64].


Vitamin D

Vitamin D is essential for efficient absorption of calcium. Only 10–15 % of dietary calcium is absorbed without vitamin D [65]. With few exceptions (oily fish), natural foods are not a significant source of vitamin $D_2$ (ergocalciferol) or $D_3$ (cholecalciferol). In some countries milk and other foods are fortified with vitamin D while in others, only infants and small children are routinely provided with supplemented products.

The essential role of vitamin D for bone health has been demonstrated by several studies. A longitudinal study of 198 children observed that when mothers had low levels of 25-hydroxyvitamin D (25OHD) during the late months of pregnancy, the children had low total-body and spine BMC at 9 years of age [42]. A 3-year longitudinal study of 171 healthy Finnish girls aged 9–15 years found that girls with severe vitamin D deficiency during puberty may fail to achieve their genetic potential for PBM, particularly at lumbar spine [66].

Vitamin D deficiency is relatively common, particularly in northern countries, in dark-skinned individuals, and in those with inadequate exposure to sunlight. Levels of 25OHD below 30 nmol/L [12 ng/ml] have been observed during winter and spring in up to 50% of children living in Denmark, Finland, Poland, Greece, Germany, and Switzerland [66–71]. Vitamin D deficiency is more common in black and Hispanic teenagers, and in winter [65–74]. Obese children and adolescents are also at increased risk, possibly due to vitamin D sequestration in body fat [74–76]. Milder forms of vitamin D deficiency are typically asymptomatic but may still compromise optimal bone growth and mineralization. Vitamin D deficiency, not sufficiently severe to cause rickets, may also lead to secondary hyperparathyroidism.

Severe vitamin D deficiency (serum 25OHD below 15 nmol/L [6 ng/ml]) causes nutritional rickets in children and osteomalacia in adults. Low intestinal calcium absorption and secondary hyperparathyroidism lead to defective mineralization of growth plates and bones, with bone deformities and high risk of fractures. Fortification of infant foods with vitamin D has greatly reduced the incidence of rickets during the first 2 years of life in developed countries [17] but this condition remains a major health problem where vitamin-D–fortified foods are not available. Severe vitamin D deficiency is also associated with reduced bone mass in adolescents [73, 77]. A prospective study of 6712 physically active girls (age 9–15 years) found that greater intake of vitamin D (not calcium or dairy foods) during childhood was associated with reduced risk of stress fractures [78].

## Protein

Adequate protein intake is necessary to build the bone matrix. Proteins also influence the secretion and action of insulin-like growth factor 1 (IGF-1), an osteogenic hormone needed to achieve optimal PBM. Inadequate protein intake adversely affects bone mass acquisition [79, 80]. A study by Chevalley et al. showed a positive correlation between protein intake and both BMC and BMD in pre-pubertal boys. With high protein intake, greater physical activity was associated with greater BMC at both axial and appendicular sites [81]. On the contrary, children with inadequate protein and caloric intake exhibited growth retardation and decreased formation of cortical bone [82].

The optimal type and quantity of protein for bone health remain to be determined [83, 84]. Milk and dairy products are probably the best sources of the calcium and proteins for bone health. Alternative sources of calcium include some vegetables, tofu, and almonds [85]. Long-term milk avoidance is associated with shorter height and lower BMC and aBMD [86–88]. Pre-pubertal children with low milk intake may be at greater risk of fractures, mainly of the distal radius [89, 90]. A 7-year study found regular intake of dairy products to be positively associated with hip and spine aBMD and greater total and cortical area at the proximal radius [91].

## Exercise

The skeleton and muscles are interrelated in a more complex way than simple locomotion. According to the "mechanostat" model of bone growth and bone loss, muscle activity and weight load (gravity) continuously apply forces to the skeleton [92, 93]. The resulting strains stimulate bone modeling and remodeling. Throughout life, the bone's cellular and biochemical reaction to mechanical strains translates into a continuous adaptation in terms of both bone mass and bone architecture that maintains and optimizes bone strength. Osteocytes imbedded in bone act as mechanosensors, transmitting signals to osteoblasts to build bone [94, 95]. Not surprisingly, muscle mass and strength are important predictors of bone strength [96–99] and conversely, prolonged immobilization and skeletal unloading lead to bone loss [100].

Regular physical activity is a major determinant of the accrual and maintenance of PBM. The type, intensity, frequency, and duration of exercise are all important. Dynamic loading seems more effective than static loading and the magnitude of the strain on bone may be more important than the number of repetitions [101]. Two observational studies of adolescent gymnasts found they had sustained increases in both BMC and aBMD [102, 103]. Several randomized controlled studies in children and adolescents reported positive effects from jumping and other high-impact activities [102–111]. Gains in hip BMC were 3.6 % greater in prepubertal children who completed a 7-month high-impact jumping program than in controls who completed non-impact stretching activities. Significant differences between the groups persisted even after 8 years (1.4 %, $p < 0.05$) [106]. A review of 22 intervention trials in children and adolescents concluded that physical activity had significant positive effects on bone, and weight-bearing exercise may enhance bone mineral gain in children, particularly during early puberty [112].

The sustained benefits of activity are mediated at least in part through changes in bone geometry. A systematic review of 14 intervention and 23 observational studies evaluated the effect of physical activity on bone structure (cross-sectional area, cortical thickness) as well as mass. Results indicated that changes in bone structure rather than bone mass were most often related to significant increase in bone strength. Prepuberty and peripuberty may be the best periods for improving bone strength through physical activity in both sexes [113].

There appear to be additive or even synergistic effects from various lifestyle factors. For example, one study found that physical activity enhanced the response to calcium supplementation at weight-bearing sites [107]. Conversely, gains from physical activity may be blunted in individuals who have inadequate intake of calcium or calories [114].

## Importance of Peak Bone Mass

PBM is recognized as a key determinant of bone health and fracture risk in adulthood and old age. After early adulthood, BMC and BMD remain stable and then inevitably decline with menopause and aging. With enough bone loss, a "bone fragility" threshold is reached where fractures are more likely. Factors that enhance early bone accrual or slow the subsequent bone loss may help reduce the risk of osteoporosis (Fig. 1.1).

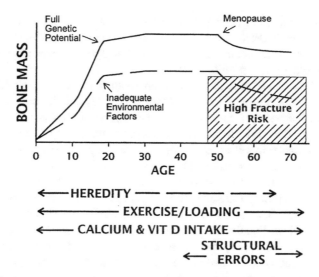

**Fig. 1.1** Diagrammatic representation of the bone mass life-line in individuals who achieve their full genetic potential for skeletal mass and in those who do not. (The magnitude of the difference between the curves is not intended to be to scale.) Along the bottom of the graph are arrayed several of the factors known to be of particular importance. (© Robert P. Heaney 1999, used with permission.) From: Heaney RP, Abrams S, Dawson-Hughes B, Looker A, Marcus R, Matkovic V, Weaver C. Peak bone mass. Osteoporosis Int 2000;11:985–1009

In older adults, the risk of fracture doubles for each standard deviation (SD) that BMD falls below the healthy young adult mean value. An intervention that results in a 10 % increase in PBM in youth (+1 SD in BMD) could thus reduce an individual's future fracture risk by 50 % [18, 23]. The magnitude of benefit from increasing PBM bone or reducing subsequent bone loss has been modeled [115]: a 10 % increase in PBM would delay by 13 years the time a woman meets criteria for osteoporosis (a BMD value of 2.5 SD or more below the young adult mean). By contrast, postponing the age at menopause or reducing the rate of age-related bone loss would delay osteoporosis by less than 2 years. In summary, optimization of nutrition and activity during childhood and adolescence can be viewed as an important and effective strategy to prevent or delay osteoporosis.

## Threats to Pediatric Bone Health

The expected gains in bone mass and geometry described above can be compromised by a number of heritable or acquired disorders as discussed in more detail in Chap. 4 [17, 116, 117]. Osteogenesis imperfecta (OI), the most common of the genetic disorders of bone, is characterized by increased bone fragility due to reduction in the quantity or quality of type 1 collagen caused by mutations in the *COL1A1* and *COL1A2* genes [118]. Loss of function mutations in the low-density lipoprotein receptor-related protein 5 (*LRP5*) gene result in reduced bone formation and low bone mass (as seen in osteoporosis-pseudoglioma syndrome) [119]. High bone mineral density syndromes including osteopetrosis and pychnodysostosis are also associated with greater bone fragility [120].

The diverse causes of secondary osteoporosis share one or more skeletal risk factors [116, 117]. For example, Crohn disease [121, 122] and the rheumatologic disorders [123] are marked by chronic inflammation, undernutrition, reduced mobility, and exposure to osteotoxic drugs. In cerebral palsy and Duchenne muscular dystrophy (DMD), reduced mobility results in narrower long bones with thinner cortices that are more vulnerable to fracture [124, 125]. In DMD, glucocorticoid therapy and delayed puberty increase the risk of vertebral fracture. Children with malignancy [126, 127] or undergoing transplantation [127, 128] are vulnerable to fracture during treatment with chemotherapy, radiation, or immunosuppression; hormone deficiencies may follow. Finally, the improved survival in patients with cystic fibrosis [129] and thalassemia [130] has been complicated by diabetes, hypogonadism, undernutrition, and reduced exercise capacity. Depending upon age at onset and disease severity, these chronic conditions can impair bone growth and mineral acquisition with or without secondary bone loss. The potential for recovery from these skeletal complications depends upon the course of the acquired disease and the age of the patient.

Even apparently healthy children and teens with a history of low-trauma forearm fractures appear to be at increased risk for future bone fragility. When compared with children without a history of forearm fracture, children who fracture have lower bone mass, increased body fat, and less physical activity [131]. They have been shown to have a greater incidence of future fracture not only during childhood [131] but as adults as well [132].

Bone densitometry is an important tool to monitor the skeletal effects of these genetic and acquired disorders. Specific indications for ordering a bone density study for patients with these conditions are discussed in detail in Chap. 4. The International Society of Clinical Densitometry (ISCD) Position Development Conference (PDC), a working group of pediatric bone experts, generated comprehensive guidelines for DXA use in 2007 [133]. These guidelines were revised in 2013 to recommend that densitometry be considered when the patient might benefit from intervention and when the densitometry results would influence management [134].

# Densitometry as a Diagnostic Tool

Bone densitometry was developed as a noninvasive means to assess skeletal status and aid in identifying patients at greatest risk for fracture, ideally before fractures occur. In older adults, densitometry has proven useful in predicting fracture risk, thus guiding clinical management. In fact, low BMD is sufficiently linked to the likelihood of fracture in post-menopausal women that it can be used as part of the diagnostic criteria for osteoporosis. Older patients with a BMD that is equal to or more than 2.5 SD below the young adult mean (T score of −2.5) are diagnosed with "osteoporosis." Densitometry results have been combined with clinical variables (including age, height, weight, prior fractures, glucocorticoid use, smoking, alcohol intake, and others) to create a Fracture Risk Assessment Tool (FRAX). FRAX may provide a more precise estimate of the risk that an adult patient will have a hip or other fracture in the next 10 years than DXA alone [135].

Accurately identifying pediatric patients at greatest risk for fracture is especially important because treatment options are limited for younger individuals [116]. However, the interpretation of DXA data is more difficult and its role in fracture prediction less certain than in adults. In part this reflects the challenges of measuring bones that are changing in size, shape, and mass throughout the first two decades of life. The tempo of skeletal development varies among individuals, depending on pubertal development and skeletal maturation, and can be altered by illness. BMD measurements by DXA are 2-dimensional (BMC/bone projection area) and the results are influenced by bone size: this means that, in the presence of equivalent "volumetric" BMD (BMC/bone volume), children with smaller bones will apparently have lower BMD by DXA than children with larger bones [134]. Therefore it is important to account not only for sex, age, and ethnicity, but also for pubertal development, skeletal maturation, and bone size when interpreting BMD, particularly if growth and puberty have been altered by chronic disease. This may include adjustment for height Z-score or for skeletal maturation (bone age) as discussed in more detail in the Chaps. 6 and 7.

The association between bone densitometry and fracture risk in pediatrics is less well established than in adults. Furthermore, there is no established FRAX tool for younger patients to consider the contribution of clinical risk factors. The 2013 ISCD PDC guidelines included a comprehensive review of the current literature linking bone densitometry to pediatric fractures [136]. Most studies to date have explored which DXA parameter(s) best correlated with fractures after low- or moderate-trauma in healthy youth, because fractures are common; 50 % of boys and 30 % of girls will sustain at least one broken bone during childhood and adolescence, most commonly in the upper limb [137]. These studies found that low whole-body BMC or BMD corrected for bone size as well as low bone area for body size, were most strongly correlated with fracture risk [138]. However, even when the best estimates of skeletal mass and size from DXA and pQCT were combined, the predictive value for fractures was limited. The area under the receiver operator curve linking fracture to various densitometry measures ranged from 0.56 to 0.59, distinguishing those with forearm fractures from controls without fractures little better than chance alone [139]. A study using high-resolution pQCT detected alterations in bone microarchitecture associated with an increased risk of low-trauma forearm fractures, suggesting that this newer 3-dimensional methodology may offer more insights into fracture risk [140].

Extrapolating from observations made in healthy youth may not be appropriate for those with chronic illness. Unlike healthy youth who are most likely to sustain upper extremity fractures, children with immobilization disorders such as cerebral palsy or DMD more commonly fracture the lower extremity [141]. For these patients, BMD measured at distal lateral femur is more predictive of fracture than spine BMD. By contrast, younger patients with acute lymphoblastic leukemia (ALL) face a greater risk of vertebral compression fractures. One study found that 16% of patients with ALL had at least one vertebral fracture at diagnosis [142] and an additional 16% sustained an incident spine fracture during the first year of chemotherapy [143]. Spine BMD was highly correlated with fracture risk with an 80% increased odds of vertebral fracture for every SD that spine BMD fell below expected mean for age [143].

After considering the limitations of densitometry to predict pediatric fractures, the 2007 PDC guidelines concluded that "the diagnosis of osteoporosis in children and adolescents should not be made on the basis of densitometry criteria alone" [133]. In 2013, criteria for the diagnosis of osteoporosis were expanded to include a child or teen who sustains one or more vertebral compression fractures without local bone disease or high-energy trauma [134]. Measuring BMD in these patients can add to the assessment but is not required. Alternatively, osteoporosis can be diagnosed in patients with a combination of low bone mass (BMC or BMD more than 2 SD below the mean for age) and a significant fracture history (two or more long bone fractures by age 10 years, or three or more long bone fractures before age 19).

Although a single BMD measurement cannot be used to diagnose osteoporosis in children, densitometry is considered a valuable part of a comprehensive skeletal health assessment. Such an evaluation includes a review of prior chronic illness, medications, nutrition, activity, fracture history, and family history which can help to identify potential risk factors for bone fragility [116]. Recommended laboratory tests include a complete blood count, sedimentation rate, serum calcium, phosphorus, alkaline phosphatase, intact parathyroid hormone, 25OHD, blood urea nitrogen (BUN), creatinine, celiac screen, and urinary calcium to creatinine ratio. In addition, measurement of sex, thyroid, and growth hormones and genetic testing for OI may be indicated depending upon the clinical situation.

## Future Directions for Densitometry

The future role of DXA in the management of pediatric patients appears promising, bolstered by advances in two areas of clinical investigation. Valuable insights have come from studies comparing DXA findings with those using the newer 3-dimensional densitometric techniques (discussed in detail in Chap. 11). Quantitative computed tomography (QCT), peripheral QCT (pQCT), and high-resolution pQCT (HRpQCT) capture elements of bone microstructure, geometry, and volumetric BMD not possible with DXA. These devices can also evaluate the trabecular and cortical compartments of bone separately. QCT, pQCT, and HRpQCT remain largely research tools because of a lack of standardized protocols for acquiring and analyzing scans, cross-calibration problems between devices, and the paucity of normative data. They have been used to investigate the process of skeletal development in both healthy youth and those with chronic illness. Comparisons of the longitudinal changes seen using 2-dimensional DXA with those detected using 3-dimensional tools enhance our interpretation of DXA findings. One study contrasted whole-body BMC and spine BMD using DXA with changes in tibial pQCT parameters 12 months following renal transplantation [144]. Changes in spine BMD correlated with changes in trabecular BMD at the tibia while whole-body BMC Z-scores correlated with tibial cortical area Z-scores. These observations suggest that DXA measures of spine BMD reflect changes in trabecular bone while whole-body BMC reflects cortical bone size but not volumetric density.

The potential for DXA to guide clinical management has also been confirmed from observational studies of pediatric patients requiring chronic glucocorticoid therapy (as described in detail in Chap. 10). Incident vertebral fractures were observed during the first year of steroid treatment in 6 % of those with rheumatologic disorders [145] and 16 % of those with ALL [143]. Children with lower spine BMD at baseline [143] and those who experienced greater decreases in BMD Z-scores during the first 6 months of steroid treatment [145] were more likely to sustain a fracture. As more data are gathered from similar observational studies, it may be possible to predict those patients at high risk for fracture with sufficient certainty to justify trials with bisphosphonates to prevent fracture before a first one occurs.

## Summary

Early skeletal development is a key determinant of lifetime bone strength or fragility. The rationale for optimizing bone acquisition is to reduce the risk of fragility fractures from osteoporosis. DXA will likely remain the recommended tool to monitor bone health in clinical practice for the foreseeable future. DXA's value in managing pediatric patients has been enhanced by improved normative data, guidelines for densitometry use, comparison of findings using DXA and 3-dimensional densitometry techniques, and studies exploring the relationship between DXA and fragility fractures in younger patients.

## Summary Points

- Peak bone mass attained by early adulthood serves as the "bone bank" for life
- Optimizing peak bone mass in childhood and adolescence is an important strategy to reduce the lifetime risk of osteoporosis
- Heritable factors determine 60–80 % of the variability in peak bone mass with hormones and modifiable factors such as diet and activity accounting for the remainder

- The expected gains in bone mass and geometry can be compromised by a number of chronic genetic or acquired disorders in childhood or adolescence
- Bone densitometry is an important tool to assess the skeletal effects of these disorders and DXA is the preferred method for clinical use
- The interpretation of bone densitometry in pediatrics requires consideration of changes in bone size, shape, and mass through the first two decades of life
- Densitometry results from pediatric patients should be compared with age, sex, and ethnicity-matched reference norms to calculate a Z-score. T-scores (using young adult reference norms) should not be used
- Criteria for the diagnosis of osteoporosis in childhood and adolescence include low BMC or BMD for age plus a history of several nonvertebral fractures or a low-trauma vertebral fracture alone.

# References

1. Bonjour JP, Theintz G, Buchs B, Slosman D, Rizzoli R. Critical years and stages of puberty for spinal and femoral bone mass accumulation during adolescence. J Clin Endocrinol Metab. 1991;73:555–63.
2. Faulkner RA, Bailey DA, Drinkwater DT, McKay HA, Arnold C, Wilkinson AA. Bone densitometry in Canadian children 8–17 years of Age. Calcif Tissue Int. 1996;59:344–51.
3. Katzman DK, Bachrach LK, Carter DR, Marcus R. Clinical and anthropometric correlates of bone mineral acquisition in healthy adolescent girls. J Clin Endocrinol Metab. 1991;73:1332–9.
4. Theintz G, Buchs B, Rizzoli R, et al. Longitudinal monitoring of bone mass accumulation in healthy adolescents: evidence for a marked reduction after 16 years of age at the levels of lumbar spine and femoral neck in female subjects. J Clin Endocrinol Metab. 1992;75:1060–5.
5. Glorieux FH, Pettifor JM, Jüppner H, editors. Pediatric bone: biology and diseases. London: Academic; 2012.
6. Bonjour JP, Theintz G, Law F, Slosman D, Rizzoli R. Peak bone mass. Osteoporos Int. 1994;4 Suppl 1:7–13.
7. Bailey DA, McKay HA, Mirwald RL, Crocker PR, Faulkner RA. A six-year longitudinal study of the relationship of physical activity to bone mineral accrual in growing children: the University of Saskatchewan bone mineral accrual study. J Bone Miner Res. 1999;14:1672–9.
8. Bass S, Delmas PD, Pearce G, Hendrich E, Tabensky A, Seeman E. The differing tempo of growth in bone size, mass, and density in girls is region-specific. J Clin Invest. 1999;104:795–804.
9. Chevalley T, Bonjour JP, Ferrari S, Hans D, Rizzoli R. Skeletal site selectivity in the effects of calcium supplementation on areal bone mineral density gain: a randomized, double-blind, placebo-controlled trial in prepubertal boys. J Clin Endocrinol Metab. 2005;90:3342–9.
10. Heaney RP, Abrams S, Dawson-Hughes B, Looker A, Marcus R, Matkovic V, Weaver C. Peak bone mass. Osteoporos Int. 2000;11:985–1009.
11. Bachrach LK. Acquisition of optimal bone mass in childhood and adolescence. Trends Endocrinol Metab. 2001;12:22–8.
12. Bailey DA, Martin AD, McKay HA, Whiting S, Mirwald R. Calcium accretion in girls and boys during puberty: a longitudinal analysis. J Bone Miner Res. 2000;15:2245–50.
13. Whiting SJ, Vatanparast H, Baxter-Jones A, Faulkner RA, Mirwald R, Bailey DA. Factors that affect bone mineral accrual in the adolescent growth spurt. J Nutr. 2004;134:696S–700.
14. Khosla S, Melton III LJ, Dekutoski MB, Achenbach SJ, Oberg AL, Riggs BL. Incidence of childhood distal forearm fractures over 30 years: a population-based study. JAMA. 2003;290:1479–85.

15. Faulkner RA, Davison KS, Bailey DA, Mirwald RL, Baxter-Jones AD. Size corrected BMD decreases during peak linear growth: implications for fracture incidence during adolescence. J Bone Miner Res. 2006;21:1864–70.
16. Kirmani S, Christen D, van Lenthe GH, Fischer PR, Bouxsein ML, McCready LK, Melton 3rd LJ, Riggs BL, Amin S, Müller R, Khosla S. Bone structure at the distal radius during adolescent growth. J Bone Miner Res. 2009;24:1033–42.
17. Bianchi ML. Osteoporosis in children and adolescents. Bone. 2007;41:486–95.
18. Rizzoli R, Bianchi ML, Garabédian M, McKay HA, Moreno LA. Maximizing bone mineral mass gain during growth for the prevention of fractures in the adolescents and the elderly. Bone. 2010;46:294–305.
19. Mora S, Goodman WG, Loro ML, Roe TF, Sayre J, Gilsanz V. Age-related changes in cortical and cancellous vertebral bone density in girls: assessment with quantitative CT. AJR Am J Roentgenol. 1994;162:405–9.
20. Trotter M, Hixon BB. Sequential changes in weight, density, and percentage ash weight of human skeleton from an early fetal period through old age. Anat Rec. 1974;179:1–18.
21. Gilsanz V, Gibbens DT, Carlson M, Boechat MI, Cann CE, Schulz EE. Peak trabecular vertebral density: a comparison of adolescent and adult females. Calcif Tissue Int. 1988;43:260–2.
22. Cooper C, Westlake S, Harvey N, Javaid K, Dennison E, Hanson M. Review: developmental origins of osteoporotic fracture. Osteoporos Int. 2006;17:337–47.
23. Bonjour JP, Chevalley T, Rizzoli R, Ferrari S. Gene–environment interactions in the skeletal response to nutrition and exercise during growth. Med Sport Sci. 2007;51:64–80.
24. Davies JH, Evans BA, Gregory JW. Bone mass acquisition in healthy children. Arch Dis Child. 2005;90:373–8.
25. Eisman JA. Genetics of osteoporosis. Endocr Rev. 1999;20:788–804.
26. Pitukcheewanont P, Austin J, Chen P, Punyasavatsut N. Bone health in children and adolescents: risk factors for low bone density. Pediatr Endocrinol Rev. 2013;10:318–35.
27. Jouanny P, Guillemin F, Kuntz C, Jeandel C, Pureel J. Environmental and genetic factors affecting bone mass: similarity of bone density among members of healthy families. Arthritis Rheum. 1995;38:61–7.
28. Albagha OME, Ralston SH. Genetic determinants of susceptibility to osteoporosis. Endocrinol Metab Clin N Am. 2003;32:65–81.
29. Alam I, Padgett LR, Ichikawa S, Alkhouli M, Koller DL, Lai D, Peacock M, Xuei X, Foroud T, Edenberg HJ, Econs MJ. SIBLING family genes and bone mineral density: association and allele-specific expression in humans. Bone. 2014;64:166–72.
30. Medina-Gomez C, Kemp JP, Estrada K, Eriksson J, Liu J, Reppe S, Evans DM, Heppe DH, Vandenput L, Herrera L, Ring SM, Kruithof CJ, Timpson NJ, Zillikens MC, Olstad OK, Zheng HF, Richards JB, St Pourcain B, Hofman A, Jaddoe VW, Smith GD, Lorentzon M, Gautvik KM, Uitterlinden AG, Brommage R, Ohlsson C, Tobias JH, Rivadeneira F. Meta-analysis of genome-wide scans for total body BMD in children and adults reveals allelic heterogeneity and age-specific effects at the WNT16 locus. PLoS Genet. 2012;8:e1002718.
31. Hopper JL, Green RM, Nowson CA, Young D, Sherwin AJ, Kaymakci B, Larkins RG, Wark JD. Genetic, common environment, and individual specific components of variance for bone mineral density in 10- to 26-year-old females: a twin study. Am J Epidemiol. 1998;147:17–29.
32. Ferrari S. Human genetics of osteoporosis. Best Pract Res Clin Endocrinol Metab. 2008;22:723–35.
33. Thakkinstian A, D'Este C, Eisman J, Nguyen T, Attia J. Meta-analysis of molecular association studies: vitamin D receptor gene polymorphisms and BMD as a case study. J Bone Miner Res. 2004;19:419–28.
34. Grant SFA, Reid DM, Blake G, Herd R, Fogelman I, Ralston SH. Reduced bone density and osteoporosis associated with a polymorphic Sp2 binding site in the collagen type Ia1 gene. Nat Genet. 1996;14:203–5.
35. Shiraki M, Shiraki Y, Aoki C, Hosoi T, Inoue S, Kaneki M, Ouchi Y. Association of bone mineral density with apolipoprotein E phenotype. J Bone Miner Res. 1996;10:S436.

36. Rivadeneira F, Styrkársdottir U, Estrada K, Halldórsson BV, Hsu YH, Richards JB, Zillikens MC, Kavvoura FK, Amin N, Aulchenko YS, Cupples LA, Deloukas P, Demissie S, Grundberg E, Hofman A, Kong A, Karasik D, van Meurs JB, Oostra B, Pastinen T, Pols HA, Sigurdsson G, Soranzo N, Thorleifsson G, Thorsteinsdottir U, Williams FM, Wilson SG, Zhou Y, Ralston SH, van Duijn CM, Spector T, Kiel DP, Stefansson K, Ioannidis JP, Uitterlinden AG, Genetic Factors for Osteoporosis (GEFOS) Consortium. Twenty bone-mineral-density loci identified by large-scale meta-analysis of genome-wide association studies. Nat Genet. 2009;41:1199–206.
37. Eisman JA, Kelly PJ, Morrison NA, Pocock NA, Yeoman R, Birmingham J, et al. Peak bone mass and osteoporosis prevention. Osteoporos Int. 1993;3 Suppl 1:56–60.
38. Seeman E, Tsalamandris C, Formica C. Peak bone mass, a growing problem? Int J Fertil Menopausal Stud. 1993;38 Suppl 2:77–82.
39. Barker DJ, Eriksson JG, Forsen T, Osmond C. Fetal origins of adult disease: strength of effects and biological basis. Int J Epidemiol. 2002;31:1235–9.
40. Holroyd C, Harvey N, Dennison E, Cooper C. Epigenetic influences in the developmental origins of osteoporosis. Osteoporos Int. 2012;23:401–10.
41. Harvey N, Dennison E, Cooper C. Osteoporosis: a lifecourse approach. J Bone Miner Res. 2014;29:1917–25.
42. Javaid MK, Crozier SR, Harvey NC, Gale CR, Dennison EM, Boucher BJ, Arden NK, Godfrey KM, Cooper C, Princess Anne Hospital Study Group. Maternal vitamin D status during pregnancy and childhood bone mass at age 9 years: a longitudinal study. Lancet. 2006;367:36–43.
43. Dennison EM, Syddall HE, Sayer AA, Gilbody HJ, Cooper C. Birth weight and weight at 1 year are independent determinants of bone mass in the seventh decade: the Hertfordshire cohort study. Pediatr Res. 2005;57:582–6.
44. Javaid MK, Eriksson JG, Kajantie E, et al. Growth in childhood predicts hip fracture risk in later life. Osteoporos Int. 2011;22:69–73.
45. Inskip HM, Godfrey KM, Robinson SM, Law CM, Barker DJ, Cooper C, SWS Study Group. Cohort profile: the Southampton Women's Survey. Int J Epidemiol. 2006;35:42–8.
46. Ay L, Jaddoe VW, Hofman A, et al. Foetal and postnatal growth and bone mass at 6 months: the Generation R Study. Clin Endocrinol (Oxf). 2011;74:181–90.
47. Golden NH, Abrams SA, Committee on nutrition. Optimizing bone health in children and adolescents. Pediatrics. 2014;134:e1229–43.
48. Wosje KS, Specker BL. Role of calcium in bone health during childhood. Nutr Rev. 2000;58:253–68.
49. Ross AC, Taylor CL, Yaktine AL, Del Valle HB, Committee to Review Dietary Reference Intakes for Vitamin D and Calcium Food and Nutrition Board; Institute of Medicine, editors. Dietary reference intakes for calcium and vitamin D. Washington, DC: The National Academies Press; 2011. Available in PDF at http://www.nap.edu/catalog.php?record_id=13050. ISBN 978-0-309-16394-1.
50. Hoppe C, Molgaard C, Michaelsen KF. Bone size and bone mass in 10-year-old Danish children: effect of current diet. Osteoporos Int. 2000;11:1024–30.
51. Ho SC, Leung PC, Swaminathan R, Chan C, Chan SS, Fan YK, Lindsay R. Determinants of bone mass in Chinese women aged 21–40 years. II. Pattern of dietary calcium intake and association with bone mineral density. Osteoporos Int. 1994;4:167–75.
52. Lee WT, Leung SS, Lui SS, Lau J. Relationship between long-term calcium intake and bone mineral content of children aged from birth to 5 years. Br J Nutr. 1993;70:235–48.
53. Zhu K, Du X, Greenfield H, Zhang Q, Ma G, Hu X, Fraser DR. Bone mass in Chinese premenarcheal girls: the roles of body composition, calcium intake and physical activity. Br J Nutr. 2004;92:985–93.
54. Kalkwarf HJ, Khoury JC, Lanphear BP. Milk intake during childhood and adolescence, adult bone density, and osteoporotic fractures in US women. Am J Clin Nutr. 2003;77:257–65.
55. van der Pols JC, Gunnell D, Williams GM, Holly JM, Bain C, Martin RM. Childhood dairy and calcium intake and cardiovascular mortality in adulthood: 65-year follow-up of the Boyd Orr cohort. Heart. 2009;95:1600–6.

56. Bonjour JP, Carrie AL, Ferrari S, Clavien H, Slosman D, Theintz G, Rizzoli R. Calcium-enriched foods and bone mass growth in prepubertal girls: a randomized, double-blind, placebo-controlled trial. J Clin Invest. 1997;99:1287–94.
57. Johnston Jr CC, Miller JZ, Slemenda CW, Reister TK, Hui S, Christian JC, Peacock M. Calcium supplementation and increases in bone mineral density in children. N Engl J Med. 1992;327:82–7.
58. Cadogan J, Eastell R, Jones N, Barker ME. Milk intake and bone mineral acquisition in adolescent girls: randomised, controlled intervention trial. BMJ. 1997;315:1255–60.
59. Huncharek M, Muscat J, Kupelnick B. Impact of dairy products and dietary calcium on bone-mineral content in children: results of a meta-analysis. Bone. 2008;43:312–21.
60. Winzenberg T, Shaw K, Fryer J, Jones G. Effects of calcium supplementation on bone density in healthy children: meta-analysis of randomised controlled trials. BMJ. 2006;333:775.
61. Bonjour JP, Chevalley T, Ammann P, Slosman D, Rizzoli R. Gain in bone mineral mass in prepubertal girls 3.5 years after discontinuation of calcium supplementation: a follow-up study. Lancet. 2001;358:1208–12.
62. Wyshak G, Frisch RE. Carbonated beverages, dietary calcium, the dietary calcium/phosphorous ratio, and bone fractures in girls and boys. J Adolesc Health. 1994;15:210–5.
63. Fitzpatrick L, Heaney RP. Got soda? J Bone Miner Res. 2003;18:1570–2.
64. Committee on Nutrition and the Council on Sports Medicine and Fitness. Sports drinks and energy drinks for children and adolescents: are they appropriate? Pediatrics. 2011;127:1182–9.
65. Holick MF. Vitamin D, deficiency. N Engl J Med. 2007;357:266–81.
66. Lehtonen-Veromaa MK, Möttönen TT, Nuotio IO, Irjala KM, Leino AE, Viikari JS. Vitamin D and attainment of peak bone mass among peripubertal Finnish girls: a 3-y prospective study. Am J Clin Nutr. 2002;76:1446–53.
67. Andersen R, Molgaard C, Skovgaard LT, Brot C, Cashman KD, Chabros E, Charzewska J, Flynn A, Jakobsen J, Karkkainen M, Kiely M, Lamberg-Allardt C, Moreiras O, Natri AM, O'Brien M, Rogalska-Niedzwiedz M, Ovesen L. Teenage girls and elderly women living in northern Europe have low winter vitamin D status. Eur J Clin Nutr. 2005;59:533–41.
68. Cheng S, Tylavsky F, Kroger H, Karkkainen M, Lyytikainen A, Koistinen A, Mahonen A, Alen M, Halleen J, Vaananen K, Lamberg-Allardt C. Association of low 25-hydroxyvitamin D concentrations with elevated parathyroid hormone concentrations and low cortical bone density in early pubertal and prepubertal Finnish girls. Am J Clin Nutr. 2003;78:485–92.
69. Lapatsanis D, Moulas A, Cholevas V, Soukakos P, Papadopoulou ZL, Challa A. Vitamin D: a necessity for children and adolescents in Greece. Calcif Tissue Int. 2005;77:348–55.
70. Hintzpeter B, Scheidt-Nave C, Muller MJ, Schenk L, Mensink GB. Higher prevalence of vitamin D deficiency is associated with immigrant background among children and adolescents in Germany. J Nutr. 2008;138:1482–90.
71. Ginty F, Cavadini C, Michaud PA, Burckhardt P, Baumgartner M, Mishra GD, Barclay DV. Effects of usual nutrient intake and vitamin D status on markers of bone turnover in Swiss adolescents. Eur J Clin Nutr. 2004;58:1257–65.
72. Gordon CM, DePeter KC, Feldman HA, Grace E, Emans SJ. Prevalence of vitamin D deficiency among healthy adolescents. Arch Pediatr Adolesc Med. 2004;158:531–7.
73. Looker AC, Dawson-Hughes B, Calvo MS, Gunter EW, Sahyoun NR. Serum 25-hydroxyvitamin D status of adolescents and adults in two seasonal subpopulations from NHANES III. Bone. 2002;30:771–7.
74. Dong Y, Pollock N, Stallmann-Jorgensen IS, et al. Low 25-hydroxyvitamin D levels in adolescents: race, season, adiposity, physical activity, and fitness. Pediatrics. 2010;125:1104–11.
75. Harel Z, Flanagan P, Forcier M, Harel D. Low vitamin D status among obese adolescents: prevalence and response to treatment. J Adolesc Health. 2011;48:448–52.
76. Turer CB, Lin H, Flores G. Prevalence of vitamin D deficiency among overweight and obese US children. Pediatrics. 2013;131(1):e152–61.
77. Cashman KD, Hill TR, Cotter AA, et al. Low vitamin D status adversely affects bone health parameters in adolescents. Am J Clin Nutr. 2008;87:1039–44.

78. Sonneville KR, Gordon CM, Kocher MS, Pierce LM, Ramappa A, Field AE. Vitamin D, calcium, and dairy intakes and stress fractures among female adolescents. Arch Pediatr Adolesc Med. 2012;166:595–600.
79. Rizzoli R, Bonjour J-P. Dietary protein and bone health. J Bone Miner Res. 2004;19:527–31.
80. Bonjour JP, Schurch MA, Chevalley T, Ammann P, Rizzoli R. Protein intake, IGF-1 and osteoporosis. Osteoporos Int. 1997;7(Suppl3):S36–42.
81. Chevalley T, Bonjour JP, Ferrari S, Rizzoli R. High-protein intake enhances the positive impact of physical activity on BMC in prepubertal boys. J Bone Miner Res. 2008;23:131–42.
82. Garn SM. The earlier gain and the later loss of cortical bone. Springfield, IL: C.C. Thomas; 1970.
83. Budek AZ, Hoppe C, Michaelsen KF, Molgaard C. High intake of milk, but not meat, decreases bone turnover in prepubertal boys after 7 days. Eur J Clin Nutr. 2007;61:957–62.
84. Dawson-Hughes B, Harris SS, Rasmussen HM, Dallal GE. Comparative effects of oral aromatic and branched-chain amino acids on urine calcium excretion in humans. Osteoporos Int. 2007;18:955–61.
85. Gueguen L, Pointillart A. The bioavailability of dietary calcium. J Am Coll Nutr. 2000;19:119S–36.
86. Black RE, Williams SM, Jones IE, Goulding A. Children who avoid drinking cow milk have low dietary calcium intakes and poor bone health. Am J Clin Nutr. 2002;76:675–80.
87. Jensen VB, Jorgensen IM, Rasmussen KB, Molgaard C, Prahl P. Bone mineral status in children with cow milk allergy. Pediatr Allergy Immunol. 2004;15:562–5.
88. Rockell JE, Williams SM, Taylor RW, Grant AM, Jones IE, Goulding A. Two-year changes in bone and body composition in young children with a history of prolonged milk avoidance. Osteoporos Int. 2005;16:1016–23.
89. Goulding A, Rockell JE, Black RE, Grant AM, Jones IE, Williams SM. Children who avoid drinking cow's milk are at increased risk for prepubertal bone fractures. J Am Diet Assoc. 2004;104:250–3.
90. Konstantynowicz J, Nguyen TV, Kaczmarski M, Jamiolkowski J, Piotrowska-Jastrzebska J, Seeman E. Fractures during growth: potential role of a milk-free diet. Osteoporos Int. 2007;18:1601–7.
91. Matkovic V, Landoll JD, Badenhop-Stevens NE, Ha EY, Crncevic-Orlic Z, Li B, Goel P. Nutrition influences skeletal development from childhood to adulthood: a study of hip, spine, and forearm in adolescent females. J Nutr. 2004;134:701S–5.
92. Frost HM. Bone's mechanostat: a 2003 update. Anat Rec A: Discov Mol Cell Evol Biol. 2003;275:1081–101.
93. Rauch F, Schoenau E. The developing bone: slave or master of its cells and molecules? Pediatr Res. 2001;50:309–14.
94. Salameh A, Dhein S. Effects of mechanical forces and stretch on intercellular gap junction coupling. Biochim Biophys Acta. 2013;1828:147–56.
95. Schnitzler CM. Childhood cortical porosity is related to microstructural properties of the bone-muscle junction. J Bone Miner Res. 2015;30:144–55.
96. Daly RM, Stenevi-Lundgren S, Linden C, Karlsson MK. Muscle determinants of bone mass, geometry and strength in prepubertal girls. Med Sci Sports Exerc. 2008;40:1135–41.
97. Rubin CT, Lanyon LE. Regulation of bone mass by mechanical strain magnitude. Calcif Tissue Int. 1985;37:411–7.
98. Khan K, McKay HA, Haapasalo H, Bennell KL, Forwood MR, Kannus P, Wark JD. Does childhood and adolescence provide a unique opportunity for exercise to strengthen the skeleton? J Sci Med Sport. 2000;3:150–64.
99. MacKelvie KJ, Khan KM, McKay HA. Is there a critical period for bone response to weight-bearing exercise in children and adolescents? A systematic review. Br J Sports Med. 2002;36:250–7.
100. Zhang P, Hamamura K, Yokota H. A brief review of bone adaptation to unloading. Genomics Proteomics Bioinformatics. 2008;6:4–7.

101. Meakin LB, Price JS, Lanyon LE. The contribution of experimental in vivo models to understanding the mechanisms of adaptation to mechanical loading in bone. Front Endocrinol (Lausanne). 2014;5:154.
102. Lehtonen-Veromaa M, Mottonen T, Irjala K, Nuotio I, Leino A, Viikari J. A 1-year prospective study on the relationship between physical activity, markers of bone metabolism, and bone acquisition in peripubertal girls. J Clin Endocrinol Metab. 2000;85:3726–32.
103. Nurmi-Lawton JA, Baxter-Jones AD, Mirwald RL, Bishop JA, Taylor P, Cooper C, New SA. Evidence of sustained skeletal benefits from impact-loading exercise in young females: a 3-year longitudinal study. J Bone Miner Res. 2004;19:314–22.
104. Fuchs RK, Bauer JJ, Snow CM. Jumping improves hip and lumbar spine bone mass in prepubescent children: a randomized controlled trial. J Bone Miner Res. 2001;16:148–56.
105. Fuchs RK, Snow CM. Gains in hip bone mass from high-impact training are maintained: a randomized controlled trial in children. J Pediatr. 2002;141:357–62.
106. Gunter K, Baxter-Jones AD, Mirwald RL, Almstedt H, Fuchs RK, Durski S, Snow C. Impact exercise increases BMC during growth: an 8-year longitudinal study. J Bone Miner Res. 2008;23:986–93.
107. Johannsen N, Binkley T, Englert V, Neiderauer G, Specker B. Bone response to jumping is site-specific in children: a randomized trial. Bone. 2003;33:533–9.
108. MacKelvie KJ, Khan KM, Petit MA, Janssen PA, McKay HA. A school-based exercise intervention elicits substantial bone health benefits: a 2-year randomized controlled trial in girls. Pediatrics. 2003;112, e447.
109. MacKelvie KJ, McKay HA, Petit MA, Moran O, Khan KM. Bone mineral response to a 7-month randomized controlled, school-based jumping intervention in 121 prepubertal boys: associations with ethnicity and body mass index. J Bone Miner Res. 2002;17:834–44.
110. McKay HA, Petit MA, Schutz RW, Prior JC, Barr SI, Khan KM. Augmented trochanteric bone mineral density after modified physical education classes: a randomized school-based exercise intervention study in prepubescent and early pubescent children. J Pediatr. 2000;136:156–62.
111. Weeks BK, Young CM, Beck BR. Eight months of regular in-school jumping improves indices of bone strength in adolescent boys and Girls: the POWER PE study. J Bone Miner Res. 2008;23:1002–11.
112. Hind K, Burrows M. Weight-bearing exercise and bone mineral accrual in children and adolescents: a review of controlled trials. Bone. 2007;40:14–27.
113. Tan VP, Macdonald HM, Kim S, Nettlefold L, Gabel L, Ashe MC, McKay HA. Influence of physical activity on bone strength in children and adolescents: a systematic review and narrative synthesis. J Bone Miner Res. 2014;29:2161–81.
114. Nattiv A, Loucks AB, Manore MM, Sanborn CF, Sundgot-Borgen J, Warren MP, American College of Sports Medicine. American College of Sports Medicine position stand. The female athlete triad. Med Sci Sports Exerc. 2007;39:1867–82.
115. Hernandez CJ, Beaupre GS, Carter DR. A theoretical analysis of the relative influences of peak BMD, age-related bone loss and menopause on the development of osteoporosis. Osteoporos Int. 2003;14:843–7.
116. Boyce AM, Gafni RI. Approach to the child with fractures. J Clin Endocrinol Metab. 2011;96:1943–52.
117. Ma NS, Gordon CM. Pediatric osteoporosis: where are we now? J Pediatr. 2012;161:983–90.
118. Marini JC, Blissett AR. New genes in bone development: what's new in osteogenesis imperfecta. J Clin Endocrinol Metab. 2013;98:3095–103.
119. Hartikka H, Makitie O, Mannikko M, Doria AS, Daneman A, Cole WG, Ala-Kokko L, Sochett EB. Heterozygous mutation in the LDL receptor-related protein 5 (LRP5) gene are associated with primary osteoporosis in children. J Bone Miner Res. 2005;20:783–9.
120. Sobacchi C, Schulz A, Coxon FP, Villa A, Helfrich MH. Osteopetrosis: genetics, treatment and new insights into osteoclast function. Nat Rev Endocrinol. 2013;9:522–36.

121. Tsampalieros A, Lam CKL, Spencer JC, Thayu M, Shults J, Zemel BS, Herskovitz RM, Baldassano RN, Leonard MB. Long term inflammation and glucocorticoid therapy impair skeletal modeling during growth in childhood Crohn disease. J Clin Endocrinol Metab. 2013;98:3438–45.
122. Ghishan FK, Kiela PR. Advances in the understanding of mineral and bone metabolism in inflammatory bowel diseases. Am J Physiol Gastrointest Liver Physiol. 2011;300:G101–201.
123. Roux C. Osteoporosis in inflammatory joint diseases. Osteoporos Int. 2011;22:421–33.
124. Henderson RC, Karalla JA, Barrington JW, Abbas A, Stevenson RC. Longitudinal changes in bone density in children and adolescents with moderate to severe cerebral palsy. J Pediatr. 2005;146:769–75.
125. King WM, Ruttencutter R, Nagaraja HN, Matkovic V, Landoll J, Hoyle C, Mendell JR, Kissel JT. Orthopedic outcomes of long-term daily corticosteroid treatment in Duchenne muscular dystrophy. Neurology. 2007;68:1607–13.
126. Van der Sluis I, van den Heuvel-Eibrink MM. Osteoporosis in children with cancer. Pediatr Blood Cancer. 2008;50:474–8.
127. Mostoufi-Moab S, Halton J. Bone morbidity in childhood leukemia: epidemiology, mechanisms, diagnosis and treatment. Curr Osteoporos Rep. 2014;12:300–12.
128. Eberling PR. Approach to the patient with transplantation-related bone loss. J Clin Endocrinol Metab. 2009;94:1483–90.
129. Sermet-Gaudelus I, Bianchi MLM, Garabedian M, Aris RM, Morton A, Hardin DS, Elkin SL, Compston JE, Conway SP, Castanet M, Wolfe S, Haworth CS. European cystic fibrosis bone mineralisation guidelines. J Cystic Fibrosis. 2011;10 Suppl 2:S16–23.
130. Vogiatzi MG, Macklin EA, Fung EB, Cheung AM, Vichinsky E, Olivieri N, Kirby M, et al. Bone disease in thalassemia: a frequent and still unresolved problem. J Bone Miner Res. 2009;24:543–57.
131. Goulding A, Jones L, Taylor RW, Manning PJ, Williams SM. More broken bones: a 4-year double cohort study of young girls with and without distal forearm fractures. J Bone Miner Res. 2000;15:2011–8.
132. Farr JN, Khosla S, Achenbach SJ, Atkinson EJ, Kirmani S, McCready LK, Melton 3rd LF, Amin S. Diminished bone strength is observed in adult women and women who sustained a mild trauma distal forearm fracture during childhood. J Bone Miner Res. 2014;29:2193–202.
133. Baim S, Leonard MB, Bianchi M-L, Hans DB, et al. Official positions of the International Society for Clinical Densitometry and executive summary of the 2007 ISCD Pediatric Position Development Conference. J Clin Densitom. 2008;11:6–21.
134. Gordon CM, Leonard MB, Zemel BS. 2013 Pediatric Position Development Conference: executive summary and reflections. J Clin Densitom. 2014;17:219–24.
135. Rubin KH, Friis-Holmberg T, Hermann AP, Abrahamsen B, Brixen K. Risk assessment tools to identify women with increased risk of osteoporotic fracture: complexity or simplicity? A systematic review. J Bone Miner Res. 2013;28:1701–17.
136. Bishop N, Arundel P, Clark E, Dimitri P, Farr J, Jones G, Makitie O, Munns CF, Shaw N. Fracture prediction and the definition of osteoporosis in children and adolescents: the ISCD 2013 Pediatric Official Positions. J Clin Densitom. 2014;17:275–80.
137. Jones IE, Williams SM, Dow N, Goulding A. How many children remain fracture-free during growth? A longitudinal study of children and adolescents participating in the Dunedin Multidisciplinary Health and Development. Osteoporos Int. 2002;13(12):990–5.
138. Clark EM, Tobias JH, Ness AR. Association between bone density and fractures in children: a systematic review and meta-analysis. Pediatrics. 2006;117:e291–7.
139. Kalkwarf HJ, Laor T, Bean JA. Facture risk in children with a forearm injury is associated with volumetric bone mineral density and cortical area (by peripheral QCT) and areal bone density (by DXA). Osteoporos Int. 2011;22:607–16.
140. Farr JN, Amin S, Melton 3rd LJ, et al. Bone strength and structural deficits in children and adolescents with a distal forearm fracture due to mild trauma. J Bone Miner Res. 2014;29:590–9.

141. Henderson RC, Gerglund LM, May R, Zemel BS, Grossberg RI, Johnson J, Plotkin H, Stevenson RD, Szalay E, Wong B, Kecskemethy HH, Harcke HT. The relationship between fractures and DXA measures of BMD in the distal femur of children and adolescent with cerebral palsy or muscular dystrophy. J Bone Miner Res. 2010;25:520–6.
142. Halton J, Gaboury I, Grant R, et al. Advanced vertebral fracture among newly diagnosed children during treatment for acute lymphoblastic leukemia: results of the Canadian Steroid-Associated Osteoporosis in the Pediatric Population (STOPP) Research Program. J Bone Miner Res. 2009;24:1326–34.
143. Alos N, Grant RM, Ramsay T, et al. High incidence of vertebral fractures in children with actue lymphoblastic leukemia 12 months after the initiation of therapy. J Clin Oncol. 2012;30:2760–7.
144. Tsampalieros A, Griffin L, Terpstra AM, Kalkwarf HJ, Shults J, Foster BJ, et al. Changes in DXA and quantitative CT measures of musculoskeletal outcomes following pediatric renal transplantation. Am J Transplant. 2014;14:124–32.
145. Rodd C, Lang B, Ramsay T, et al. Incident vertebral fractures among children with rheumatic disorders 12 months after glucocorticoid initiation: a national observational study. Arthritis Care Res. 2012;64:122–31.

# Chapter 2
# Tools for Measuring Bone in Children and Adolescents

Kate A. Ward, Thomas M. Link, and Judith E. Adams

## Introduction

This chapter provides an overview of the current densitometry techniques that are used in children. Dual energy X-ray absorptiometry (DXA) is discussed only briefly as other chapters concentrate in detail on this technique. The strengths and limitations of each of the techniques are discussed and a technical overview is provided in Table 2.1. Comparative radiation doses for other imaging modalities and natural background radiation are given in Table 2.2. Table 2.3 provides a summary of published pediatric normative data for each of the densitometry methods discussed. Table 2.4 summarises what each technique measures in relation to the biological organisation of bone and Table 2.5 gives the advantages and limitations of the techniques described in this chapter.

K.A. Ward, Ph.D.
MRC Human Nutrition Research, Cambridge, Cambridge CB1 9NL and MRC Lifecourse Epidemiology Unit, University of Southampton, Southampton, S016 6YD, UK
e-mail: kate.ward@mrc-hnr.cam.ac.uk

T.M. Link, M.D., Ph.D.
Department of Radiology and Biomedical Imaging, UCSF,
400 Parnassus Ave, A-367, San Francisco, CA 94143, USA
e-mail: Thomas.Link@ucsf.edu

J.E. Adams, M.B.B.S., F.R.C.R., F.R.C.P. (✉)
Radiology & Manchester Academic Health Science Centre, Central Manchester University Hospitals NHS Foundation Trust, University of Manchester,
Oxford Road, Manchester, Lancashire M13 9WL, UK
e-mail: judith.adams@manchester.ac.uk

© Springer International Publishing Switzerland 2016
E.B. Fung et al. (eds.), *Bone Health Assessment in Pediatrics*,
DOI 10.1007/978-3-319-30412-0_2

**Table 2.1** A technical overview of currently available bone densitometry techniques

| Technique | Approximate costs[a] | Sites | Clinical/research | Radiation dose (μSv) | Precision (CV %) |
|---|---|---|---|---|---|
| DXA (including iDXA) | $72–180 K £39–99 K €59–147 K | Lumbar spine | Both | 0.4–4 | <1 |
| | | Total body | Both | 0.02–5 | 1–2 |
| | | Proximal femur | Both | 0.15–5.4[c] | 0.15–5.4 |
| | | Lateral spine[b] | | 12 | NA |
| Axial QCT | Scanner *(Software)* $630–900 K *(18–22 K)* £345–493 K *(10–12 K)* €516–736 *(15–18 K)* | Spine | Both | 3D: 0.59–1.09 mSv 2D: 55 microSv | 0.8–1.5 [126] |
| | | Femur | Research | 3000 [127] | <1 [128] |
| Peripheral QCT | $76–251 K £42 K €37 K | Radius | Research | <1.5–4 per scan | 0.8–1.5 |
| | | Tibia | Research | | 3.6–7.8 3–5 year olds [61] 0.5–2.8 12 year olds [129] |
| | | Femur | Research | | 1.2–4 [130] |
| HRpQCT | $450–500 K £250 K–280 K €370–420 | Radius | Research | <3 per scan | Not available |
| | | Tibia | Research | | |
| MRI | Scanner *(Software)* $1.8–2.7 million *(18–22 K)* £1–1.5 million *(10–12 K)* €1.5–2.2 million *(15–18 K)* | Tibia Humerus Femur | Research | None | 0.12–1.02 [97] 0.55–3.63 |

[a]Calculated from US Dollar $ at conversion rate $1 USD=£0.55 GBP, € 0.82 Euros. These figures are subject to currency fluctuations and prices are approximations
[b]GE-Lunar iDXA only
[c]Not including Lunar Expert

# What is Being Measured by Bone Densitometry?

Bone densitometry offers a tool with which pediatric bone status can be assessed. As the child grows, the skeleton will increase in size and mineral content, and bones will change in shape. When interpreting measurements from bone densitometry scanners, it is imperative that these changes in bone size, shape and mass are taken into account [1]. For example, changes in bone mineral density over time could reflect changes in bone size, mineral content or a combination of these. The

**Table 2.2** An overview of radiation exposures for comparison with bone densitometry techniques

|  | Effective dose (µSv) |
|---|---|
| Return (round trip) transatlantic flight [131] | 80 µSv |
| Annual naturally occurring background radiation [132] |  |
| North America | 3000 µSv |
| UK | 2000 µSv |
| Australia | 1500 µSv |
| Hand radiograph [133] | 0.17 µSv |
| Chest radiograph [134] | 12–20 µSv |
| Lumbar spine radiograph [134] | 700 µSv |
| Radioisotope bone scan [135] | 3000 µSv |

**Table 2.3** An overview of reference data currently available with machines

| Technique | Reference data | Source | N = | Age range (years) |
|---|---|---|---|---|
| DXA | Spine | • Hologic, [136, 137][a], [138][b], [139–142]<br>• GE Lunar [4, 143–147] & unpublished manufacturer data<br>• Norland [148, 149] | 218[c], 666<br><br>1444<br>>1100<br>778 | 1–19, 8–17, 3–20 3 month - 19<br><br>2–20 |
|  | Proximal femur | • Hologic [137][a] [138][b] [139–142]<br>• GE Lunar [4, 143–147] and unpublished manufacturer data<br>• Norland [148, 149] | 892, 1047<br>>1100<br>778 | 8–17, 5–20<br>4–27<br>2–20 |
|  | Total body | • Hologic [137][a] [138][b] [139–142]<br>• GE Lunar [4, 143–147] and unpublished manufacturer data<br>• Norland Argentina, [148, 149] | 977, 1948<br>>1100<br>778 | 8–17, 3–20, 5–19<br>4–27<br>2–20 |
|  | Forearm | • Hologic [17, 138–140, 142] |  |  |
| QCT | Spine | • GE CT 9800[d] [39] [30, 31] |  |  |
|  | Radius | • Stratec XCT-2000 [55, 64, 76] |  |  |
|  | Tibia | • Stratec XCT-2000 [75] |  |  |

*NB*: databases provided above are those, which are currently provided by the manufacturer, there are many other databases derived from research groups for own ethnic and population specific purposes. In certain cases, use of these may be appropriate but caution should be taken regarding the machine type, origin of data and in longitudinal studies the same database should always be used

[a]only provided with IRB in US

[b]Version 12.1 onwards

[c]These data are not gender specific

[d]Cross calibration performed [150], reference data provided with Mindways software for Philips SR4000 and newer generation CT scanners

**Table 2.4** A summary of what each technique '[a]measures' in relation to the bone's biological organisation [2]

| Method | BMD$_{material}$ | BMD$_{compartment}$ | | BMD$_{total}$ |
| | | Cortical | Trabecular | |
| --- | --- | --- | --- | --- |
| DXA | No | Yes | No | Yes |
| QCT central, peripheral | No | Yes | Yes | Yes |
| HR pQCT | Yes (cortical) | Yes | Yes | Yes |

[a]MRI does not measure BMD, but provides measurement of parameters related to the structure of the bone but not BMD by definition

**Table 2.5** A summary of the main advantages and limitations of each of the bone measurement techniques in children discussed in this chapter

| Technique | Advantages | Limitations |
| --- | --- | --- |
| DXA | 1. Speed<br>2. Cost<br>3. Precision<br>4. Availability of reference data<br>5. Low-radiation dose<br>6. Clinical applications established<br>7. Body composition measurement | 1. Size dependence<br>2. Sensitive to body composition changes<br>3. Software and reference data changes<br>4. Integral measurement of trabecular and cortical bone |
| QCT | 1. Size independent<br>2. Separate measure of cortical and trabecular bone<br>3. Measurements of bone geometry<br>4. Imaging of trabecular bone structure feasible<br>5. Measurement of muscle and fat<br>6. Applicable to central and peripheral sites | 1. Radiation dose<br>2. Cost<br>3. Access for bone densitometry<br>4. Skilled staff<br>5. Specialist acquisition and analysis software limited<br>6. Limited reference data |
| Peripheral QCT | 1. 1–5 as axial QCT above<br>2. Low-radiation dose<br>3. Lower cost than axial | 1. Scan time<br>2. Only applicable to peripheral sites<br>3. Difficulties in re-positioning in follow-up scans |
| HR pQCT | 4. 1–4 as axial<br>5. Assessment and estimation of trabecular and cortical microstructure<br>6. In-vivo assessment of cortical BMD$_{material}$ | 4. Cost<br>5. Susceptibility to movement artefact<br>6. Only applicable to peripheral sites |
| MRI | 1. Non-ionising, non invasive<br>2. Size independent<br>3. Imaging in multiple planes<br>4. Applicable to axial and peripheral sites<br>5. Measurement of muscle and fat | 1. Noisy<br>2. Long scan time<br>3. Claustrophobia in ~10% people<br>4. Parents cannot be in room with children |

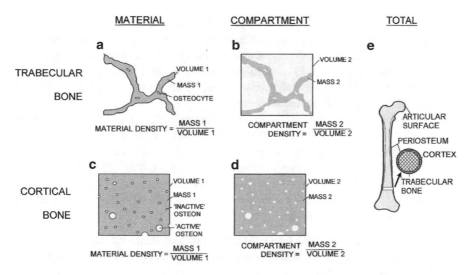

**Fig. 2.1** A model based on the biological organisation of bone proposed by Rauch and Schonau [2] to help in understanding and interpreting the measurements obtained from bone densitometry and to relate these changes to the physiological changes that occur during bone development. The model describes separate definitions for the material, compartment and total densities of bone

quantitative measures that can be obtained from most two-dimensional densitometry techniques include bone area (BA, cm²), bone mineral content (BMC, g) and areal bone mineral density (BMD, g/cm²).

A model based upon the biological organisation of bone was proposed by Rauch to help in understanding and interpreting the measurements obtained from bone densitometry and relating these changes to the physiological changes that occur during bone development [2]. The model describes separate definitions for the 'material', 'compartment' and 'total' densities of bone (Fig. 2.1) and each of these will be discussed briefly:

1. *Material mineral density*: This reflects the degree of mineralization of the organic bone matrix. Material density can be determined only within a very small volume occupied only by bone matrix exclusive of marrow spaces, osteonal canals, lacunae and canaliculi. Until recently, the resolution required to measure $BMD_{material}$ was not possible with current non-invasive densitometric techniques. The spatial resolution of high-resolution peripheral quantitative computed tomography makes possible the measurement of cortical $BMD_{material}$ at distal, peripheral sites. $BMD_{material}$ can be determined from specimens taken at bone biopsy, which is an invasive procedure. These specimens can be analysed by mineral/ash weight, contact radiography, backscatter electron microscopy or laser ablated mass spectrometry. Measurement of $BMD_{material}$ is not routinely assessed in clinical practice.

2. *Compartment mineral density*: The $BMD_{compartment}$ is the amount of mineral contained within the trabecular, or the cortical, compartments i.e. the mass of mineral per unit volume of trabecular or cortical bone. Quantitative computed

tomography (QCT) measures cortical and trabecular bone separately and can therefore measure $BMD_{compartment}$ in both types of bone. DXA measurements are a composite of integral (trabecular and cortical) bone, and so the technique is not able to separate the two components at most sites. $BMD_{compartment}$ can be determined by DXA in skeletal sites such as the diaphyses of the femur or radius which are comprised of cortical bone.

3. *Total mineral density*: $BMD_{total}$ is the mineral density of all the material contained within the periosteal envelope and articular surfaces of a bone. QCT and DXA measure $BMD_{total}$. Calculations are required to estimate bone volume from DXA scans since this technique measures areal density only. Bone mineral apparent density (BMAD) is an example of a volumetric density calculated using $BMD_{total}$ [3–5]. This density is sometimes inappropriately referred to in the literature as 'true bone density'.

Table 2.4 summarises which of the aforementioned BMD measurements can be determined using the densitometry techniques discussed in this chapter; QUS and MRI do not measure BMD.

## Dual Energy X-Ray Absorptiometry (DXA)

Dual energy X-ray absorptiometry (DXA) has been available since the late 1980's and is now used extensively for diagnosis and monitoring of osteoporosis in adults (Tables 2.1 and 2.2) [6–8]. The fundamental principle of DXA is to measure the transmission of X-rays through the body at high and low energies. The use of two energies allows discrimination between soft tissue and bone; low-energy photons are attenuated by soft tissue and the high-energy photons by bone and soft tissue. By subtracting the soft tissue from soft tissue and bone, it is possible to quantify the amount of bone within the X-ray scan path. Pixel-by-pixel attenuation values are converted to 'areal' bone mineral density (aBMD [g/cm²]) by comparison to a bone mineral phantom. Bone area (BA [cm²]) is calculated by summing the pixels within the bone edges as defined by software algorithms. Bone mineral content (BMC [g]) is calculated by multiplying mean aBMD by BA. DXA may be applied to the whole body or skeletal regions of interest, for example the spine, proximal femur and radius.

One of the important technical developments in DXA over the past decade is the ability to image the whole spine for Vertebral Fracture Assessment (VFA) [9] at considerably lower radiation doses (40 microSv) than is the case with spinal radiographs (700–2000 microSv). Because of the high-radiation dose paediatricians were reluctant to perform spinal radiographs and so the prevalence of vertebral fractures in children with some chronic diseases was consequently underestimated. Recent studies confirm the prevalence of vertebral fractures in children with diseases treated with glucocorticoids ranged between 7 and 16% [10–12]. DXA VFA is used increasingly in adults and children to identify vertebral fractures [13, 14] and so improve management of osteoporosis and reduce future fracture risk [15]. Both major DXA companies (Hologic Inc. Bedford MA and General Electric Healthcare:

Lunar, Madison, WI) have improved image quality generally by the use of more sensitive detectors and small increases in radiation dose. Dual energy images give superior visualisation of vertebrae in the thoracic region. To acquire lateral VFA images the major DXA manufactures use different techniques: GE Lunar acquire single- (SE) and dual-energy (DE) images simultaneously and rapidly (less than 2 min) and Hologic acquire such images separately, with a rapid 10 s SE scan which is what is usually performed but the DE acquisition which is superior for visualisation of vertebrae in the thoracic spine may take up to 5–8 min depending on the size of the patient. The latter DE scan acquisition is impractical in children due to respiratory movement artefact. The GE-Lunar iDXA makes more feasible the assessment of lateral spine images for fracture identification in children (Fig. 2.2), which improves diagnosis in children with chronic conditions [11, 16] in which such fractures are more common than was thought previously [17, 18].

DXA is the most widely available bone densitometry technique for measurement of bone status in children [19]. The advantages and limitations of the technique are discussed more extensively in subsequent chapters. The advantages of DXA include rapid scan times (less than a minute, low-ionising radiation dose and the availability

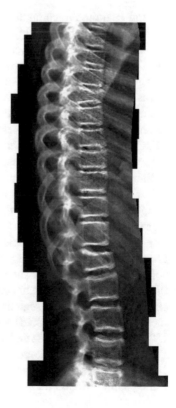

**Fig. 2.2** Lateral DXA vertebral Fracture Assessment (VFA) image (dual energy) in a child of 16 years with osteogenesis imperfect obtained on a GE Lunar iDXA scanner. Vertebrae from T3 to L5 are visualised with vertebral fractures at T6 and L1. The vertebral endplates are dense as occurs with bisphosphonate therapy. The jagged edge to the field of view is due to the use of SmartScan which minimises ionising radiation dose as appropriate in children

of pediatric reference data). The cost of running a DXA service is also relatively inexpensive. DXA can be used to assess body composition and is currently the only technique that can be applied to the hip region in children.

Whilst DXA has many advantages, the limitations of the method must be considered. BMD measurements provided by DXA are size dependent, since they are based on two-dimensional projections of three-dimensional structures which do not adjust for the depth of the bone. As a consequence BMD in small children will be under-estimated and over-estimated in children with large bones. Growth between scans should be taken into account when interpreting longitudinal data. There are several methods to correct DXA data for size dependence [3, 4, 20–25] as discussed further in Chaps. 3 and 6. DXA measurements are also influenced by changes in body composition and due consideration must be given to such changes when interpreting data. Overall, DXA remains the primary bone densitometry tool for clinical pediatric bone assessments and an important research tool.

## Quantitative Computed Tomography (QCT)

### Central

Central quantitative computed tomography (QCT) of the spine was first described in the late 1970s [26], and became more widely used during the 1980s [27]. With the introduction of dual energy X-ray absorptiometry (DXA) in 1988 the use of QCT declined. However, there has been renewed interest in QCT as investigators recognise the importance of bone size and geometry in assessing pediatric bone status. QCT is particularly useful in children since it measures volumetric density $(g/cm^3)$, which is not as size dependent as areal density $(g/cm^2)$ measured by DXA. Recent technical developments (such as spiral and spiral multi-detector MDCT) add to the potential information available from QCT. While QCT for clinical and research purposes may increase in the future, it should be noted that the radiation dose from QCT is substantially higher than that of DXA, but lower than in CT of the torso used for other clinical indications [28–32].

QCT of the spine requires that the patient lie supine on the scanner table with the legs flexed and supported on a pad to flatten out the natural lumbar lordosis (Fig. 2.3a). The height of the scanner table should be kept constant. A bone mineral equivalent phantom is placed under the patient in the site to be scanned (Fig. 2.3b). A water or soft tissue equivalent pad should be placed between the patient and the phantom if there is a significant air gap (Fig. 2.3b). Solid hydroxyapatite calibration phantoms are currently used with regions of varying density that allow the transformation of measurements in Hounsfield units (HU) to bone mineral equivalents in $mg/cm^3$. Some CT manufacturers provide their own software and phantoms (e.g. Siemens Healthcare, Erlangen, Germany); alternatively software and phantoms can be purchased (e.g. Mindways, Austin, Texas, USA). For comparable results in longitudinal studies the same phantom (and scanner) should be used. Similar to DXA instrumentation [33,

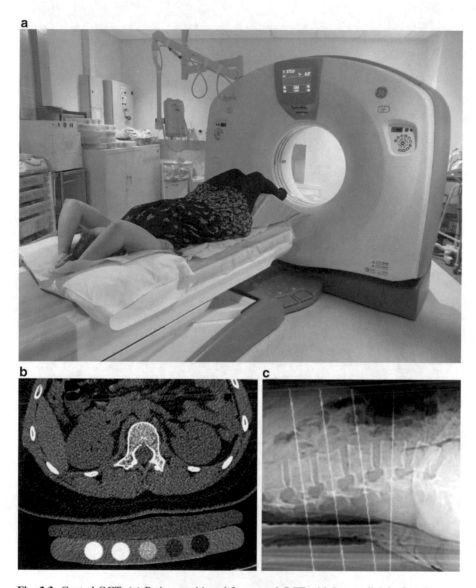

**Fig. 2.3** Central QCT: (**a**) Patient positioned for central QCT with knees slightly flexed over a moulded support to flatten lumbar lordosis. (**b**) cross section through mid-plane of lumbar vertebra with patient lying on the bone reference phantom from Mindways with cylinders of fat, water and 50, 100, and 200 mg of hydroxyapatite, and gel cushion between phantom and patient to reduce artefacts. The defect in the posterior cortical margin of the vertebral body is the entry of the basi-vertebral vein indicating the middle of the vertebral body. (**c**) 2D single slice technique: lateral scout projection radiograph (*scout view*) with the plane of the mid vertebral body sections of L1 to L4 indicated where volumetric BMD will be measured. (**d**) 3D volumetric technique: acquired with MDCT - midline sagittal (*middle images*) and coronal (*lower images*) reformats through L1 to L3 with mid-plane lines through each vertebra and oval region of interest of analysis placed in trabecular region to provide vBMD (*upper images*). (**e**) Lateral CT scout view: which should be scrutinised for vertebral fractures; grade 2 moderate vertebral fracture of T12 (*arrow*)

d

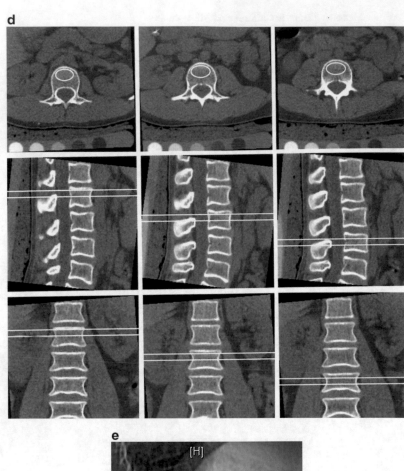

e

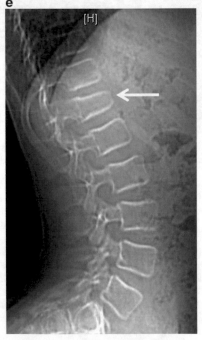

**Fig. 2.3** (continued)

34] if scanners or phantoms have to be changed during longitudinal studies then cross-calibration with patients and a phantom, such as the European Spine Phantom (ESP) [35], must be undertaken to make results comparable, although the ionising radiation involved makes duplicate measurements in children problematic (Table 2.2).

For two-dimensional (2D) spine measurements, an initial lateral scan projection radiograph is obtained (Fig. 2.3c). A 10 mm section is then performed through the mid plane of the vertebrae to be measured and parallel to the vertebral endplates. The section is confirmed to be in the correct plane when the area of the basi-vertebral vein is identified (Fig. 2.3b). For 2D QCT in adults, generally three vertebrae are scanned (L1 to L3) to ensure that at least 2–3 vertebrae are available for analysis at follow-up scans, should it be necessary to exclude vertebrae that have fractured between measurements. Since vertebral fractures occur less commonly in children and to minimise ionising radiation dose, generally only two adjacent vertebrae (between L1 to L3) are scanned. Vertebrae should be matched to those scanned in the reference database used, because BMD differs between vertebrae. If longitudinal studies are performed it is essential to scan the identical vertebrae examined at baseline.

QCT results are expressed as a mean volumetric bone mineral density (vBMD) in mg/cm$^3$. The trabecular vBMD measured by QCT is a composite of the amount of bone and marrow per voxel. The reason for this is the relatively small size of trabeculae compared to the voxel, resulting in marrow being included in the measurement. Because marrow fat is limited in children, age related marrow changes in fat composition should not confound spinal vBMD measurements in children as significantly as they do in adults [36].

Over the past two decades advances in CT technology and the introduction of multi-detector spiral CT (MDCT) enable rapid scanning so that several vertebral bodies are imaged within less than a minute. This technology has been used for volumetric QCT, which provides 3-D volume analysis of the vertebral bodies (mostly L1-L3). These developments improve precision (coefficients of variation of better than 1 %) and have advantages in children by reducing movement artefacts. In 3D MDCT sagittal midline reformatted images are obtained to define the mid-plane section to be analysed (Fig. 2.3d). Then, on the selected mid-plane cross-sectional image an oval region of interest (ROI) is placed in the central trabecular bone of the vertebral body at the site of the entry posteriorly of the basi-vertebral vein. The ROI should be as large as possible but not include the cortical rim of bone. As quantitative skeletal assessment does not require the optimisation of image quality needed for conventional CT, a low-dose technique can be employed to minimise radiation dose [37, 38] (Table 2.2). The results are expressed as standard deviations (SD) from the mean for appropriate age-, race- and sex-matched reference data (Z-score). The most frequently used normative data for spinal QCT were reported by Gilsanz and colleagues in 2009 [30, 31, 39, 40] (Table 2.3).

QCT offers several advantages as a densitometric technique. Whereas DXA measures integral (cortical and trabecular) BMD, QCT provides separate measures of cortical and trabecular BMD. As trabecular bone is generally more metabolically active than cortical bone, trabecular vBMD as measured by QCT is more sensitive to change in BMD [41]. The BMD provided is volumetric and less influenced by bone size than DXA, which provides an 'areal' density (g/cm²). CT also provides true morphometric dimensions of bones, and in the shafts can measure cross-sectional area of bone, cortical thickness and density, and periosteal and endosteal circumference. These parameters can be used to calculate estimates of biomechanical bone strength including moment of inertia. QCT also has the potential to be applied to peripheral skeletal sites such as radius, tibia and mid femur with lower associated radiation exposure than spinal QCT [30, 42, 43]. In addition QCT studies can be used to perform finite element analysis allowing the calculation of bone strength [44].

The limitations of QCT include the substantially greater dose of ionising radiation than DXA for spine scans (Table 2.2). For single slice (2D) QCT low-dose protocols using 80 kVp (or 120 kVp) and 120 mAs (or 150–200 mAs) result in effective doses of less than 200 µSv [32]. Felsenberg et al. described a low-energy, low-dose protocol with 80 kVp and 146 mAs resulting in effective doses down to 50–60 µSv, including the preliminary scan projection (scoutview) radiograph [45]. In comparison DXA has radiation doses in the range of 5–13 µSv for the lumbar spine and 9 µSv for the hip while an AP lumbar spine radiograph has a dose of 700 µSv and a standard abdominal CT has an exposure dose of approximately 8000 µSv [46]. For volumetric (3D) MDCT QCT radiation doses are higher and have been estimated to be as high as 1.5 mSv for the spine and 2.5–3 mSv for the hip [47]. Access to QCT may be problematic because many radiology departments lack the appropriate phantoms and software to perform bone densitometry studies. Furthermore, CT equipment is in great demand for other clinical diagnostic purposes. Currently there is a dearth of commercial analysis packages for QCT that can be purchased which require little set-up (for example Mindways, Austin, Texas, USA), Therefore, some centres have resorted to developing their own analysis software [48]. As with other bone densitometry techniques, QCT requires skilled and dedicated technical staff to perform the scans and optimise precision. Finally, there are far fewer published pediatric reference data for QCT than for DXA (Table 2.3) [30, 39].

More recently Habashy et al. investigated the feasibility and potential limitations of estimating BMD from standard diagnostic CT studies. They compared BMD measurements obtained with and without an external calibration phantom and found that phantomless QCT adds clinically useful BMD information to standard diagnostic CT studies [49]. The preliminary scout view should always be scrutinised for the presence of vertebral fractures (Fig. 2.3e).

In summary, and based on the general consensus of the ISCD QCT Task Force and working group [30]: the most common sites scanned on whole body CT scanners are the lumbar spine (L1 to L3), mid femoral shaft and the tibia. In the long bones, a metaphyseal and diaphyseal site should be scanned, and ideally in longitudinal studies the whole bone using 3D MDCT QCT should be scanned. This will enable results from similar anatomical sites to be compared which may be problematic in growing bones in 2D pQCT. Also, lying on the table of a general purpose scanner may afford easier positioning of children with disability (e.g. cerebral palsy,

Duchenne muscular dystrophy) and rapid scanning (20 s) reduces movement arte-fact. The proximal femur (hip) should not be scanned as it is in adults as the ionising radiation dose is high (3 mSv). Currently, adult scan protocols are being used in children, and there is an urgent need for development of pediatric protocols to mini-mise radiation dose. More robust reference data and analysis tools are required for the wider applicability of the technique.

## Peripheral Quantitative Computed Tomography (PQCT)

Peripheral quantitative computed tomography (pQCT) first became commercially available in the early 1990's [50–52]. The most commonly used pQCT scanner (XCT 2000, Stratec, Pforzheim, Germany) utilises the original rotate-translate CT technology, which generates only single 2D slices (1–2 mm thick) and requires a long acquisition time of about 1 min to obtain a single slice.

The sites of measurement are the radius, tibia and femur. For clinical assessment of a child's bone, the most commonly used site is the distal 4 % of the forearm or tibia length proximal to the distal growth plate. Peripheral QCT is most commonly applied to the non-dominant forearm. The forearm length is measured as the dis-tance between the tip of the ulnar styloid and the olecranon. The forearm is placed pronated in the pQCT gantry with the elbow resting on a block and the hand grip-ping the hand fixture and the arm is secured with Velcro straps to prevent movement (Fig. 2.4a and b). In children it is important to avoid the section including the growth plate, which produces falsely high measures due to the zone of provisional calcifica-tion. To locate the appropriate scan slice, a scanogram is performed (Fig. 2.4c and d). A reference line is placed to bisect the medial border of the end of the distal radius in adults. In children if the growth plate is visible, the reference line is posi-tioned to bisect the medial border of the distal dense metaphysis (Fig. 2.4c). If the distal radial growth plate has fused, the reference line is placed to bisect the medial border of the distal articular surface of the radius (Fig. 2.4d). For the tibia the refer-ence line location varies but is usually placed on the metaphysis and again the scan-ner moves to the measurement site from this point (Fig. 2.5). Upon closure of the growth plate at skeletal maturity the distal surface of the epiphysis joint margin is used for placement of the reference line. Radial abnormalities such as Madelung's deformity (disturbance of growth of the medial component of the distal end of the radius which causes reduction in the carpal angle) may cause difficulties in posi-tioning the reference line. In children treated with bisphosphonates, the reference line should be positioned to try to ensure that the growth arrest lines (residue of the provisional zone of calcification) are avoided in the measurement which will be artefactually elevated [53, 54].

The low-radiation dose of pQCT allows multiple site measurements to be made. Often research protocols include sections taken at 4 %, 14 %, 20 %, 38 %, 66 % of the leg length, in the forearm sections 4 % 50 % and 65 % of the forearm length. Multiple site measurements allow site-specific changes in bone and soft tissue to be

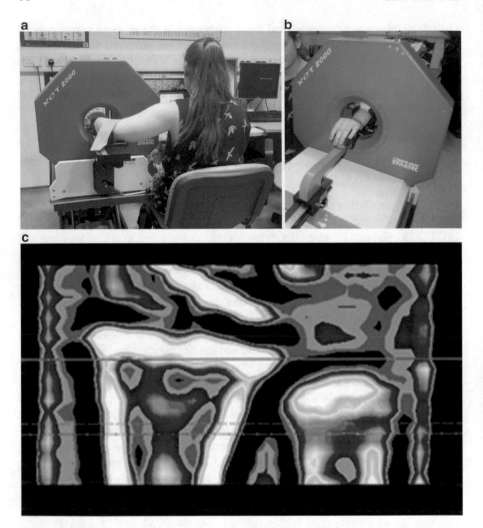

**Fig. 2.4** Peripheral QCT Radius: before scanning the forearm length is measured from ulna styloid to olecranon with arm flexed. (**a**) Child positioned in Stratec XCT 2000 pQCT scanner for scanning of non-dominant radius with forearm pronated in gantry and held securely with Velcro strap and (**b**) hand on moulded support. (**c**) Scout view: when the growth plate is unfused the reference line is placed to bisect the corner of the medial metaphysis of the distal radius (*single line*); the scan plane is then 4 % proximal to this reference line (*double line*). (**d**) Scout view: when the growth plates have fused in older children the reference line has to be placed to bisect the corner of the medial border of the distal articular surface of the radius. Cross-section at (**e**) 4 % distal radial site showing central trabecular bone and outer cortical bone (*white*) at which vBMD can be measured and (**f**) 50 % mid diaphyseal site at which bone geometry, density, strength and muscle area and 'density' can be measured

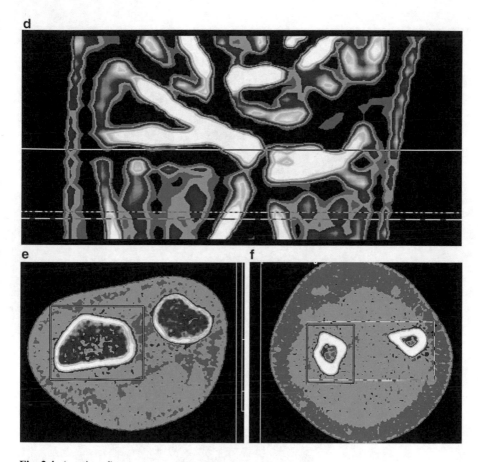

**Fig. 2.4** (continued)

studied. The scan time is approximately 1 min per slice; typically a single slice is obtained at each site. Therefore the technique is more successful in older children who are able to remain still during the relatively long scan procedure; good quality scans are difficult to obtain in children under 5 years.

Peripheral QCT offers the same benefits as central QCT (Tables 2.4 and 2.5). Volumetric BMD is measured which is not size-dependent and therefore will be less affected by growth [55, 56]. pQCT is able to separate trabecular from cortical bone. As the technique is only applicable to the peripheral skeleton, these measurements are obtained at much lower cost and radiation exposure (Table 2.1) than central QCT. pQCT also allows assessments of bone geometry, parameters related to bone strength, and muscle cross-sectional area and muscle density (surrogates for muscle strength). In order to measure these parameters, the sites of measurement by pQCT are optimised. The 4 % site at the distal end of the radius or tibia assesses total and trabecular vBMD (Figs. 2.4e and 2.5b). In the mid-diaphyseal portion of the bone,

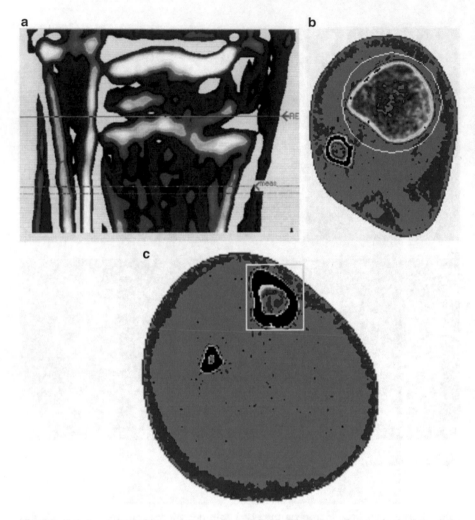

**Fig. 2.5** Peripheral QCT Tibia: (**a**) Scout view of distal tibia with unfused growth plate so the reference line is placed to bisect the lateral corner of the metaphysis of the distal tibia (*single line*); the scan plane is then 4 % proximal to this reference line (*double line*). (**b**) Section through the distal tibial shaft and (**c**) through the tibial diaphysis. At the distal site total and trabecular vBMD is measured. In the diaphysis bone geometry, density, strength and muscle area and 'density' can be measured

measurements are made of cortical vBMD, bone area, cortical thickness, periosteal circumference, endosteal circumference and muscle cross-sectional area (Figs. 2.4f and 2.5c). Parameters related to bone strength are also measured at the mid-diaphyseal site, the axial moment of inertia (AMI) and the stress–strain index (SSI). The AMI is the distribution of bone material around the centre of the bone and the SSI is a combination of AMI and the vBMD of the cortex; both parameters relate well to the fracture load [57, 58]. The study of the adaptation of bone to loading from muscle can be made using pQCT. By calculating the ratio of bone to muscle it is possible to investigate whether the bones have adapted adequately to the mechanical stresses to which they are exposed, and whether this may be a cause for increased bone fragility [59].

Peripheral QCT has been used in pediatric research to assess bone development in healthy children [2, 55, 60–67], response to pharmacological and non-pharmacological interventions and in those at risk for poor bone health [30, 68–74]. At present, pQCT is an FDA approved device but is used primarily for research, rather than clinical, studies for several reasons. There have been challenges in achieving adequate precision, controversies related to the optimum site of scanning of bone for pediatric studies, and a paucity of pediatric reference data. There are three studies reporting pediatric reference data in children of European ancestry which can be used [64, 75, 76], whilst ensuring protocols are carefully replicated, to calculate age-, height- and gender-matched Z-scores in accordance with ISCD recommendations [30, 77]. Finally, a model for the use of pQCT in the assessment of clinical conditions has been proposed to assess whether bone fragility results from a bone, muscle or mixed-bone and muscle deficit [59]. This is based on the principle that loading by muscles is the driver of postnatal bone development and is described by the mechanostat theory [78]. The 'mechanostat' model is also applicable to DXA measurements of lean mass and BA or BMC [20, 21]. Despite the increased use of pQCT there remains a lack of evidence for fracture prediction of the measurements; most consistently significantly lower trabecular or total vBMD at distal sites is reported [30, 67, 79].

Whereas general purpose CT scanners are calibrated to water being 0HU, so that trabecular bone does not have a negative value related to marrow fat, Stratec pQCT scanners add a constant of 60 mg/cm$^3$ to the calibrated BMD values. As a consequence results from scanners calibrated with this fat offset correction and those from scanners calibrated to water are not comparable.

## High-Resolution Peripheral Quantitative Computed Tomography (HR-PQCT)

The High-resolution pQCT (HR-pQCT) scanner is produced by a single manufacturer (XtremeCT, Scanco Medical AG, Brüttisellen, Switzerland) (Fig. 2.6a) and has higher spatial resolution compared to standard pQCT, MD-CT and MRI [80]. While the reconstructed voxel size is 82 μm for the standard patient HR-pQCT protocol, the actual spatial resolution of the image is approximately 130 μm near the centre of the field of view, and somewhat less off-centre (140–160 μm) [81]. Newer generation HR-pQCT systems have a voxel size down to 41 μm. The effective radiation dose is low at <3 microSv.

The system allows acquisition of BMD, trabecular and cortical bone architecture at the distal radius and tibia in a standardised fashion (Fig. 2.6b). Based on a semi-automated contouring and segmentation process, the trabecular and cortical compartments are segmented automatically for subsequent densitometric, morphometric and biomechanical analyses (Fig. 2.6c). Morphometric indices analogous to classical histomorphometry as well as connectivity, structure model index (a measure of the rod

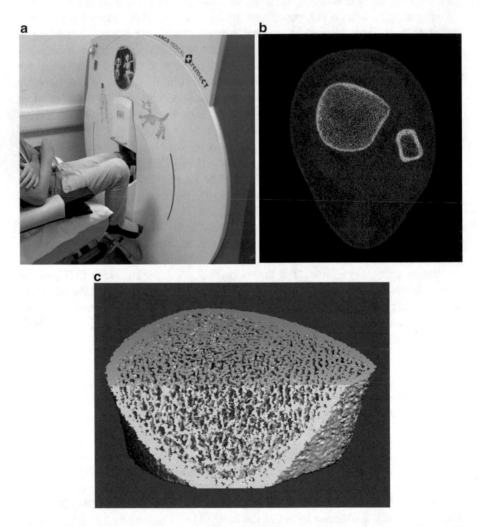

**Fig. 2.6** High-resolution peripheral QCT: (**a**) Child having scan of left distal tibia in an XtremeCT scanner (Scanco Medical AG, Brüttisellen, Switzerland). (**b**) Section through the distal tibia with high spatial resolution (130 μm) enabling acquisition of vBMD, and trabecular and cortical bone architecture. (**c**) Based on a semi-automated contouring and segmentation process, the trabecular and cortical compartments are segmented automatically for subsequent densitometric, morphometric, and biomechanical analyses

or plate-like appearance of the structure) and anisotropy can be calculated from the binary images of the trabecular bone. In addition finite element analysis (FEA) can be applied to these datasets and apparent biomechanical properties (e.g. stiffness, elastic modulus) can be computed by decomposing the trabecular bone structure into small cubic elements (i.e. the voxels) with assumed mechanical properties [82, 83].

However, the application of HR-pQCT in pediatric clinical and research studies has been limited to date and only a small number of studies have been published. In an initial feasibility study Burrows et al. investigated the bone microstructure of the distal radius in 328 children (9–21 years old) and standardised scanning parameters [84]. From the scout view images they determined that a ROI in the distal radius at 7 % of bone length excluded the radial growth plate in 100 % of participants. Liu et al. compared bone architecture between the distal radius and distal tibia and found substantial variations between the two sites [85]. Clinical studies to date using HR-pQCT focused on physical activity [86], bone assessment in chronic kidney disease [87] and childhood obesity [88]. As with other QCT methods it is imperative to reproduce exactly scanning and measurement protocols when using data from healthy children as a comparator. Adjustment for limb-length should also be made in protocols otherwise comparisons will be made between different anatomical sites [63, 89].

As a fixed bone mineralization of 1200 mg/cm³ is assumed, any disease or treatment which alters mineralisation (e.g. rickets) will cause inaccuracies in all the parameters measured [90]. As the bone cortex is thinner in children than in adults, partial volume averaging and different spatial resolution of CT scanners result in cortical assessment being more problematic [91].

## Magnetic Resonance Imaging

Magnetic resonance imaging (MRI) is the most recently developed technique for skeletal assessment in children. Quantification of an MRI scan is based upon the resonance and relaxation of protons in lipids and water; different tissues will have varying quantities of water and lipid, thus allowing imaging and differentiation of various anatomical structures. In bone, the marrow provides the signal with little contribution from bone; therefore the image formed shows marrow as white and bone as black (Fig. 2.7). In MRI varying sequences can be used but in all (T1 or T2 weighted) bone has low/absent signal and muscle intermediate signal. In validation studies bone quantification using MRI has been shown to correlate well to ash weight and 3D-QCT scans [92].

MRI offers several potential advantages. The technique provides a volumetric measure of bone without using ionising radiation. Imaging in multiple anatomical planes is possible, without having to reposition the subject (Fig. 2.7c and d). Simultaneous scanning of several limbs is also feasible. Similar to QCT, MRI distinguishes trabecular from cortical bone compartments and provides measures of bone morphometry from which parameters of bone strength can be calculated. By

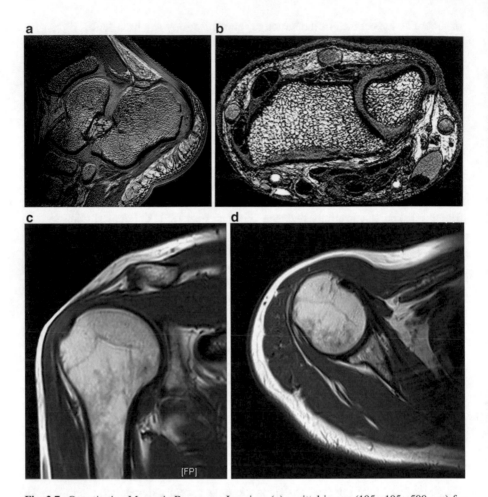

**Fig. 2.7** Quantitative Magnetic Resonance Imaging: (**a**) sagittal image (195×195×500 μm) for assessment of calcaneus trabecular bone structure in a 7-year-old boy; (**b**) trabecular structure of the distal radius acquired on a 3T scanner using the Mayo wrist coil; from these images histomorphometric parameters can be extracted. The multi-planar capabilities of MRI shown by (**c**) coronal and (**d**) axial images of the shoulder. Images can also be taken in the sagittal plane. Bone has no signal (*black*), muscle has an intermediate signal (*dark grey*), and fat, a high signal (*white*). Images are normally performed in the midshaft of the long bones for bone geometry and muscle analysis

scanning whole bones MRI offers the possibility to study comprehensively the differential growth patterns of the bones [93, 94]. The technique is applicable to both the central [95] and appendicular skeleton [93, 94, 96–98].

There are a few limitations of MRI. During the measurement, the scanning equipment is noisy which can be uncomfortable for the subject being scanned; additionally, the scan time is lengthy, taking as long as 20–30 min with positioning and scout scans depending on the imaging sequences used. Lying in the long-narrow horizontal gantry of the scanner can be distressing to claustrophobic individuals (1–2 % of subjects). Furthermore, keeping children still without sedation may be problematic. However, in published research studies, sedation was not used and the children tolerated the scan process well [94, 98, 99]. The environment of the scanner room is also not as child-friendly as other densitometry techniques and parents cannot remain with the child during scanning. Accurate in vivo measurement of trabecular bone structure (trabecular thickness is 0.05–0.2 mm) is technically challenging and still being developed [100–107]. The optimisation of sequence, field strength and receiver coils are imperative for the quality of imaging required. To date, MRI has been used only in research protocols; its applicability in clinical practice has yet to be assessed.

## Relationships of Peripheral to Central (Axial) Techniques in Children

In adults, measurements of BMD at both central and peripheral sites have been proven to predict future osteoporotic fracture [108]. In older adults, osteoporosis is defined in terms of bone densitometry as a T score (SD from mean of ethnic- and sex-matched peak BMD) of −2.5 or below, using central DXA in the lumbar spine, proximal femur and distal 1/3 radius. The agreement in classification by the various densitometric techniques has been studied in adults [109–111] and each performs well in differentiating osteoporosis or osteopenia from normal bone status. However, each technique identifies different people as osteoporotic/osteopenic and hence the diagnostic agreement between the methods is poor (Kappa[1] score 0.4). As an exception to the rule, several studies have shown that the agreement between lumbar spine trabecular vBMD (measured by QCT) and lateral DXA BMD has a kappa score 0.75 [111]. The reasons for poor agreement between various bone density methods and at different sites are likely to include differences in the cortical/trabecular content, the ability of the technique to measure integral or separate cortical and trabecular bone [112, 113], differing patterns of regional bone loss (e.g. spine versus distal 1/3 radius) and differential disease-specific effects on bone. Differences in scanner technology will also be relevant in contributing to the poor agreement between methods. Whether BMD is measured in adults or in children, the agreement between different techniques is likely to be of similar magnitude (r between 0.4 and 0.9). For example in children with juvenile idiopathic arthritis, who are most likely to suffer a vertebral crush fracture [114, 115] measurement of spinal trabecular bone should be a priority. Therefore, any measurement, which does not include the spine, is less likely to be sensitive to the bone changes that occur. Diagnostic agreement between

---

[1] A kappa score is a measurement of agreement between two methods when the measurements are measured on a categorical scale. The methods being tested have to rate or classify using the same scale, for example z-scores. Degree of agreement ranges from 0 to 1 with 1 being excellent, 0.8 good, etc.

central and peripheral skeletal sites may also differ depending on the child's phase of skeletal development. A large change in DXA spine BMD, with no change in radius trabecular BMD, may be due to the increase in bone size due to the pubertal growth spurt rather than change in volumetric bone mineral density. To date, there are limited studies investigating the relationship between the peripheral and central bone densitometry techniques and fracture prediction in children [14, 116].

Several studies have been performed which investigate the ability of peripheral measurement to predict osteoporotic fracture in adults [108, 117, 118]. Site-specific measurements have proven to be the best predictors of fractures at that site; for example, hip BMD will predict hip fracture better than radius or spine BMD measurements. However, BMD by peripheral techniques do predict spine and hip fracture in adults, thus providing useful information and if central BMD measurement is not available.

The forearm is the most common site of fracture in children. Goulding et al. have shown that children who have suffered fractures have generally lower aBMD in the whole skeleton [119]. Others have confirmed this observation for all upper limb fractures [120], whereas other data show low hip and spine BMD measurements in children who have suffered fractures but not whole body deficits [121, 122]. Low aBMD as measured by central DXA was predictive of the likelihood of a child to re-fracture within 4 years of initial fracture date [123]. Similarly, the largest prospective cohort study to date showed total body less head size-adjusted BMC was predictive of fracture in healthy children [124]. Together the findings of fracture studies in children suggest that low BMD may be a contributing factor to childhood fracture, just as it is in adults. However, there are insufficient data to establish a "fracture threshold" in children and young adults. The ISCD make recommendations for the diagnosis of osteoporosis in children based on low BMD (total body less head or spine) and a clinically significant fracture history [125]. Furthermore, comparisons between different scanning techniques for childhood fractures have not yet been made.

# Summary

DXA is currently the most widely available and accepted clinical tool for the assessment of bone status in children. With appropriate use and consideration of its limitations, DXA provides valuable information of the bone status of an individual child. The following chapters give details regarding the acquisition, interpretation and reporting of DXA in children to provide the best possible clinical service. The other densitometry techniques discussed in this chapter remain predominantly research tools. However, their use in clinical practice is likely to increase in future as a means of assessing bone geometry and the site specific effects of diseases. It should be remembered that all bone densitometry techniques were designed for use in adults; the application and interpretation of all of the methods described in this chapter are much more difficult in children and adolescents.

## Summary Points

- X-rays have been used in many different imaging modalities from simple radiographic images to highly sophisticated spiral, multi-detector computed tomography, which can provide 2D cross-sectional and 3D volume images of the body and its organs.
- The absorption of X-rays by tissues is determined by the energy (or wavelength) of the radiation and the composition (electron density and atomic number) of the tissue though which the X-rays pass.
- In longitudinal bone densitometry changes to scanner, phantom, reference data or software should always be made with caution; guidance for appropriate procedures is provided in other chapters in this book.
- Table 2.5 presents the advantages and limitations of each of the techniques discussed in this chapter
- DXA is currently the most accepted and widely used bone densitometry technique for clinical application in children
- QCT and MRI, applied to peripheral and central sites, provide additional complimentary important research information on bone size, shape, density and structure which gives insights into the effect of disease and therapies on the skeleton

## References

1. Nelson D, Koo W. Interpretation of absorptiometric bone mass measurements in the growing skeleton: issues and limitations. Calcif Tissue Int. 1999;65:1–3.
2. Rauch F, Schonau E. Changes in bone density during childhood and adolescence: an approach based on bone's biological organization. J Bone Miner Res. 2001;16(4):597–604.
3. Carter D, Bouxsein M, Marcus R. New approaches for interpreting projected bone densitometry data. J Bone Miner Res. 1992;7:137–45.
4. Kroger H, Kontaniemi A, Vainio P, Alhava E. Bone densitometry of the spine and femur in children by dual-energy x-ray absorptiometry. Bone miner. 1992;17(1):75–85.
5. Fewtrell MS, Gordon I, Biassoni L, Cole TJ. Dual X-ray absorptiometry (DXA) of the lumbar spine in a clinical paediatric setting: does the method of size-adjustment matter? Bone. 2005;37(3):413–9.
6. Mazess RB, Barden HS. Bone densitometry for diagnosis and monitoring osteoporosis. Proc Soc Exp Biol Med. 1989;191(3):261–71.
7. Compston JE, Cooper C, Kanis JA. Fortnightly review: bone densitometry in clinical practice. BMJ. 1995;310(6993):1507–10.
8. Genant HK, Engelke K, Fuerst T, Gluer CC, Grampp S, Harris ST, et al. Noninvasive assessment of bone mineral and structure: state of the art. J Bone Miner Res. 1996;11(6):707–30.
9. Adams JE. Advances in bone imaging for osteoporosis. Nat Rev Endocrinol. 2013;9(1):28–42.
10. LeBlanc CM, Ma J, Taljaard M, Roth J, Scuccimarri R, Miettunen P, et al. Incident vertebral fractures and risk factors in the first three years following glucocorticoid initiation among pediatric patients with rheumatic disorders. J Bone Miner Res. 2015;30(9):1667–75.
11. Huber AM, Gaboury I, Cabral DA, Lang B, Ni A, Stephure D, et al. Prevalent vertebral fractures among children initiating glucocorticoid therapy for the treatment of rheumatic disorders. Arthritis Care Res (Hoboken). 2010;62(4):516–26.

12. Halton J, Gaboury I, Grant R, Alos N, Cummings EA, Matzinger M, et al. Advanced vertebral fracture among newly diagnosed children with acute lymphoblastic leukemia: results of the Canadian Steroid-Associated Osteoporosis in the Pediatric Population (STOPP) research program. J Bone Miner Res. 2009;24(7):1326–34.
13. Kyriakou A, Shepherd S, Mason A, Faisal AS. A critical appraisal of vertebral fracture assessment in paediatrics. Bone. 2015;81:255–9.
14. Crabtree NJ, Hogler W, Cooper MS, Shaw NJ. Diagnostic evaluation of bone densitometric size adjustment techniques in children with and without low trauma fractures. Osteoporos Int. 2013;24(7):2015–24.
15. Kuet KP, Charlesworth D, Peel NF. Vertebral fracture assessment scans enhance targeting of investigations and treatment within a fracture risk assessment pathway. Osteoporos Int. 2013;24(3):1007–14.
16. Rodd C, Lang B, Ramsay T, Alos N, Huber AM, Cabral DA, et al. Incident vertebral fractures among children with rheumatic disorders 12 months after glucocorticoid initiation: a national observational study. Arthritis Care Res (Hoboken). 2012;64(1):122–31.
17. Crabtree NJ, Arabi A, Bachrach LK, Fewtrell M, El-Hajj Fuleihan G, Kecskemethy HH, et al. Dual-energy X-ray absorptiometry interpretation and reporting in children and adolescents: the revised 2013 ISCD Pediatric Official Positions. J Clin Densitom. 2014;17(2):225–42.
18. Crabtree NJ, Chapman S, Hogler W, Shaw NJ. Is vertebral fracture assessment by DXA more useful in a high fracture risk paediatric population than in a low-risk screening population. Bone Abstracts (2013) 2 P135. DOI:10.1530/boneabs.2.P135
19. Adams JE, Shaw N, editors. A practical guide to bone densitometry in children. 1st ed. Bath, UK: National Osteoporosis Society; 2004.
20. Crabtree NJ, Kibirige MS, Fordham JN, Banks LM, Muntoni F, Chinn D, et al. The relationship between lean body mass and bone mineral content in paediatric health and disease. Bone. 2004;35(4):965–72.
21. Hogler W, Briody J, Woodhead HJ, Chan A, Cowell CT. Importance of lean mass in the interpretation of total body densitometry in children and adolescents. J Pediatr. 2003;143(1):81–8.
22. Molgaard C, Thomsen B, Prentice A, Cole T, Michaelsen K. Whole body bone mineral content in healthy children and adolescents. Arch Dis Child. 1997;76:9–15.
23. Prentice A, Parsons T, Cole T. Uncritical use of bone mineral density in absorptiometry may lead to size-related artifacts in the identification of bone mineral determinants. Am J Clin Nutr. 1994;60:837–42.
24. Warner J, Cowan F, Dunstan F, Evans W, Webb D, Gregory J. Measured and predicted bone mineral content in healthy boys and girls aged 6–18 years: adjustment for body size and puberty. Acta Paediatr. 1998;87:244–9.
25. Nevill A, Holder R, Maffulli N, Cheng J, Leung S, Lee W, et al. Adjusting bone mass for differences in projected bone area and other confounding varaibles: an allometric perspective. J Bone Miner Res. 2002;17(4):703–8.
26. Isherwood I, Rutherford R, Pullan B, Adams P. Bone mineral estimation by computed assisted transverse axial tomography. Lancet. 1976;2:712–5.
27. Guglielmi G, Lang T, Cammisa M, Genant H. Quantitative computed tomography at the axial skeleton. In: Genant H, Guglielmi G, Jergas M, editors. Bone densitometry and osteoporos. Berlin Heidelberg: Springer Verlag; 1998. p. 335–47.
28. Van Rijn R, van der Sluis I, Link T, Grampp S, Guglielmi G, Imhof H, et al. Bone densitometry in children: a critical appraisal. Eur Radiol. 2003;13:700–10.
29. Mughal M, Ward K, Adams J. Assessment of bone status in children by densitometric and quantitative ultrasound techniques. In: Carty H, editor. Imaging in children. 2nd ed. Edinburgh: Elsevier Science; 2004. pp 477–486.
30. Adams JE, Engelke K, Zemel BS, Ward KA. Quantitative computer tomography in children and adolescents: the 2013 ISCD Pediatric Official Positions. J Clin Densitom. 2014;17(2):258–74.
31. Gilsanz V, Perez FJ, Campbell PP, Dorey FJ, Lee DC, Wren TA. Quantitative CT reference values for vertebral trabecular bone density in children and young adults. Radiology. 2009;250(1):222–7.

32. Link TM, Lang TF. Axial QCT: clinical applications and new developments. J Clin Densitom. 2014;17(4):438–48.
33. Faulkner K, McClung M. Quality control of DXA instruments in multicentre trials. Osteoporos Int. 1995;5:218–27.
34. Genant H, Grampp S, Gluer C, Faulkner K, Jergas M, Engelke K, et al. Universal standardization for dual energy X-ray absorptiometry: patient and phantom cross-calibration results. J Bone Miner Res. 1994;9:1503–14.
35. Kalender W, Felsenberg D, Genant H, Fischer M, Dequeker J, Reeve J. European Spine Phantom - a tool for standardization and quality control in spinal bone mineral measurements by DXA and QCT. Eur J Radiol. 1995;20:83–92.
36. Gilsanz V. Bone density in children: a review of the available techniques and indications. Eur J Radiol. 1998;26:177–82.
37. Cann C. Low dose CT scanning for quantitative spinal bone mineral analysis. Radiology. 1981;140:813–5.
38. Kalender W. Effective dose values in bone mineral measurements by photon absorptiometry and computed tomography. Osteoporos Int. 1992;2:82–7.
39. Gilsanz V, Gibbens D, Roe T, Carlson M, Senac M, Boechat M, et al. Vertebral bone density in children: effect of puberty. Radiology. 1988;166(3):847–50.
40. Mora S, Gilsanz V, editors. Bone densitometry in children. Berlin Heidelberg: Springer Verlag; 1998.
41. Genant H, Cann C, Ettinger B, Gordan G. Quantitative computed tomography of vertebral spongiosa: a sensitive method for detecting early bone loss after oophorectomy. Ann Intern Med. 1982;97:699–705.
42. Ward K, Alsop C, Caulton J, Rubin C, Adams J, Mughal Z. Low magnitude mechanical loading is osteogenic in children with disabling conditions. J Bone Miner Res. 2004;19(3):360–9.
43. Caulton JM, Ward KA, Alsop CW, Dunn G, Adams JE, Mughal MZ. A randomised controlled trial of standing programme on bone mineral density in non-ambulant children with cerebral palsy. Arch Dis Child. 2004;89(2):131–5.
44. Kopperdahl DL, Aspelund T, Hoffmann PF, Sigurdsson S, Siggeirsdottir K, Harris TB, et al. Assessment of incident spine and hip fractures in women and men using finite element analysis of CT scans. J Bone Miner Res. 2014;29(3):570–80.
45. Felsenberg D, Gowin W. Bone densitometry by dual energy methods. Radiologe. 1999;39(3):186–93.
46. Damilakis J, Adams JE, Guglielmi G, Link TM. Radiation exposure in X-ray-based imaging techniques used in osteoporosis. Eur Radiol. 2010;20(11):2707–14.
47. Engelke K, Adams JE, Armbrecht G, Augat P, Bogado CE, Bouxsein ML, et al. Clinical use of quantitative computed tomography and peripheral quantitative computed tomography in the management of osteoporosis in adults: the 2007 ISCD official positions. J Clin Densitom. 2008;11(1):123–62.
48. Lang T, LeBlanc A, Evans H, Lu Y, Genant H, Yu A. Cortical and trabecular bone mineral loss from the spine and hip in long-standing spaceflight. J Bone Miner Res. 2004;19:1006–12.
49. Habashy AH, Yan X, Brown JK, Xiong X, Kaste SC. Estimation of bone mineral density in children from diagnostic CT images: a comparison of methods with and without an internal calibration standard. Bone. 2011;48(5):1087–94.
50. Schneider P, Borner W. Peripheral quantitative computed tomography for bone mineral measurement using a new special QCT-scanner. Methodology, normal values, comparison with manifest osteoporosis. Rofo. 1991;154(3):292–9.
51. Ruegsegger P, Durand E, Dambacher MA. Localization of regional forearm bone loss from high resolution computed tomographic images. Osteoporos Int. 1991;1(2):76–80.
52. Ruegsegger P, Durand EP, Dambacher MA. Differential effects of aging and disease on trabecular and compact bone density of the radius. Bone. 1991;12(2):99–105.
53. Rauch F, Travers R, Munns C, Glorieux FH. Sclerotic metaphyseal lines in a child treated with pamidronate: histomorphometric analysis. J Bone Miner Res. 2004;19(7):1191–3.

54. Sarraf KM. Images in clinical medicine. Radiographic zebra lines from cyclical pamidronate therapy. N Engl J Med. 2011;365(3), e5. July 21, 2011. DOI: 10.1056/NEJMicm1014009

55. Neu C, Manz F, Rauch F, Merkel A, Schonau E. Bone densities and bone size at the distal radius in healthy children and adolescents: a study using peripheral quantitative computed tomography. Bone. 2001;28(2):227–32.

56. Fujita T, Fujii Y, Goto B. Measurement of forearm bone in children by peripheral computed tomography. Calcif Tissue Int. 1999;64:34–9.

57. Schiessl H, Ferretti J, Tysarczyk-Niemeyer G, Willnecker J. Noninvasive bone strength index as analyzed by peripheral quantitative computed tomography (pQCT). In: Schoenau E, editor. Paediatric osteology: new developments in diagnostics and therapy, International Congress Series, vol. 1105. Amsterdam: Elsevier; 1996.

58. Augat P, Iida H, Jiang Y, Diao E, Genant HK. Distal radius fractures: mechanisms of injury and strength prediction by bone mineral assessment. J Orthop Res. 1998;16:629–35.

59. Schonau E, Neu C, Beck B, Manz F, Rauch F. Bone mineral content per muscle cross-sectional area as an index of the functional muscle-bone unit. J Bone Miner Res. 2002;17(6):1095–101.

60. Schonau E. The development of the skeletal system in children and the influence of muscular strength. Horm Res. 1998;47:27–31.

61. Binkley T, Specker B. pQCT measurement of bone parameters in young children - validation of technique. J Clin Densitom. 2000;3(1):9–14.

62. Schonau E, Neu C, Rauch F, Manz F. Gender-specific pubertal changes in volumetric cortical bone mineral density at the proximal radius. Bone. 2002;31(1):110–3.

63. Leonard MB, Shults J, Elliott DM, Stallings VA, Zemel BS. Interpretation of whole body dual energy X-ray absorptiometry measures in children: comparison with peripheral quantitative computed tomography. Bone. 2004;34(6):1044–52.

64. Ashby RL, Ward KA, Roberts SA, Edwards L, Mughal MZ, Adams JE. A reference database for the Stratec XCT-2000 peripheral quantitative computed tomography (pQCT) scanner in healthy children and young adults aged 6–19 years. Osteoporos Int. 2009;20(8):1337–46.

65. Ashby RL, Adams JE, Roberts SA, Mughal MZ, Ward KA. The muscle-bone unit of peripheral and central skeletal sites in children and young adults. Osteoporos Int. 2011;22(1):121–32.

66. Wetzsteon RJ, Zemel BS, Shults J, Howard KM, Kibe LW, Leonard MB. Mechanical loads and cortical bone geometry in healthy children and young adults. Bone. 2011;48(5):1103–8.

67. Kalkwarf HJ, Laor T, Bean JA. Fracture risk in children with a forearm injury is associated with volumetric bone density and cortical area (by peripheral QCT) and areal bone density (by DXA). Osteoporos Int. 2011;22(2):607–16.

68. Schonau E, Matkovic V. The functional muscle-bone unit in health and disease. In: Schonau E, Matkovic V, editors. Paediatric osteology prevention of osteoporosis - a paediatric task, International Congress Series, vol. 1154. Singapore: Elsevier; 1998. p. 191–202.

69. Schweizer R, Martin DD, Schwarze CP, Binder G, Georgiadou A, Ihle J, et al. Cortical bone density is normal in prepubertal children with growth hormone (GH) deficiency, but initially decreases during GH replacement due to early bone remodelling. J Clin Endocrinol Metab. 2003;88(11):5266–72.

70. Lima EM, Goodman WG, Kuizon BD, Gales B, Emerick A, Goldin J, et al. Bone density measurements in pediatric patients with renal osteodystrophy. Pediatr Nephrol. 2003;18(6):554–9.

71. Moyer-Mileur LJ, Dixon SB, Quick JL, Askew EW, Murray MA. Bone mineral acquisition in adolescents with type 1 diabetes. J Pediatr. 2004;145(5):662–9.

72. Brennan BM, Mughal Z, Roberts SA, Ward K, Shalet SM, Eden TO, et al. Bone mineral density in childhood survivors of acute lymphoblastic leukemia treated without cranial irradiation. J Clin Endocrinol Metab. 2005;90(2):689–94.

73. Roth J, Palm C, Scheunemann I, Ranke MB, Schweizer R, Dannecker GE. Musculoskeletal abnormalities of the forearm in patients with juvenile idiopathic arthritis relate mainly to bone geometry. Arthritis Rheum. 2004;50(4):1277–85.

74. Bechtold S, Ripperger P, Bonfig W, Pozza RD, Haefner R, Schwarz HP. Growth hormone changes bone geometry and body composition in patients with juvenile idiopathic arthritis requiring glucocorticoid treatment: a controlled study using peripheral quantitative computed tomography. J Clin Endocrinol Metab. 2005;90(6):3168–73.

75. Moyer-Mileur LJ, Quick JL, Murray MA. Peripheral quantitative computed tomography of the tibia: pediatric reference values. J Clin Densitom. 2008;11(2):283–94.
76. Rauch F, Schoenau E. Peripheral quantitative computed tomography of the proximal radius in young subjects--new reference data and interpretation of results. J Musculoskelet Neuronal Interact. 2008;8(3):217–26.
77. Zemel B, Bass S, Binkley T, Ducher G, Macdonald H, McKay H, et al. Peripheral quantitative computed tomography in children and adolescents: the 2007 ISCD pediatric official positions. J Clin Densitom. 2008;11(1):59–74.
78. Frost H. Bone "mass" and the "mechanostat": a proposal. Anat Rec. 1987;219(1):1–9.
79. Cheng S, Xu L, Nicholson PH, Tylavsky F, Lyytikainen A, Wang Q, et al. Low volumetric BMD is linked to upper-limb fracture in pubertal girls and persists into adulthood: a seven-year cohort study. Bone. 2009;45(3):480–6.
80. Krug R, Burghardt AJ, Majumdar S, Link TM. High-resolution imaging techniques for the assessment of osteoporosis. Radiol Clin North Am. 2010;48(3):601–21.
81. Cheung AM, Adachi JD, Hanley DA, Kendler DL, Davison KS, Josse R, et al. High-resolution peripheral quantitative computed tomography for the assessment of bone strength and structure: a review by the Canadian Bone Strength Working Group. Curr Osteoporos Rep. 2013;11(2):136–46.
82. Burghardt AJ, Kazakia GJ, Ramachandran S, Link TM, Majumdar S. Age- and gender-related differences in the geometric properties and biomechanical significance of intracortical porosity in the distal radius and tibia. J Bone Miner Res. 2010;25(5):983–93.
83. Liu XS, Zhang XH, Sekhon KK, Adams MF, McMahon DJ, Bilezikian JP, et al. High-resolution peripheral quantitative computed tomography can assess microstructural and mechanical properties of human distal tibial bone. J Bone Miner Res. 2010;25(4):746–56.
84. Burrows M, Liu D, McKay H. High-resolution peripheral QCT imaging of bone microstructure in adolescents. Osteoporos Int. 2010;21(3):515–20.
85. Liu D, Burrows M, Egeli D, McKay H. Site specificity of bone architecture between the distal radius and distal tibia in children and adolescents: an HR-pQCT study. Calcif Tissue Int. 2010;87(4):314–23.
86. Gabel L, McKay HA, Nettlefold L, Race D, Macdonald HM. Bone architecture and strength in the growing skeleton: the role of sedentary time. Med Sci Sports Exerc. 2015;47(2):363–72.
87. Bacchetta J, Boutroy S, Vilayphiou N, Ranchin B, Fouque-Aubert A, Basmaison O, et al. Bone assessment in children with chronic kidney disease: data from two new bone imaging techniques in a single-center pilot study. Pediatr Nephrol. 2011;26(4):587–95.
88. Dimitri P, Jacques RM, Paggiosi M, King D, Walsh J, Taylor ZA, et al. Leptin may play a role in bone microstructural alterations in obese children. J Clin Endocrinol Metab. 2015;100(2):594–602. jc20143199.
89. Ward KA, Riddell AR, Prentice A. Re: 'Compromised bone microarchitecture and estimated bone strength in young adults with cystic fibrosis' by Putman et al. J Clin Endocrinol Metab. 2015;100(1):L8. doi: 10.1210/jc.2014–3933.
90. Donnelly E. Methods for assessing bone quality: a review. Clin Orthop Relat Res. 2011;469(8):2128–38.
91. Ward KA, Adams JE, Hangartner TN. Recommendations for thresholds for cortical bone geometry and density measurement by peripheral quantitative computed tomography. Calcif Tissue Int. 2005;77(5):275–80.
92. Hong J, Hipp JA, Mulkern RV, Jaramillo D, Snyder BD. Magnetic resonance imaging measurements of bone density and cross-sectional geometry. Calcif Tissue Int. 2000;66(1):74–8.
93. Hogler W, Blimkie CJ, Cowell CT, Kemp AF, Briody J, Wiebe P, et al. A comparison of bone geometry and cortical density at the mid-femur between prepuberty and young adulthood using magnetic resonance imaging. Bone. 2003;33(5):771–8.
94. Macdonald HM, Heinonen A, Khan K, MacKelvie K, Sievanen H, Whittall K, editors. Geometric characteristics of the developing tibia in early pubertal girls a quantitative MRI study. J Bone Miner Res 2003;18(suppl 1): S66, abstract #F091.
95. Kroger H, Vainio P, Nieminen J, Kotaniemi A. Comparison of different models for interpreting bone mineral density measurements using DXA and MRI technology. Bone. 1995;17(2):157–9.

96. Heinonen A, McKay H, Whithall K, Forster B, Khan K. Muscle cross-sectional area is associated with specific site of bone in prepubertal girls: a quantitative magnetic resonance imaging study. Bone. 2001;29(4):388–92.
97. Bass SL, Saxon L, Daly RM, Turner CH, Robling AG, Seeman E, et al. The effect of mechanical loading on the size and shape of bone in pre-, peri-, and postpubertal girls: a study in
tennis players. J Bone Miner Res. 2002;17(12):2274–80.
98. Daly RM, Saxon L, Turner CH, Robling AG, Bass SL. The relationship between muscle size
and bone geometry during growth and in response to exercise. Bone. 2004;34(2):281–7.
99. McKay HA, Sievanen H, Petit MA, MacKelvie KJ, Forkheim KM, Whittall KP, et al.
Application of magnetic resonance imaging to evaluation of femoral neck structure in growing girls. J Clin Densitom. 2004;7(2):161–8.
100. Herlidou S, Grebe R, Grados F, Leuyer N, Fardellone P, Meyer ME. Influence of age and
osteoporosis on calcaneus trabecular bone structure: a preliminary in vivo MRI study by
quantitative texture analysis. Magn Reson Imaging. 2004;22(2):237–43.
101. Boutry N, Cortet B, Dubois P, Marchandise X, Cotten A. Trabecular bone structure of the
calcaneus: preliminary in vivo MR imaging assessment in men with osteoporosis. Radiology.
2003;227(3):708–17.
102. Link TM, Vieth V, Stehling C, Lotter A, Beer A, Newitt D, et al. High-resolution MRI vs
multislice spiral CT: which technique depicts the trabecular bone structure best? Eur Radiol.
2003;13(4):663–71.
103. Newitt DC, van Rietbergen B, Majumdar S. Processing and analysis of in vivo high-resolution
MR images of trabecular bone for longitudinal studies: reproducibility of structural measures and micro-finite element analysis derived mechanical properties. Osteoporos Int.
2002;13(4):278–87.
104. Laib A, Newitt DC, Lu Y, Majumdar S. New model-independent measures of trabecular bone
structure applied to in vivo high-resolution MR images. Osteoporos Int. 2002;13(2):130–6.
105. Wehrli FW, Hilaire L, Fernandez-Seara M, Gomberg BR, Song HK, Zemel B, et al. Quantitative
magnetic resonance imaging in the calcaneus and femur of women with varying degrees of
osteopenia and vertebral deformity status. J Bone Miner Res. 2002;17(12):2265–73.
106. Wehrli FW, Saha PK, Gomberg BR, Song HK, Snyder PJ, Benito M, et al. Role of magnetic
resonance for assessing structure and function of trabecular bone. Top Magn Reson Imaging.
2002;13(5):335–55.
107. Wehrli FW, Leonard MB, Saha PK, Gomberg BR. Quantitative high-resolution magnetic
resonance imaging reveals structural implications of renal osteodystrophy on trabecular and
cortical bone. J Magn Reson Imaging. 2004;20(1):83–9.
108. Marshall D, Johnell O, Wedel H. Meta-analysis of how well measures of bone mineral density predict occurence of osteoporotic fractures. BMJ. 1996;312:1254–9.
109. Martin JC, Campbell MK, Reid DM. A comparison of radial peripheral quantitative computed tomography, calcaneal ultrasound, and axial dual energy X-ray absorptiometry measurements in women aged 45–55 yr. J Clin Densitom. 1999;2(3):265–73.
110. Kroger H, Lunt M, Reeve J, Dequeker J, Adams JE, Birkenhager JC, et al. Bone density reduction in various measurement sites in men and women with osteoporotic fractures of spine and
hip: the European quantitation of osteoporosis study. Calcif Tissue Int. 1999;64(3):191–9.
111. Grampp S, Genant HK, Mathur A, Lang P, Jergas M, Takada M, et al. Comparisons of noninvasive bone mineral measurements in assessing age-related loss, fracture discrimination,
and diagnostic classification. J Bone Miner Res. 1997;12(5):697–711.
112. Eastell R, Wahner HW, O'Fallon WM, Amadio PC, Melton 3rd LJ, Riggs BL. Unequal
decrease in bone density of lumbar spine and ultradistal radius in Colles' and vertebral fracture syndromes. J Clin Invest. 1989;83(1):168–74.
113. Faulkner KG, Gluer CC, Majumdar S, Lang P, Engelke K, Genant HK. Noninvasive measurements of bone mass, structure, and strength: current methods and experimental techniques.
AJR Am J Roentgenol. 1991;157(6):1229–37.
114. Elsasser U, Wilkins B, Hesp R, Thurnham D, Reeve J, Ansell B. Bone rarefaction and crush
fractures in juvenile chronic arthritis. Arch Dis Child. 1982;57:377–80.

115. Varonos S, Ansell B, Reeve J. Vertebral collapse in juvenile chronic arthritis: its relationship with glucocorticoid therapy. Calcif Tissue Int. 1987;41(2):75–8.
116. Crabtree NJ, Hogler W, Shaw NJ. Fractures in children with chronic inflammatroy and/or disabling conditions: The SNAP study. Osteoporos Int. 2014;25 Suppl 6:S670.
117. Black D, Cummings S, Genant H, Nevitt M, Palermo L, Browner W. Axial and appendicular bone density predict fractures in older women. J Bone Miner Res. 1992;7:633–8.
118. Gardsell P, Johnell O, Nilsson BE. Predicting fractures in women by using forearm bone densitometry. Calcif Tissue Int. 1989;44:235–42.
119. Goulding A, Cannan R, Williams S, Gold E, Taylor R, Lewis-Barnes N. Bone mineral density in girls with forearm fractures. J Bone Miner Res. 1998;13(1):143–8.
120. Ma D, Jones G. The association between bone mineral density, metacarpal morphometry, and upper limb fracctures in children: a population-based case–control study. J Clin Endocrinol Metab. 2003;88:1486–91.
121. Kalkwarf H, Laor T, Bean J. Bone mass, density, and dimensions and forearm fracture risk among injured children. Bone. 2005;36(S2):S40.
122. Mobley S, Ha E, Landoll J, Badenhop-Stevens N, Clairmont A, Goel P, et al. Children and bone fragility fractures have reduced bone mineral areal density at the forearm and hip and higher percent body fat. J Bone Miner Res. 2005;20(S1).
123. Goulding A, Jones I, Taylor R, Manning P, Williams S. More broken bones: a 4-year double cohort study of young girls with and without distal forearm fractures. J Bone Miner Res. 2000;15(10):2011–8.
124. Clark EM, Ness AR, Bishop NJ, Tobias JH. Association between bone mass and fractures in children: a prospective cohort study. J Bone Miner Res. 2006;21(9):1489–95.
125. Bishop N, Arundel P, Clark E, Dimitri P, Farr J, Jones G, et al. Fracture prediction and the definition of osteoporosis in children and adolescents: the ISCD 2013 Pediatric Official Positions. J Clin Densitom. 2014;17(2):275–80.
126. Gilsanz V, Boechat M, Roe T, Loro M, Sayre J, Goodman W. Gender differences in vertebral body sizes in children and adoloescents. Radiology. 1994;190:673–7.
127. Hangartner T, Gilsanz V. Evaluation of cortical bone by computed tomography. J Bone Miner Res. 1996;11(10):1518–25.
128. Kovanlikaya A, Loro M, Hantgartner T, Reynolds R, Roe T, Gilsanz V. Osteopenia in children: CT assessment. Radiology. 1996;198(3):781–4.
129. Moyer-Mileur L, Xie B, Pratt T, editors. Peripheral quantitative computed tomography: assessment of tibial bone mass change in preadolescent girls. Federation of American Societies for Experimental Biology, Experimental Biology 2000; San Diego, CA; 2000.
130. Sievanen H, Koskue V, Rauhio A, Kannus P, Heinonen A, Vuori I. Peripheral quantitative computed tomography in human long bones: evaluation of in vitro and in vivo precision. J Bone Miner Res. 1998;13(5):871–82.
131. NRPB. Living with radiation. Oxon: National Oncologic Protection Board.
132. Radiation and The Nuclear Fuel Cycle. World Nuclear Association, 2004 March. Report No.
133. Huda W, Gkanatsios N. Radiation dosimetry for extremity radiographs. Health Phys. 1998;75(6):492–9.
134. Hart D, Wall B. Radiation exposure of the UK population from medical and dental X-ray examinations. Oxon: National Radiological Protection Board, 2002 March 2002. Report No.: ISBN 0 85951 468 4.
135. ARSAC. Notes for guidance on the clinical administration of radiopharmaceuticals and use of sealed radioactive sources. National Radiological Protection Board: Oxon; 1998.
136. Southard R, Morris J, Mahan J, Hayes J, Torch M, Sommer A, et al. Bone mass in healthy children: measurement with quantitative DXA. Radiology. 1991;179:735–8.
137. Faulkner RA, Bailey DA, Drinkwater DT, McKay HA, Arnold C, Wilkinson AA. Bone densitometry in Canadian children 8–17 years of Age. Calcif Tissue Int. 1996;59(5):344–51.
138. Zemel B, Leonard M, Kalkwarf H, Specker B, Moyer-Mileur L, Shepherd J, et al. Reference data for the whole body, lumbar spine and proximal femur for american children relative to age, gender and body size. Am Soc Bone Min Res. 2004;19(S1):S231.

139. Arabi A, Nabulsi M, Maalouf J, Choucair M, Khalife H, Vieth R, et al. Bone mineral density by age, gender, pubertal stages, and socioeconomic status in healthy Lebanese children and adolescents. Bone. 2004;35(5):1169–79.
140. Kalkwarf HJ, Zemel BS, Gilsanz V, Lappe JM, Horlick M, Oberfield S, et al. The bone mineral density in childhood study: bone mineral content and density according to age, sex, and race. J Clin Endocrinol Metab. 2007;92(6):2087–99.
141. Ward KA, Ashby RL, Roberts SA, Adams JE, Zulf MM. UK reference data for the Hologic QDR Discovery dual-energy x ray absorptiometry scanner in healthy children and young adults aged 6–17 years. Arch Dis Child. 2007;92(1):53–9.
142. Zemel BS, Kalkwarf HJ, Gilsanz V, Lappe JM, Oberfield S, Shepherd JA, et al. Revised reference curves for bone mineral content and areal bone mineral density according to age and sex for black and non-black children: results of the bone mineral density in childhood study. J Clin Endocrinol Metab. 2011;96(10):3160–9.
143. Kroger H, Kotaniemi A, Kroger L, Alhava E. Development of bone mass and bone density of the spine and femoral neck--a prospective study of 65 children and adolescents. Bone Miner. 1993;23(3):171–82.
144. Lu PW, Briody JN, Ogle GD, Morley K, Humphries IR, Allen J, et al. Bone mineral density of total body, spine, and femoral neck in children and young adults: a cross-sectional and longitudinal study. J Bone Miner Res. 1994;9(9):1451–8.
145. Matkovic V, Jelic T, Wardlaw GM, Ilich JZ, Goel PK, Wright JK, et al. Timing of peak bone mass in Caucasian females and its implication for the prevention of osteoporosis. Inference from a cross sectional model. J Clin Invest. 1994;93(2):799–808.
146. Boot AM, de Ridder MAJ, Pols HAP, Krenning EP, de Muinck K-SSMPF. Bone mineral density in children and adolescents: relation to puberty, calcium intake, and physical activity. J Clin Endocrinol Metab. 1997;82(1):57–62.
147. Maynard LM, Guo SS, Chumlea WC, Roche AF, Wisemandle WA, Zeller CM, et al. Total-body and regional bone mineral content and areal bone mineral density in children aged 8–18 y: the Fels Longitudinal Study. Am J Clin Nutr. 1998;68(5):1111–7.
148. Zanchetta JR, Plotkin H, Filgueira MLA. Bone mass in children: normative values for the 2-20-year-old population. Bone. 1995;16(4):393S–9.
149. Plotkin H, Nunez M, Alvarez Filgueira ML, Zanchetta JR. Lumbar spine bone density in Argentine children. Calcif Tissue Int. 1996;58(3):144–9.
150. Cann C. Quantitative CT, applications: comparison of current scanners. Radiology. 1987; 162:257–61.

# Chapter 3
# Dual-Energy X-Ray Absorptiomery Technology

John Shepherd and Nicola J. Crabtree

## History

Early attempts at bone densitometry used conventional X-rays with a step wedge made from an aluminum or ivory phantom included in the field of view as a means of calibration. The bone density was calculated by a visual comparison of the density of the bone and the known densities of the each of the steps on the phantom.

The next advancement in the field of bone density was the invention of single-photon absorptiometry (SPA) by Cameron and Sorenson in 1963 [1]. This technique used a radioactive source of either iodine (I-125) or americium (Am-241), with energies of 27 keV and 60 keV, respectively. The subject placed his or her arm in a water bath to provide a uniform path length through which the gamma rays would pass. This process allowed the calculation of the amount of bone tissue in the region scanned by means of subtraction of the photons attenuated by the soft tissue from the photons attenuated by bone and soft tissue. This technique proved to be very useful in terms of bone quantification, but it was limited to a peripheral site.

To measure bone density at axial sites (i.e., the spine or hip), in which the soft tissue is of variable thickness, gamma rays of two different energies are required to distinguish soft tissue from bone. Dual-photon absorptiometry (DPA) allowed this, providing the simultaneous transmission of gamma rays with photon energies of 44 and 100 keV from gadolinium-153 [2]. Estimates of bone and soft tissue were then derived using algebraic equations.

J. Shepherd, Ph.D. (✉)
Department of Radiology and Biomedical Imaging, University of California, San Francisco,
1 Irving Street, Suite A-C108, San Francisco, CA 94930, USA
e-mail: john.shepherd@ucsf.edu

N.J. Crabtree, Ph.D.
Department of Endocrinology, Birmingham Children's Hospital,
Steelhouse Lane, Birmingham, West Midlands B4 6NH, UK
e-mail: Nicola.crabtree@bch.nhs.uk

© Springer International Publishing Switzerland 2016
E.B. Fung et al. (eds.), *Bone Health Assessment in Pediatrics*,
DOI 10.1007/978-3-319-30412-0_3

Since the late 1980s, the expensive and potentially hazardous radioactive sources used in both SPA and DPA have been superseded by single X-ray absorptiometry (SXA) [3] and dual-energy X-ray absorptiometry (DXA). Similarly to DPA, the fundamental principle of DXA is the measurement of the transmission of X-rays, produced from a stable X-ray source, at high and low energies. The advantages of using X-rays instead of SPA or DPA include a shorter acquisition time and improved accuracy and precision due to the increased photon flux. Improvements in precision and resolution have been coupled with a decrease in radiation exposure [4]. With the increased availability of DXA, there has been a dramatic rise in its use in pediatric research and clinical practice.

## Principles of DXA

The X-rays used in diagnostic imaging and densitometry must have sufficient energy to pass through the body and still be detectable by sensors after passage. X-ray beam energy is attenuated or reduced with the passage through tissue. The extent of attenuation varies with the energy of the photons and the density and thickness of the material through which they pass.

Attenuation will follow an exponential pattern often observed in other biological situations. For monoenergetic radiation (i.e., from photons with the same energy) this pattern of attenuation can be described using the following formula:

$$I = I_0 e^{-\mu M}$$

where $I$ = measured intensity of the X-ray
$I_0$ = initial intensity of the X-ray beam
$\mu$ = mass attenuation coefficient ($cm^2 g^{-1}$)
$M$ = area density ($g/cm^2$))

In other words, for a given beam intensity level, each tissue will have a unique attenuation property such that the attenuation is a function of a constant (i.e., the mass attenuation coefficient) specific to that tissue and the tissue's mass. Because bone is surrounded by soft tissue, a more complex model is required to be able to distinguish the density of the bone from the surrounding tissue.

The fundamental principle of DXA is the measurement of transmission of X-rays with high and low energy photons through the body. The mathematics used to calculate bone density values can be explained using an exponential equation that assumes the body to be a two-compartment model consisting of bone mineral and soft tissue. Bone mineral is a physically dense material mainly made up of phosphorus and calcium molecules that have relatively high atomic numbers. Soft tissue is a mixture of muscle, fat, skin, and water. It has a lower physical density and a lower effective atomic number since its main chemical constituents are hydrogen, carbon, and oxygen. To further simplify the mathematics, we also assume that the low- and high-energy X-ray sources are monochromatic at two different energies. At the same photon energy, soft tissue and bone will have quite different mass attenuation coefficients ($\mu$, so the exponential equation becomes:

$$I = I_0 \exp\left(-\mu_B M_B + \mu_S M_S\right)$$

Where B = bone
  S = soft tissue
For the different X-ray energies, the mass attenuation coefficient will be different, leading to two equations, one for low-energy photons and one for high-energy photons:

$$I^L = I^L_{\ 0} \exp\left(-\mu_B^{\ L} M_B + \mu_S^{\ L} M_S\right)$$

$$I^H = I^H_{\ 0} \exp\left(-\mu_B^{\ H} M_B + \mu_S^{\ H} M_S\right)$$

where L = low-energy photons
  H = high-energy photons
These equations are solved for $M_B$ (i.e., the area density of bone)

$$M_B = \frac{\mathrm{Ln}\left(I^L_{\ 0} / I^L\right) - k\mathrm{Ln}\left(I^H_{\ 0} / I^H\right)}{\mu^L_{\ B} - k\mu^H_{\ B}}$$

where $k = \mu^L_S / \mu^H_S$
    The ratio $k$ can be derived from the patient measurement by measuring the transmitted intensity of the beam at points at which there is no bone (i.e., at which $M_B = 0$). Once the ratio $k$ is determined, the equation can be solved to calculate the area bone density, $M_B$.
    The bone density is determined for each point, or each pixel, of the area being scanned. As the source and detector move linearly across the scanned area, a bone profile is generated on a pixel-by-pixel basis. The bone density image is then made up of many linear passes.
    After acquisition, the machine's software employs an edge-detection algorithm to evaluate the bone profile and to identify the pixels that represent where the bone edge begins and ends within the area scanned. The bone density is then calculated as the average $M_B$ across the bone profile (Fig. 3.1). From the pixel-by-pixel density image, the software sums the number of pixels containing bone to calculate the bone area (BA) that was scanned. Using the mean bone density value (BMD) and the BA, it is possible to calculate the actual amount of bone mineral content (BMC) within the image:

$$\mathrm{BMC}(\mathrm{g}) = \mathrm{BMD}\left(\mathrm{g} / \mathrm{cm}^2\right) \times \mathrm{BA}\left(\mathrm{cm}^2\right)$$

    DXA is a projectional technique in which three-dimensional objects are analyzed as two-dimensional. DXA provides an estimate of areal BMD in g/cm². This BMD is not a measure of volumetric density (in g/cm³) because it provides no information about the depth of bone. Given two bones of identical volumetric BMD, the smaller bone will have a lower areal BMD than the larger one because the influence of bone thickness is not factored. This would mean that areal BMD in a small child

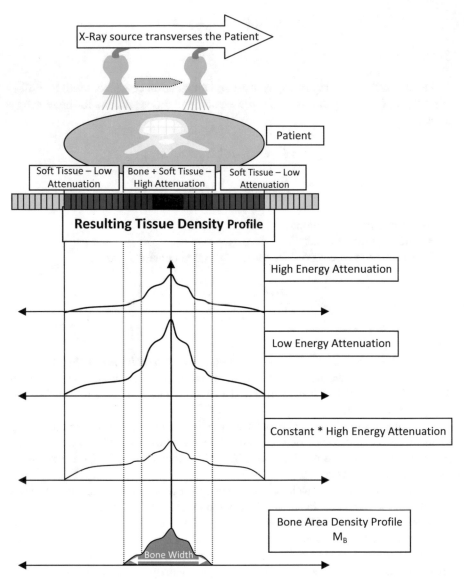

**Fig. 3.1** Bone profile, observed as the X-ray moves linearly across the patient, and the corresponding tissue density profiles

would be lower than areal BMD in a taller child even if they had identical volumetric bone densities. Numerous strategies have been proposed to estimate volumetric BMD from areal BMD results [5, 6]; these are described elsewhere in this book.

DXA measurements represents the sum of cortical and trabecular bone within the projected bone area, concealing the distinct structural characteristics. Therefore, the influence of disease processes or medications that differentially affect cortical versus trabecular bone may be obscured or difficult to detect by DXA.

Other potential problems arise when the DXA software is unable to detect the difference between bone and soft tissue. This typically occurs in patients with undermineralized bones, as may occur in younger or sicker children. Bone densitometry manufacturers have tried to tackle this issue with the introduction of low-density software for better edge detection of the bone [7]. As detailed in Sect. 6.3, it is important to recognize the limitations of this software and the potential for further underestimation of BMD.

# Development

Since the introduction of clinical DXA, there have been changes in the technique for acquiring the information required to calculate bone density. New technology has allowed more-stable X-ray units to be made and more-sensitive detectors to be utilized. However the most significant change has been the introduction of the fan beam and narrow fan beam systems.

## *Pencil Beam Versus Fan Beam Scanners*

Originally, the scanners used a highly collimated beam of X-rays in conjunction with sequential detectors or a single detector that moved in a raster pattern (i.e., in a series of thin parallel lines) across the patient. This pencil beam system produces the most geometrically correct information, with little or no magnification of the area being scanned.

The current fan beam systems use a slit collimator to generate a beam that diverges in two directions in conjunction with a linear array of solid-state detectors, so bone measurements can be made with a single sweep of the X-ray arm. The fan beam systems use higher energy photon intensities and a greater photon flux, thus producing a better-resolution image considerably faster than the older pencil beam machines. The lumbar spine can be scanned in 30 s or less with the fan beam, as compared with the 3–10 min required for the pencil beam system.

The trade off for improved image resolution with the fan beam is a higher radiation exposure. Additionally, the geometry associated with this technique leads to magnification of the image in one direction [8, 9]. The degree of magnification will depend on the distance of the bone or tissue away from the source: the closer the body part is to the source, the greater the magnification.

Fan beam systems can create either wide or narrow x-ray beam profiles depending on the make and model. The narrowest fan beam systems scan in a rectilinear raster fashion to cover the scan area, much like the original pencil beam machines. However, since the beam is wider than the original pencil beam machine, it can cover the body in a much faster time, typically 30 s. Wide fan beam systems can cover the scan areas of hip, spine, and forearm systems in one pass. Cross-calibration studies demonstrated no detectable magnification effect between the old-generation pencil beam scanner and the new narrow fan beam machine [10] (Fig. 3.2).

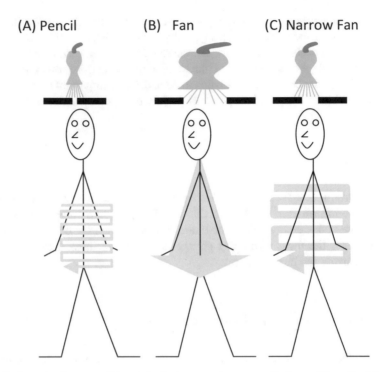

**Fig. 3.2** Scanning by a, pencil beam; b, fan beam; and c, narrow fan beam. The path of the X-ray beams is represented with the *arrow*

## Radiation

The amount of radiation exposure in DXA is extremely low compared to many other X-ray imaging techniques. It has been difficult to estimate the degree of risk of harms associated with these very low levels of radiation except by extrapolation from studies that involved distinctly higher levels of radiation exposure. Presently, studies have not been able to establish a link between health risk and the low levels of radiation exposure that are typical of DXA. According to the Health Physics Society, the risks of health effects for exposures less than 5–10 REM "are either too small to be observed or are nonexistent [11]."

Health effects of radiation have been demonstrated at doses above 5–10 REM (greater than 50,000–100,000 μSv) [11]. The principal risk due to radiation is random X-ray interactions with the body, which can result in carcinogenic or genetic effects. Typically, carcinogenic effects will not manifest in an individual for several decades following an exposure [12]. This is an important consideration when scanning children since they have a longer amount of time for expression of an effect than adults [12]. Because the majority of the children scanned will still be fertile, the potential genetic effects of radiation exposure are a theoretical consideration

[13]. However, as shown in Table 3.1, radiation exposures from DXA are approximately 10,000 times less than the radiation doses at which health effects occur.

Estimates of risk from radiation exposure are expressed in terms of effective dose, in units of sieverts or REMs, where 1 milliREM (mREM) equals 10 microsieverts (10 $\mu$Sv). The effective dose is calculated from the magnitude of exposure, the type of radiation causing the exposure, the organs exposed, and their relative radiosensitivities. The resulting value can be compared to other scanning techniques (Table 3.1), to naturally occurring background radiation (8 $\mu$Sv/day), or to a round trip transatlantic flight (80 $\mu$Sv).

**Table 3.1** Effective dose and entrance surface doses for the commonly available bone densitometers

| Make | Model | Region | Scan mode | Entrance surface dose ($\mu$Gy) | Effective dose, adult ($\mu$Sv) | Effective dose, 15 year old ($\mu$Sv) | Effective dose, 5 year old ($\mu$Sv) |
|---|---|---|---|---|---|---|---|
| Hologic [16] | Discovery/ horizon | Spine | Fast | 156.0 | 6.7 | 8.5 | 24.1 |
| | | | Express | 104.0 | 4.4 | 5.6 | 16.1 |
| | | Whole body | A model | 13.0 | 4.2 | 4.2 | 5.2 |
| | | | W model | 26.1 | 8.4 | 8.4 | 10.5 |
| Norland [17] | XR-46 | Spine | | 4.7 | | | |
| | | Whole body | | 0.2 | | | |
| | XR-26 | Spine | | 44.0 | | | |
| | | Whole body | | 0.5 | | | |
| General electric [18] | Prodigy | Spine | thin | 9 | 0.18 | | |
| | | | standard | 37.0 | 0.7 | | |
| | | | thick | 83.0 | 1.4 | | |
| | | Whole body | thin | 0.37 | 0.5 | | 0.2(17b) |
| | | | standard | 0.37 | 0.5 | | 0.2(17b) |
| | | | thick | 0.74 | 1.0 | | |
| | iDXA | Spine | thin | 37.0 | 0.8 | | |
| | | | standard | 146.0 | 3.4 | | |
| | | | thick | 329.0 | 6.8 | | |
| | | Whole body | thin | 3.0 | 0.9 | | 1.2 |
| | | | standard | 3.0 | 0.96 | | |
| | | | thick | 6.0 | 1.92 | | |

Note: Effective dose estimations are for individuals with functioning reproductive organs
1 mREM = 10 $\mu$Sv; 1 mrad = 10 $\mu$Gy

The more commonly cited unit of radiation exposure is the entrance surface dose, or ESD, in units of gray (Gy); 10 μGy = 1 mrad (i.e., 1 Gy = 100 rad). ESD is a measure of the radiation on the surface of the patient, before it passes through and is absorbed by the body. It is an easier measure to obtain as it requires only a simple measure of the X-ray output detected at the skin surface. It will be approximately the same for any patient scanned at any one exposure level, irrespective of the region scanned. The ESD will be higher than the effective dose since only a fraction of the X-rays are stopped by the patient. Although ESD gives the operator an indication of the exposure levels, it does not take into account the organs being exposed and the relative radiosensitivities of the irradiated organs.

Table 3.1 lists both the effective and entrance surface doses of ionizing radiation doses associated with the more commonly used densitometers. The doses in the table refer to estimates for either adults, children aged 15, or children aged 5 years old when available.

Movement of the patient during the DXA scan acquisition is a common problem encountered by DXA technologist. If a scan contains movement or some other removable quality issues, it is common practice to attempt the scan again. If an error-free scan is not acquired in three attempts, one should abort that exam to limit the dose exposure to the child.

In summary, the radiation exposure associated with DXA is acceptable for pediatric use. However, efforts should always be made to minimize lifetime radiation exposure through the judicious selection of patients and skeletal sites for DXA scanning and through optimal densitometry technique.

## Precision

The precision of a diagnostic test such as DXA is an indication of the expected reproducibility of replicate measurements in patients. Precision determines the certainty about the initial quantitative measurements as well as the ability to detect small changes with future measurements. The precision of DXA measurements is determined by factors related to the machine (machine precision), the software's ability to precise find bone (analysis precision), and the operator's ability to position the patient (operator precision). Precision can determined for short-term and long-term replicate measurements. It is expressed either as the percent coefficient of variation (%CV) or as a standard deviation (SD). Percent coefficient of variation is the percentage of variation of the measurement compared to the mean value for replicate measurements.

$$\%CV = \frac{100 \left( \text{Standard Deviation} \left[ \text{SD} \right] \text{of the Measurement} \right)}{\text{Mean Value of the Measurements}}$$

## Short-Term Machine Precision

Machine precision is calculated from repeated scanning of a single phantom, without moving the phantom between scans. The usual protocol for the measurement of machine precision requires scanning a phantom ten times on the same day. For newer DXA models, the %CV for this procedure is typically less than 1 %.

## Long-Term or Temporal Machine Precision

Long-term precision is measured by repeatedly scanning a phantom daily or weekly over months to years to monitor any temporal changes in the machine. These measurements can be used to assess the long-term stability of a scanner; since the measurements from a phantom should theoretically be the same each day, any drift or change would therefore be due to the machine.

$$CV\% = \frac{100\left(\text{Standard Error in the Estimate}\left[\text{SEE}\right]\right)}{\text{Mean Change}}$$

## In Vivo Short-Term Precision

In vivo short-term precision is calculated by repeated scanning of subjects a minimum of two times on the same day or within a short time interval. To achieve statistical power, BMD testing must be done three times in each of 15 individuals or twice in each of 30 subjects. The standard deviation for each patient is calculated, and then the root mean square standard deviation for the group is calculated. A good explanation for these calculations can be found on the website of the International Society for Clinical Densitometry (http://www.iscd.org). The ISCD also provides an online calculator for quantifying your precision values. Because this procedure requires two scans and twice the radiation exposure, in vivo precision testing is considered by some to be clinical research. Regardless of interpretation, all participants should provide written informed consent.

The precision estimates reflect both machine precision and operator precision. For this reason, in vivo precision is worse (greater %CV) than the machine precision alone, but in vivo precision is representative of the real scanning situation. The best precision will be achieved if the patients are scanned and analyzed by an operator that has been trained in the positioning and analysis of patients. An excellent metric for training is certification from a program specializing in DXA operation.

Precision studies should be performed in the population to be scanned most often since precision can vary as a function of body size [14]. However, precision measured in mature individuals may differ from that measured in children due to the latter's smaller size and variable ability to cooperate. The ability of the software to detect the edges of smaller bones may also affect precision in children. Ideally, pediatric data should be gathered when possible. One multicenter study of DXA precision in 155 children, ages 6–15 years, demonstrated coefficient of variation values of 0.64–1.03 for spine and 0.66–1.20 for whole body BMD, depending on the age range [15].

## Long-Term In Vivo Precision

This measure is obtained by repeat scanning of a group of patients over a period of time. It is harder to evaluate since, unlike a phantom, which maintains stable bone density over time, the patient's bone density may increase or decrease. For children, this is particularly difficult to estimate due to the expected changes in bone measures in growing children.

## Least Significant Change (LSC)

The least significant change (LSC) is the smallest percent difference that can be detected by the technique from repeat measurement of a patient. The value usually expressed for LSC is 2.8 × precision where the precision can be in the form of the %CV or SD. However, there are a few caveats. First, both measurements should be acquired on the same DXA system. Second, The DXA system should be known to be stable in its calibration between the two measurements. Third, the LSC defines how much change has to occur to have 95 % confidence that any real change in the bone density has occurred at all. The correct way to report change in bone density would be to report the measured difference ± the %LSC. For example, with a measured decrease of 4 % between two DXA scans and a precision of 1 %, the LSC would be 2.8 %. The report should state there was a decrease 4 ± 2.8 % in bone density. If the decrease had only been 2 %, then it would be appropriate to report that no significant change in bone density has occurred.

## Strengths of DXA

All bone assessments have strengths and limitations compared to one another. DXA's strengths include the following; first, multiple bone sites can be measured on children including spine, hip, forearm, distal femur [19], and total body. Second, total body also provide the ability to quantify soft tissue composition. Third, the dose to the patient is low compared to quantitative computed tomography. However, DXA has limitations as well that include the need for fairly extensive training to operate DXA systems, the need to hold still from anywhere from 30 s (hip and spine scans) to 10 min (whole body scans), and this can be difficult for young children.

## Accessibility

Although availability of DXA may vary from country to country, this technique is now widely available in both general hospitals and academic medical centers. In some areas, mobile units are also available, reducing the need for the patient to travel long distances to the nearest machine.

## Radiation Dose

Although any radiation exposure results in a degree of risk to the patient, DXA has one of the lowest effective doses of all the ionizing radiation imaging techniques, being equivalent to approximately less than one day's naturally occurring radiation in most cases. The low dose of DXA is a strength, since there are no alternatives to measure bone density with lower dose. Quantitative CT is used in children but has at least six times or higher dose.

## Precision

Much work has been done by the manufacturers of DXA machines to produce a stable X-ray source and an efficient detector system, thereby making DXA a precise technique for measuring bone. The average coefficient of variation for a spine DXA scan is 1.5 % or less, compared to as much as 5 % for an average calcaneus ultrasound scan [20]. Additionally, sophisticated analysis software packages are used, which, for a large proportion of DXA scans, require little or no operator intervention, thus further improving precision.

## Short Scan Time

Current generation DXA fan-beam systems and hardware have drastically shortened scan times and offer a definite advantage to older pencil beam systems. Whole body DXA scans can be completed in from 3 to 10 min, and spine scans, in as short a time as 30 s, which minimizes the possibility of movement artifacts in young children.

## Normative Data

As a result of the wide availability and relatively low radiation dose, DXA data have been collected on samples of healthy infants, children, and adolescents in several countries. Table 3.2 is a survey of selected reference data for a variety of makes and

**Table 3.2** Summary of normative data for DXA in pediatric subjects on contemporary bone densitometers

| Year of Publication (Ref) | DXA | Subject Number | Age, years | Ethnicity | Sites Measured |
|---|---|---|---|---|---|
| 2002 [22] | Hologic 4500A | 231 | 5–22 | White (American) | Total Body |
| 2004[a] [23, 24] | Hologic 4500A | 363 | 10–17 | Arab (Lebanese) | Spine, femoral neck, total body, forearm |
| 2004 [b] [25] | Hologic 4500 W | 422 | 12–18 | White, Black (American) | Spine, Femoral neck |
| 2007 [a] [26] | Hologic 4500A | 442 | 6-17 | White (British) | Spine, femoral neck, total body |
| 2007 [27] | Hologic 4500A | 1554 | 7–17 | White, black, Hispanic (American) | Spine, femoral neck, total body, forearm |
| 2007 [28] | Hologic 4500A | 179 | 3–18 | White (Canadian) | Spine, femoral neck, total body |
| 2007[c] [29] | Hologic 4500 W | 1155 | 15–39 | Chinese | Spine, femoral neck, total femur |
| 2009[a] [30] | Hologic 4500A | 7398 | 8–20 | White, black, Hispanic (American) | Total body |
| 2009 [31] | Hologic 4500A | 821 | 5–18 | White, black (American) | Distal lateral femur |
| 2010 [32] | Hologic 4500A/ GE Lunar DPX/ Prodigy | 439 | 16–24 | White (Canadian) | Spine, femoral neck, total hip |
| 2010 [d] [33] | Hologic 4500A | 5173 | 8–25 | White, black, Asian, Hispanic (American & Canadian) | Spine, femoral neck, whole body |
| 2010 [a] [34] | Hologic 4500A | 2014 | 5–23 | Black, non-black (American) | Spine, femoral neck, total body, forearm |
| 2013 [35] | Hologic 4500A | 307 | 1–36 months | White, black, Asian (American) | Spine |
| 2011 [a] [36] | GE Lunar Pro | 920 | 5–17 | Asian (Indian) | Spine, femoral neck, total body |
| 2013 [a] [37] | GE lunar Prodigy & iDXA | 3300 | 5–18 | White, black, Asian | Spine, femoral neck, total body |
| 2007 [38] | GE Lunar Prodigy | 877 | 5–13 | Asian (Chinese) | Total body |

(continued)

**Table 3.2**   (continued)

| Year of Publication (Ref) | DXA | Subject Number | Age, years | Ethnicity | Sites Measured |
|---|---|---|---|---|---|
| 2007 [39] | GE Lunar Pixi | 664 | 7–17 | Asian (Indian) | Forearm, Calcaneum |
| 2010 [40] | GE Lunar Pixi | 1115 | 9–29 | Asian (Korean) | Forearm, Calcaneum |
| 1995 [17] | Norland XR-26 | 778 | 2–20 | White (Argentinean) | Spine, femoral neck, total body, forearm |
| 1998 [41] | Norland XR-26 | 179 | 12–13 | Asian (Chinese) | Spine, forearm |
| 2004 [42] | Norland XR-35 | 102 | 3–15 | Turkish | Spine, femoral neck |

Abbreviation: *DXA* dual-energy X-ray absorptiometry

Notes: For reference data on older-generation bone densitometers, the reader is referred to the previous International Society for Clinical Densitometry Pediatric guidelines publication [43] Hologic 4500A, 4500 W (Hologic Inc.; Bedford, MA); GE Lunar DPX/Prodigy, Pro, Prodigy & iDXA, Pixi (GE Lunar Corp.; Madison WI); Norland XR-26, XR-35 (Norland Corp.; Norland Corporation, White Plains, NY)

Taken with Permission from Crabtree NJ, Arabi A, Bachrach LK, et al. Dual-energy X-ray absorptiometry interpretation and reporting in children and adolescents: the revised 2013 ISCD Pediatric Official Positions. J Clin Densitom. 2014;17(2):225–42 (Reference #21)

[a]Size adjustment available

[b]Females only

[c]Males only

[d]Includes longitudinal "x"

countries [21]. With respect to data available by the manufacturers on their systems, reference data for spine and total body BMD is available for GE and Hologic down to 5 years for GE and 3 years for Hologic. These data have been used clinically as reference values to identify children with "normal" versus "abnormal" bone density.

However, caution should be used in applying these reference data for several reasons: (1) the manufacturer, model, and software version will affect DXA results, so data on healthy children used for comparison should all be acquired and analyzed in a similar fashion; (2) these data are derived from convenience samples that may not provide adequate representation of all age and gender groups; (3) reference data that do not provide gender-specific norms are likely to overestimate bone deficits in boys compared to girls [44]; and (4) most reference data provide means and standard deviations relative to age, and there are no guidelines on how to account for children with delayed skeletal age or altered body size. These issues are discussed in further detail in Chap. 6.

## *Interpretation of DXA Results*

DXA is widely accepted as a quantitative measurement technique for assessing skeletal status. In elderly adults, DXA BMD is also a sufficiently robust predictor of osteoporotic fractures, that it can be used to define the disease. The World Health Organization criteria for the diagnosis of osteoporosis in adults is based on a T-score, the comparison of a measured BMD result with the average BMD of young adults at the time of peak bone mass [45]. A T-score ≤–2.5 SD below the mean peak bone mass is used for the diagnosis of osteoporosis, and a T-score ≤–2.5 SD with a history of a low-impact fracture is classified as severe osteoporosis.

In adults, each standard deviation decrease in the T-score is associated with an average increase of fracture risk by 1.5–3-fold [46]. Measurements of BMD in anatomic regions that are likely to fracture—such as the spine, hip, or forearm—provide the best prediction of risk of fracture at that site. For example, the Study of Osteoporotic Fractures showed that at the femoral neck, each SD decrease in bone density increased the age-adjusted risk of hip fracture 2.6 times (95 % confidence interval [CI] 1.9, 3.6). Low hip bone density was a stronger predictor of hip fracture than bone density measurements of the spine, radius, or calcaneus [47].

Ongoing epidemiological studies in adults have demonstrated that the relationship between T-score and fracture risk is age-dependent; for a given T-score, the risk of fracture increases with age [48]. In addition, other risk factors, such as previous fracture, maternal history of hip fracture, greater height, impaired cognition, slower walking speed, nulliparity, Type II diabetes mellitus, Parkinson's disease, and poor depth perception also contribute independently to the risk of hip fracture in older women [49]. These observations reflect the fact that bone mass is only one factor contributing to the risk of fracture in adults. Bone quality and geometry and the risk of falling also contribute to the likelihood of bone fracture. In children, less is known about the risk factors for fractures and whether they are age-dependent.

Because of the predictive value of the T-score in adults, it is a standard component of DXA BMD reporting software. However, it is clearly inappropriate to compare the bone mineral status of a child with adults who have reached peak bone mass. Instead, the bone density of children should be expressed as a Z-score, the number of standard deviations from the mean for age and gender. Additional adjustments for body size or body composition are recommended by some, as discussed in Chap. 6. Despite the growing body of published normative data utilizing DXA in children, there are no evidence-based guidelines for the definition of osteoporosis, osteopenia, or fracture risk based upon BMD in children. Further discussion of this important consideration and the relationship between DXA BMD and fracture risk can be found in Chaps. 4 and 6.

# Limitations of DXA

## *Confounding by Bone Size*

DXA provides only two-dimensional measurements of bone mineral content and bone area for the three-dimensional bone. Thus, BMD is not a measure of volumetric density (g/cm³) because it provides no information about bone depth. Bones of larger width and height are also thicker. As shown in Fig. 3.3, the BMD of bones with identical volumetric BMD but varying size will differ substantially in areal BMD. Smaller bones will have a lower areal BMD than larger bones because bone thickness is not factored into DXA results. The lower areal BMD of children when compared with adults is due, in part, to their smaller bone size. In addition, children who are small for their age will have a lower areal BMD than their same-age peers, even if their volumetric BMD is identical.

Because of the confounding by bone size, several investigators have suggested that the use of bone mineral content adjusted for body size is preferable to conventional units of areal BMD, especially in children [50–53]. Others have suggested that volumetric bone mineral density can be estimated from the bone mineral content and bone area values obtained from DXA by calculating bone mineral apparent density [5, 54, 55]. For whole body DXA scans, bone area relative to height may provide additional information about bone dimensions and strength [51, 53]. The clinical utility of these approaches remains to be determined.

## *Projection Artifacts*

An additional limitation of DXA is that it may introduce artifacts into the measurement of bone size (i.e., the projected area) and density in children with abnormal body composition [9, 56]. Hologic scanners are configured such that the fan beam

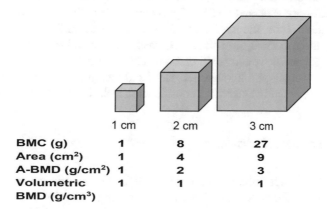

|  | 1 cm | 2 cm | 3 cm |
|---|---|---|---|
| BMC (g) | 1 | 8 | 27 |
| Area (cm²) | 1 | 4 | 9 |
| A-BMD (g/cm²) | 1 | 2 | 3 |
| Volumetric BMD (g/cm³) | 1 | 1 | 1 |

**Fig. 3.3** The difference between volumetric and areal BMD in differently sized bones, as assessed by DXA

is projected from below the patient, with a linear array of detectors above the patient. The portion of the body that is closest to the source of the beam is magnified more than if the same region were closer to the detector. Subsequently, thinner individuals will appear to have a disproportionately greater bone area and BMC. This has important implications for longitudinal studies because children will increase in length and thickness as they grow. Moreover, increases in soft-tissue thickness associated with glucocorticoid therapy may result in the erroneous impression of decreased BMC and bone area as the bone is lifted further from the X-ray source. The fan beam is projected from above the patient on GE Lunar scanners; it has in the opposite effect of the Hologic scanners.

Changes in the surrounding soft tissues may also impact bone detection algorithms. Given that many children for whom poor bone mineral accrual is a concern also have altered body size and composition, these effects are likely important but have not been quantified. For adults, the effects of weight and body composition changes on the estimation of total body BMC, bone area, and BMD have been evaluated using in vivo and in vitro models. The direction and magnitude of the effects depend on the manufacturer and software version [57, 58]. For example, with a 16 % weight loss in obese adult women, the GE Lunar DPX system operating in the standard software mode showed losses of 5.3 %, 3.2 %, and 2.3 % for BMC, bone area, and BMD estimations, respectively. For the Hologic 1000 W, a 12 % weight loss in obese adult women resulted in losses of 8.3, 6.8, and 1.6 % for BMC, bone area, and BMD estimations [57]. Measurements of whole body phantoms wrapped in lard confirmed that these observed changes with weight loss in adults were attributable, at least in part, to changes in surrounding soft tissue and distance from the X-ray source and not to actual changes in bone size and density. Across all scanners evaluated, the effects of weight and body composition changes are more pronounced for total body BMC and bone area than they are for BMD. Similar results have been noted for estimation of BMC, bone area, and BMD of the spine as well [57, 59].

For children with weight and body composition in the normal range, it is fair to assume that the effects of normal growth-related changes in weight and body composition on BMC, bone area, and BMD will be comparable to those occurring in the reference population. Thus, the interpretation of reference-based Z-scores should not be affected by these normal, growth-related changes. For children experiencing rapid shifts in weight and body composition, for example, with intentional weight loss regimens or with weight gain through glucocorticoid therapy, the measurement artifacts described above should be taken into consideration in the interpretation of DXA results.

## Bone Detection Algorithms

Pediatric DXA images often could not be analyzed with early-generation software due to failure of the bone edge detection algorithm to identify and measure completely all bones. In one series, the DXA lumbar spine scan could not be analyzed using standard software (QDR 2000, Hologic, Waltham, MA, USA) in 40 % of chronically ill children less than 12 years of age and in younger healthy children, particularly those less than 6 years of age [7]. Although it is possible to use visual inspection to fill in the regions missed by standard software, this reduces precision by introducing greater operator-related variability. It resulted in loss of the systematic algorithm's threshold definition of bone edge and led to inaccuracies in measurements of bone mineralization.

In an effort to address this limitation, software modifications were developed to improve detection of low-density bone in children and severely osteopenic adults (Hologic, GE Lunar). Although the new software performed well, these modifications increased the detection of low-density bone. Since the bone map included areas of less dense bone (not detectable by standard software), low-density software resulted in a systematic decrease in the BMD measurement compared with the standard analysis [7]. Comparable effects were seen with whole body pediatric software analyses [60]. Because results acquired using standard and low density software analyses differed by as much as 9–11 %, these two software options could not be used interchangeably in studies of BMD in children. For the same reason, reference data must be acquired in the same analysis mode as that used to examine the patient.

More recent software modifications include methods to adjust bone detection thresholds based upon the subject's weight [61] and techniques for improved bone detection in the lumbar spine based on anatomical assumptions. Future studies are needed to evaluate the utility of these new approaches in longitudinal studies and in children with altered body composition. Although these techniques illustrate the advancements that are being made in bone mineral analysis, it must also be remembered that proper comparison to a reference population requires that the same methods be used in subjects and controls.

## Lack of Standardized Reference Data

The ability to interpret DXA measurements has also been influenced by the lack of standardized reference data. As noted above, DXA results vary by manufacturer, model number, and software version. In particular, manufacturers and software versions vary in how the lower BMD of children is detected. Cross-calibration of DXA machines from different manufacturers has been performed and published (1995–1997), to establish a set of equations to convert bone mineral density (BMD) on each machine to a "standardized BMD" (sBMD) [62]. These formulae are based on measurements from instruments that are now 20 years old, and all were performed in adult subjects. Further research is needed to determine if these equations remain applicable with newer instruments, and in pediatric patients. Consequently, careful selection of pediatric reference data that matches the manufacturer, model, and software version is essential.

In addition, utilizing reference data that are based on adequate numbers of children within each age and gender group is crucial for characterizing bone mineral status. Currently, the U.S. National Institutes of Health is conducting a large, mixed longitudinal multiethnic multicenter study, the Bone Mineral Density in Children Study (BMDCS) to establish national norms for bone mineral density [63]. This data of over 1500 children followed annually for 6 years has been published and is available for spine, hip, whole body, and forearm regions. Tables are provided that allow one to calculate both Z-scores and Height-Adjusted Z-scores for all regions [34].

Pediatric studies of healthy children have identified numerous factors influencing bone mineral density. BMC and BMD are largely influenced by body size (height, weight, and body mass index [BMI, weight/height$^2$]) [51, 55, 64–69]. Gender, sexual maturation [55, 64–71], ethnicity [54, 55, 69, 72, 73], body composition [64, 65, 74], nutrient intake [75, 76], physical activity [77, 78], skeletal age [65, 79], and genetics [73, 80, 81] are also important factors. Age, body size and composition, and sexual maturation explain up to 88 % of the variability in DXA measures of BMD, especially when study samples consist of children of widely varying ages [65, 67, 68, 82].

Although it is recognized that these are important covariates of bone density, it is unclear how they should be used clinically. For adults, the International Society of Clinical Densitometry recommends the use of a uniform Caucasian reference database for evaluating bone density for all ethnic groups [83]. The reasons are that (1) it is not always possible to identify patient ethnicity, and reference data are not available for all ethnic groups; (2) there is insufficient evidence linking BMD to fracture risk in other ethnic groups; and (3) use of Caucasian reference data in African Americans results in a lower prevalence of osteoporosis, which is in accordance with the lower rates of fracture among African Americans. A useful discussion of this topic can be found at the website of the International Society for Clinical Densitometry (http://www.iscd.org/Visitors/positions/official.cfm). Among children, it is unclear if reference norms should follow similar guidelines since even less is known about BMD and fracture risk across different ethnic groups. Similarly, evidence-based pediatric recommendations for adjusting for body size, body composition, and skeletal and sexual maturation are lacking.

## Summary Points

- The fundamental principle of dual-energy X-ray absorptiometry (DXA) is the measurement of transmission of X-rays, produced from a stable X-ray source, at high and low energies.
- Since the introduction of DXA, there has been an exponential increase in pediatric research and clinical practice of bone densitometry in pediatrics.
- DXA is a projectional technique in which three-dimensional objects are analyzed as two-dimensional. Problems may arise when the dimensions of the area scanned change with time, as is the case in a growing child.
- DXA technology has numerous strengths as a clinical tool in the field of pediatric densitometry, including its availability, short scan times, minimal radiation exposure, and excellent precision.
- There remain a number of factors that must be considered carefully when interpreting DXA results in pediatrics, including size and projection artifacts, bone detection limitations, and the lack of standardized normative data for children and adolescents.

# References

1. Cameron JR, Sorenson J. Measurement of bone mineral in vivo: an improved method. Science. 1963;11:230–2.
2. Madsen M, Peppler W, Mazess RB. Vertebral and total body bone mineral content by dual photon absorptiometry. Calcif Tissue Res. 1976;21(Suppl):361–4.
3. Kelly TL, Crane G, Baran D. Single X-ray absorptiometry of the forearm: precision, correlation, and reference data. Calcif Tissue Int. 1994;53:212–8.
4. Kelly TL, Slovik D, Schoenfeld DA, Neer RM. Quantitative digital radiography versus dual photon absorptiometry of the lumbar spine. J Clin Endocrinol Metab. 1988;67:839–44.
5. Carter DR, Bouxsein ML, Marcus R. New approaches for interpreting projected bone densitometry data. J Bone Miner Res. 1992;7:137–45.
6. Kroger H, Vainio P, Nieminen J, Kotaniemi A. Comparison of different models for interpreting bone mineral density measurements using DXA and MRI technology. Bone. 1995;17:157–9.
7. Leonard MB, Feldman HI, Zemel BS, Berlin JA, Barden EM, Stallings VA. Evaluation of low density spine software for the assessment of bone mineral density in children. J Bone Miner Res. 1998;13:1687–90.
8. Cole JH, Scerpella TA, van der Meulen MC. Fan-beam densitometry of the growing skeleton: are we measuring what we think we are? J Clin Densitom. 2005;8:57–64.
9. Pocock NA, Noakes KA, Majerovic Y, Griffiths MR. Magnification error of femoral geometry using fan beam densitometers. Calcif Tissue Int. 1997;60:8–10.
10. Oldroyd B, Smith AH, Truscott JG. Cross-calibration of GE/Lunar pencil and fan-beam dual energy densitometers—Bone mineral density and body composition studies. Eur J Clin Nutr. 2003;57:977–87.
11. Position Statement of the Health Physics Society, "Radiation Risk Perspective." Adopted 1996, Reissued, 2004. http://hps.org/documents/radiationrisk.pdf
12. Board statement on diagnostic medical exposures to ionizing radiation during pregnancy and estimates of late radiation effects to the U.K. population. Documents of NRPB4, No 4, 1993.
13. Annals of the ICRP. 1990 Recommendations of the International Commission on Radiological Protection. ICRP Publication 60. 1991; Volume 21: No. 1–3.
14. Powers C, Fan B, Borrud LG, Looker AC, Shepherd JA. Long-term precision of dual-energy X-ray absorptiometry body composition measurements and association with their covariates. J Clin Densitom. 2015;18(1):76–85.
15. Shepherd JA, Wang L, Fan B, Gilsanz V, Kalkwarf HJ, Lappe J, et al. Optimal monitoring time interval between DXA measures in children. J Bone Min Res. 2011;26(11):2745–52.
16. Blake GM, Naeem M, Boutros M. Comparison of effective dose to children and adults from dual X-ray absorptiometry examinations. Bone. 2006;38(6):935–42.
17. Zanchetta JR, Plotkin H, Alvarez Filgueira ML. Bone mass in children: normative values for the 2–20-year-old population. Bone. 1995;16:393S–9.
18. Damilakis J, Solomou G, Manios GE, Karantanas A. Pediatric radiation dose and risk from bone density measurements using a GE Lunar Prodigy scanner. Osteoporos Int. 2013;24(7):2025–31.
19. Henderson RC, Berglund LM, May R, Zemel BS, Grossberg RI, Johnson J, et al. The relationship between fractures and DXA measures of BMD in the distal femur of children and adolescents with cerebral palsy or muscular dystrophy. J Bone Miner Res. 2010;25(3):520–6.
20. Nejh CF, Hans D, Li J, Fan B, Fuerst T, He YQ, et al. Comparison of six calcaneal quantitative ultrasound devices: precision and hip fracture discrimination. Osteoporos Int. 2000;11(12):1051–62.
21. Crabtree NJ et al. Dual-energy X-ray absorptiometry interpretation and reporting in children and adolescents: the revised 2013 ISCD Pediatric Official Positions. J Clin Densitom. 2014;17(2):225–42.
22. Binkley TL, Specker BL, Wittig TA. Centile curves for bone density measurements in healthy males and females ages 5–22 yr. J Clin Densitom. 2002;5:343–53.
23. Arabi A, Nabulsi M, Maalouf J, et al. Bone mineral density by age, gender, pubertal stages, and socioeconomic status in healthy Lebanese children and adults. Bone. 2004;35:1169–79.

24. Arabi A, Tamim H, Nabulsi M, et al. Sex differences in the effect of body-composition variables on bone mass in healthy children and adolescents. Am J Clin Nutr. 2004;80:1428–35.
25. Cromer BA, Binkovitz L, Ziegler J, et al. Reference values for bone mineral density in 12- to 18-year-old girls categorized by weight, race, and age. Pediatr Radiol. 2004;34:787–92.
26. Ward KA, Ashby RL, Roberts SA, et al. UK reference data for the Hologic QDR Discovery dual-energy x ray absorptiometry scanner in healthy children and young adults aged 6–17 years. Arch Dis Child. 2007;92:53–9.
27. Kalkwarf HJ, Zemel BS, Gilsanz V, et al. The bone mineral density in childhood study (BMDCS): bone mineral content and density according to age, sex and race. J Clin Endocrinol Metab. 2007;92(6):2087–99.
28. Sala A, Webber CE, Morrison J, et al. Whole-body bone mineral content, lean body mass, and fat mass as measured by dual-energy x-ray absorptiometry in a population of healthy Canadian children and adolescents. Can Assoc Radiol J. 2007;58(1):46–52.
29. Tan LJ, Lei SF, Chen XD, et al. Establishment of peak bone mineral density in Southern Chinese males and its comparisons with other males from different regions of China. J Bone Miner Metab. 2007;25:114–21.
30. Kelly TL, Wilson KE, Heymsfield SB. Dual energy X-ray absorptiometry body composition reference values from NHANES. PLoS One. 2009;4(9):e7038.
31. Zemel BS, Stallings VA, Leonard MB, et al. Revised pediatric reference data for the lateral distal femur measured by Hologic Discovery/Delphi dual-energy X-ray absorptiometry. J Clin Densitom. 2009;12(2):207–18.
32. Zhou W, Langsetmo L, Berger C, et al. CaMos Research Group. Normative bone mineral density z-scores for Canadians aged 16 to 24 years: the Canadian Multicenter Osteoporosis Study. J Clin Densitom. 2010;13(3):267–76.
33. Baxter-Jones AD, Burrows M, Bachrach LK, et al. International longitudinal pediatric reference standards for bone mineral content. Bone. 2010;46(1):208–16.
34. Zemel BS, Kalkwarf HJ, Gilsanz V, et al. Revised reference curves for bone mineral content and areal bone mineral density according to age and sex for black and non-black children: results of the bone mineral density in childhood study. J Clin Endocrinol Metab. 2011;96(10):3160–9.
35. Kalkwarf HJ, Zemel BS, Yolton K, Heubi JE. Bone mineral content and density of the lumbar spine of infants and toddlers: influence of age, sex, race, growth, and human milk feeding. J Bone Miner Res. 2013;28(1):206–12.
36. Khadilkar AV, Sanwalka NJ, Chiplonkar SA, et al. Normative data and percentile curves for dual energy X-ray absorptiometry in healthy Indian girls and boys aged 5–17 years. Bone. 2011;48(4):810–9.
37. Crabtree NJ, Machin M, Bebbington NA, et al. 2013 The Amalgamated Paediatric Bone Density Study (the ALPHABET Study): the collation and generation of UK based reference data for paediatric bone densitometry. Bone Abstr 2. doi:10.1530/boneabs.2.OC1.
38. Xu H, Chen JX, Gong J, et al. Normal reference for bone density in healthy Chinese children. J Clin Densitom. 2007;10(3):266–75.
39. Marwaha RK, Tandon N, Reddy DH, et al. Peripheral bone mineral density and its predictors in healthy school girls from two different socioeconomic groups in Delhi. Osteoporos Int. 2007;18(3):375–83.
40. Min JY, Min KB, Paek D, et al. Age curves of bone mineral density at the distal radius and calcaneus in Koreans. J Bone Miner Metab. 2010;28(1):94–100.
41. Cheng JCY, Leung SSSF, Lee WTK, et al. Determinants of axial and peripheral bone mass in Chinese adolescents. Arch Dis Child. 1998;78:524–30.
42. Hasanoglu A, Tumer L, Ezgu FS. Vertebra and femur bone mineral density values in Turkish children. Turk J Pediatr. 2004;46:298–302.
43. Gordon CM, Bachrach LK, Carpenter TO, et al. Dual energy X-ray absorptiometry interpretation and reporting in children and adolescents: the 2007 ISCD Pediatric Official Positions. J Clin Densitom. 2008;11(1):43–58.

44. Leonard MB, Propert KJ, Zemel BS, Stallings VA, Feldman HI. Discrepancies in pediatric bone mineral density reference data: potential for misdiagnosis of osteopenia. J Pediatr. 1999;135:182–8.
45. WHO. The WHO Study Group: Assessment of fracture risk and its application to screening for postmenopausal osteoporosis. Geneva, Switzerland, 1994.
46. Marshall D, Johnell O, Wedel H. Meta-analysis of how well measures of bone mineral density predict occurrence of osteoporotic fractures. BMJ. 1996;312:1254–9.
47. Cummings SR, Black DM, Nevitt MC, Browner W, Cauley J, Ensrud K, et al. Bone density at various sites for prediction of hip fractures. The Study of Osteoporotic Fractures Research Group. Lancet. 1993;341:72–5.
48. Kanis JA, Johnell O, Oden A, Dawson A, De Laet C, Jonsson B. Ten year probabilities of osteoporotic fractures according to BMD and diagnostic thresholds. Osteoporos Int. 2001;12:989–95.
49. Taylor BC, Schreiner PJ, Stone KL, Fink HA, Cummings SR, Nevitt MC, et al. Long-term prediction of incident hip fracture risk in elderly white women: study of osteoporotic fractures. J Am Geriatr Soc. 2004;52:1479–86.
50. Prentice A, Parsons TJ, Cole TJ. Uncritical use of bone mineral density in absorptiometry may lead to size-related artifacts in the identification of bone mineral determinants. Am J Clin Nutr. 1994;60:837–42.
51. Molgaard C, Thomsen BL, Prentice A, Cole TJ, Michaelsen KF. Whole body bone mineral content in healthy children and adolescents. Arch Dis Child. 1997;76:9–15.
52. Heaney RP. Bone mineral content, not bone mineral density, is the correct bone measure for growth studies. Am J Clin Nutr. 2003;78:350–2.
53. Leonard MB, Shults J, Elliott DM, Stallings VA, Zemel BS. Interpretation of whole body dual energy X-ray absorptiometry measures in children: comparison with peripheral quantitative computed tomography. Bone. 2004;34:1044–52.
54. Bachrach LK, Hastie T, Wang MC, Narasimhan B, Marcus R. Bone mineral acquisition in healthy Asian, Hispanic, black, and Caucasian youth: a longitudinal study. J Clin Endocrinol Metab. 1999;84:4702–12.
55. Wang MC, Aguirre M, Bhudhikanok GS, Kendall CG, Kirsch S, Marcus R, et al. Bone mass and hip axis length in healthy Asian, black, Hispanic, and white American youths. J Bone Miner Res. 1997;12:1922–35.
56. Blake GM, Parker JC, Buxton FM, Fogelman I. Dual X-ray absorptiometry: a comparison between fan beam and pencil beam scans. Br J Radiol. 1993;66:902–6.
57. Tothill P, Laskey MA, Orphanidou CI, Van Wijk M. Anomalies in dual energy X-ray absorptiometry measurements of total-body bone mineral during weight change using Lunar, Hologic and Norland instruments. Br J Radiol. 1999;72:661–9.
58. Tothill P. Dual-energy X-ray absorptiometry measurements of total-body bone mineral during weight change. J Clin Densitom. 2005;8(1):31–8.
59. Tothill P, Avenill A. Anomalies in the measurement of changes in bone mineral density of the spine by dual-energy X-ray absorptiometry. Calcif Tissue Int. 1998;63:126–33.
60. Zemel BS, Leonard MB, Stallings VA. Evaluation of the Hologic experimental pediatric whole body analysis software in healthy children and children with chronic disease (Abstract). J Bone Miner Res. 2000;15(15(Supp 11)):S400.
61. Kelly TL. Pediatric whole body measurements. J Bone Miner Res 2002;17(Suppl 1): Abstract#S296.
62. Hui SL, Gao S, Zhou XH, Johnston Jr CC, Lu Y, Gluer CC, et al. Universal standardization of bone density measurements: a method with optimal properties for calibration among several instruments. J Bone Miner Res. 1997;12:1463–70.
63. Kalkwarf HJ, Zemel BS, Gilsanz V, Lappe JM, Horlick M, Oberfield S, et al. The bone mineral density in childhood study: bone mineral content and density according to age, sex, and race. J Clin Endocrinol Metab. 2007;92(6):2087–99.

64. del Rio L, Carrascosa A, Pons F, Gusinye M, Yeste D, Domenech FM. Bone mineral density of the lumbar spine in white Mediterranean Spanish children and adolescents: changes related to age, sex, and puberty. Pediatr Res. 1994;35:362–6.
65. Glastre C, Braillon P, David L, Cochat P, Meunier PJ, Delmas PD. Measurement of bone mineral content of the lumbar spine by dual energy X-ray absorptiometry in normal children: correlations with growth parameters. J Clin Endocrinol Metab. 1990;70:1330–3.
66. Katzman DK, Bachrach LK, Carter DR, Marcus R. Clinical and anthropometric correlates of bone mineral acquisition in healthy adolescent girls. J Clin Endocrinol Metab. 1991;73:1332–9.
67. Lu PW, Briody JN, Ogle GD, Morley K, Humphries IR, Allen J, et al. Bone mineral density of total body, spine, and femoral neck in children and young adults: a cross-sectional and longitudinal study. J Bone Miner Res. 1994;9:1451–8.
68. Southard RN, Morris JD, Mahan JD, Hayes JR, Torch MA, Sommer A, et al. Bone mass in healthy children: measurement with quantitative DXA. Radiology. 1991;179:735–8.
69. Horlick M, Wang J, Pierson Jr RN, Thornton JC. Prediction models for evaluation of total-body bone mass with dual-energy X-ray absorptiometry among children and adolescents. Pediatrics. 2004;114:337–45.
70. Plotkin H, Nunez M, Alvarez Filgueira ML, Zanchetta JR. Lumbar spine bone density in Argentine children. Calcif Tissue Int. 1996;58:144–9.
71. Theintz G, Buchs B, Rizzoli R, Slosman D, Clavien H, Sizonenko PC, et al. Longitudinal monitoring of bone mass accumulation in healthy adolescents: evidence for a marked reduction after 16 years of age at the levels of lumbar spine and femoral neck in female subjects. J Clin Endocrinol Metab. 1992;75:1060–5.
72. Nelson DA, Simpson PM, Johnson CC, Barondess DA, Kleerekoper M. The accumulation of whole body skeletal mass in third- and fourth-grade children: effects of age, gender, ethnicity, and body composition. Bone. 1997;20:73–8.
73. Parfitt AM. Genetic effects on bone mass and turnover-relevance to black/white differences. J Am Coll Nutr. 1997;16:325–33.
74. Pietrobelli A, Faith MS, Wang J, Brambilla P, Chiumello G, Heymsfield SB. Association of lean tissue and fat mass with bone mineral content in children and adolescents. Obes Res. 2002;10:56–60.
75. Chan GM, Hoffman K, McMurry M. Effects of dairy products on bone and body composition in pubertal girls. J Pediatr. 1995;126:551–6.
76. Sentipal JM, Wardlaw GM, Mahan J, Matkovic V. Influence of calcium intake and growth indexes on vertebral bone mineral density in young females. Am J Clin Nutr. 1991;54:425–8.
77. Slemenda CW, Christian JC, Williams CJ, Norton JA, Johnston CC. Genetic determinants of bone mass in adult women: a reevaluation of the twin model and the potential importance of gene interaction in heritability estimates. J Bone Miner Res. 1991;6:561–7.
78. Bailey DA, McKay HA, Mirwald RL, Crocker PR, Faulkner RA. A six-year longitudinal study of the relationship of physical activity to bone mineral accrual in growing children: The University of Saskatchewan bone mineral accrual study. J Bone Miner Res. 1999;14:1672–9.
79. Magarey AM, Boulton TJ, Chatterton BE, Schultz C, Nordin BE, Cockington RA. Bone growth from 11 to 17 years: relationship to growth, gender and changes with pubertal status including timing of menarche. Acta Paediatr. 1999;88:139–46.
80. Seeman E. From density to structure: growing up and growing old on the surfaces of bone. J Bone Miner Res. 1997;12:509–21.
81. Seeman E, Hopper JL, Young NR, Formica C, Goss P, Tsalamandris C. Do genetic factors explain associations between muscle strength, lean mass, and bone density? A twin study. Am J Physiol. 1996;270:E320–7.
82. Bachrach LK. Acquisition of optimal bone mass in childhood and adolescence. Trends Endocrinol Metab. 2001;12:22–8.
83. Leib ES, Lewiecki EM, Binkley N, Hamdy RC. Official positions of the International Society for Clinical Densitometry. J Clin Densitom. 2004;7:1–6.

# Chapter 4
# Indications for DXA in Children and Adolescents

**Sarah Pitts and Catherine M. Gordon**

The demand for bone mineral density assessments in children and adolescents continues to grow. The importance of considering early bone health for osteoporosis prevention is well established [1, 2]. Achieving a high peak bone mass early in life predicts a higher bone mass and greater fracture protection later in life [1]. Genetic factors, malnutrition, hormonal disorders, medications, immobilization, and chronic illness during childhood and adolescence may compromise bone size, mineral content accrual, and bone quality [1–3]. If not reversed, the accrual of peak bone mass may be impaired, thereby increasing the lifetime risk for osteoporotic fracture. In severely affected individuals, low-impact or fragility fractures can even occur during childhood [4, 5].

Given the widespread availability, speed, high precision, and safety of dual-energy x-ray absorptiometry (DXA), there is abundant research to inform its clinical use in pediatrics. This chapter will review current evidence and expert opinion regarding which children and adolescents warrant DXA screening, how often these studies should be repeated, and how the results should be used to guide clinical management.

S. Pitts, M.D. (✉)
Divisions of Adolescent Medicine and Endocrinology, Harvard Medical School,
Boston Children's Hospital, 300 Longwood Avenue, Boston, MA 02115, USA
e-mail: sarah.pitts@childrens.harvard.edu

C.M. Gordon, M.D., M.Sc.
Division of Adolescent and Transition Medicine, Cincinnati Children's Hospital
Medical Center, University of Cincinnati College of Medicine, Cincinnati, OH, USA
e-mail: Catherine.Gordon@cchmc.org

© Springer International Publishing Switzerland 2016
E.B. Fung et al. (eds.), *Bone Health Assessment in Pediatrics*,
DOI 10.1007/978-3-319-30412-0_4

# The Rationale for DXA and Challenges in Pediatrics

Bone densitometry is performed in adults to measure bone mass, a surrogate measure of bone strength and resistance to fracture. These results are used to determine if deficits in bone mineral are present, to predict the risk of osteoporotic fracture, to help identify which patients warrant therapy, and to monitor the response to treatment. The rationale for performing DXA measurements in pediatrics is similar, although the reliability, interpretation, and clinical significance of bone densitometry in growing children and adolescents are more challenging, as reviewed in Chaps. 5 and 6.

Regarding fracture prediction, the association between low bone mineral density (BMD) and fracture in older adults is sufficiently robust such that the World Health Organization (WHO) has developed criteria for "osteopenia" and "osteoporosis" based upon BMD T-scores alone (i.e., standard deviations above or below the mean for healthy young adults) [6]. However, the WHO criteria are not appropriate for use in children, adolescents, and young adults who have not yet achieved peak bone mass as they will normally have negative T-scores [7]. Additionally, there are insufficient data to determine a specific risk of fragility fracture, or a "fracture threshold," based solely on bone mass in pediatrics and young adult populations. Even in adults, bone quality, rates of bone turnover, and the nature of trauma contribute to fracture risk. Collecting the evidence to define the relationship between bone mass and fracture risk in children and adolescents is a difficult goal given the overall low incidence of fractures and requirement for a large study cohort.

Despite these limitations, DXA has clinical utility in the bone health evaluation of any child or adolescent who may be at increased risk for low bone mass and/or significant fracture [8]. Establishing a baseline BMD Z-score (i.e., standard deviation above or below the mean for an age-matched individual) for any patient who may be at risk for poor bone health allows subsequent DXA measurements to inform the success of therapeutic interventions or to identify evidence of disease progression. The International Society for Clinical Densitometry (ISCD) recently endorsed a BMD Z-score of −2 SD as indicative of a significant low bone mass for age [7]. Children or adolescents identified as having bone mass in this range would warrant close monitoring for fractures.

# Potential Candidates for DXA

Candidates for DXA screening measurements include children and adolescents with genetic disorders or chronic diseases associated with low bone mass, with significant mild to moderate impact fractures, and/or with "osteopenia" noted on a standard radiograph (Table 4.1) [8, 9]. This list should not be interpreted as a mandate for screening all young people with these diagnoses; clinical judgment is needed to determine when DXA studies will influence clinical care for a given patient.

**Table 4.1** Clinical indications for DXA studies in pediatrics [8, 9, 11]

The decision to perform a DXA in an individual patient with any of the following disorders should be influenced by disease severity and other clinical risk factors for poor bone health:
- "Osteopenia" diagnosed on conventional radiograph
- A significant fracture history defined below, occurring as a result of clinically defined "mild-moderate" trauma:
  - Two or more long bone fractures by age 10 years
  - Three or more long bone fractures by age 19 years
  - Vertebral compression (or crush) fracture
- Chronic disease
  - Primary bone and connective tissue disorders
  - Chronic inflammatory diseases (e.g., Crohn disease)
  - Endocrinopathies (e.g., hypogonadism, anorexia nervosa)
  - Disorders resulting in impaired mobility (e.g., myopathies, cerebral palsy)
  - Hematologic diseases (e.g., thalassemia)
  - Disease processes requiring prolonged systemic glucocorticoid therapy
- Therapeutic monitoring

## *"Osteopenia" on Conventional X-Ray*

Standard radiographs are an insensitive tool for evaluating bone mineralization; an estimated decrease of 20–40 % must occur before reduced bone mass, or "osteopenia," is detected [10]. While the term "osteopenia" is commonly used to describe an appearance suggestive of low bone mass on radiographs, it is not a recommended term for describing actual low bone mass by DXA in a pediatric population [7, 8]. The appearance of low bone mass may be an incidental finding on a chest or abdominal x-ray taken for nonskeletal indications or reported on a radiograph ordered due to bone pain or trauma. Such patients thought to have low bone mass on a standard radiograph should have subsequent DXA measures of bone density, especially if there are other identifiable risk factors for poor bone health.

## *Childhood Fractures*

Fractures occur in otherwise normal children. As many as half of all boys and one-third of girls will fracture by age 18, and one-fifth will sustain 2 or more fractures [11]. Most childhood fractures affect the forearm. Since peak bone growth precedes peak bone mineral accrual by 6–12 months, in early adolescence the skeleton may be relatively under-mineralized and more susceptible to fracture upon exposure to trauma. Several studies have compared the bone mineral density of "normal" children and adolescents who have sustained fractures to that of age-matched controls without fractures. Most [12–15], but not all [16, 17], studies have found the mean BMD to be significantly lower in children with forearm fractures than in controls. In a longitudinal study, Goulding et al. [13] found that 29 % of the subjects with a fracture at study entry had at least one subsequent fracture during the next 4 years as compared with only 8 % of control subjects. This being said, given the high prevalence of fractures among children it is not recommended that DXA measures be performed on all children who sustain a forearm fracture.

Recurrent fractures and those that occur in the setting of mild to moderate trauma warrant investigation with DXA. A detailed history of the nature of the injury is important, to assess the direction and magnitude of the force associated with the fracture [18]. For example, some fractures from a standing height, such as those that occur while is child is playing soccer or other vigorous sports, involve significant impact or torsion and may not qualify as mild trauma.

Vertebral compression fractures are far less common than extremity fractures during childhood. Spine fractures may indicate a marked deficit in bone quality, quantity, or both, particularly if other risk factors such as chronic glucocorticoid exposure are present. Recently, the ISCD noted that the presence of a compression (or crush) fracture in a child or adolescent constitutes a diagnosis of osteoporosis [8]. Bone densitometry is warranted in these patients to measure bone mass at non-vertebral sites and to establish a baseline DXA measure prior to treatment. However, bone mineral density may be increased in areas of compression as an artifact of the collapsed vertebrae. For this reason, areas of compression should be excluded when analyzing a DXA measure of the spine. With the availability of higher resolution bone densitometers, vertebral fracture assessments (VFA) by DXA has proven to be a useful tool for the diagnosis of moderate and severe vertebral fractures in children and adolescent, and radiation exposure is markedly less than with standard radiographs (see Chap. 10) [7, 19]. However, the "gold standard" for diagnosing vertebral fractures continues to be lateral spine x-rays.

## Genetic Disorders and Chronic Diseases

Table 4.2 expands upon the genetic and acquired disorders that have been reported to be associated with low bone mass and fragility fractures in children and adolescents. Most of the conditions listed have been examined only in small convenience samples, many of which failed to consider delayed growth or maturity in interpreting the results. Because of these limitations, it is not possible to predict the risk of low bone mass or fractures in each condition with certainty. It is beyond the scope of this chapter to provide a detailed discussion for each of these disorders, but several are highlighted below, reviews are available in the literature [9], and additional disease-specific references are cited in Table 4.2.

Bone fragility in most of the heritable disorders results from defects in the bone matrix that can affect the entire skeleton [20–22]. Osteogenesis imperfecta, a primary bone disorder, exemplifies this point. With variable expressivity of the associated genetic defects, there is a wide range of skeletal effects and disease severity. Some patients show only asymptomatic low bone mass, whereas others progress to chronic bone pain, recurrent fractures, and progressive skeletal deformity. Others may have dentinogenesis imperfecta, hyperextensible joints, or other physical manifestations of the disorder. In patients with fibrous dysplasia, total bone

**Table 4.2** Disorders associated with low bone mass and/or mild to moderate impact fractures in children and adolescents [9]

*Genetic bone/connective tissue disorders* [20–22]
• Ehlers-Danlos syndrome
• Fibrous dysplasia
• Gaucher's disease
• Galactosemia
• Glycogen storage diseases
• Homocystinuria
• Hypophosphatasia
• Marfan's syndrome
• Menke's kinky hair syndrome
• Osteogenesis imperfecta
*Chronic disease* [4, 19, 23–25, 33, 35, 36, 41–43, 49–51]
• Systemic inflammatory diseases (i.e., inflammatory bowel disease, rheumatologic diseases)
• Malnutrition/malabsorptive disorders (i.e., anorexia nervosa, celiac disease, inflammatory bowel disease, cystic fibrosis)
• Hematologic diseases (i.e., thalassemia and sickle cell anemia)
• Malignancy (leukemia)
• Chronic kidney disease
*Idiopathic juvenile osteoporosis* [26–28]
*Idiopathic adolescent scoliosis* [48]
*Endocrine disorders* [29–31, 34]
• Glucocorticoid excess (endogenous or iatrogenic as seen in the treatment of nephrotic syndrome, malignancy, inflammatory bowel disease, rheumatologic diseases, solid organ transplant and hematopoietic stem cell transplant)
• Hypothyroidism
• Hyperparathyroidism
• Sex steroid deficiency or resistance
• Type I diabetes (poorly controlled and/or with concurrent celiac disease)
*Neuromuscular diseases/immobilization* [37–40]
• Cerebral palsy
• Muscular dystrophies
• Paraplegia/spinal cord injury

mass is not diminished, but fragility fractures and pain occur at sites of lytic or cystic lesions. Idiopathic juvenile osteoporosis (IJO) is another primary bone disease process, highlighted in more depth below.

Myriad acquired diseases have been associated with a low bone mass, as noted in Table 4.2. In most of these diverse disorders, there is more than one threat to skeletal health. Malnutrition, vitamin D insufficiency, inadequate calcium intake or retention, immobility, deficiency of or resistance to sex steroids or growth hormone, and increased cytokines associated with these disorders can complicate the clinical picture [2]. Glucocorticoids, chemotherapeutic agents, and radiation therapy used to treat these disorders contribute to impaired bone health [9]. Therefore, severity of deficits in bone quantity and quality in chronic disease varies by diagnosis and disease course. For example, children with cystic fibrosis with marked disease severity and malnutrition may have markedly reduced bone mass and low-trauma fractures [23, 24]. By contrast, some, but not all, well-nourished children with mild cystic fibrosis have normal BMD for age [25]. Therefore, the decision to order DXA scans must be based upon clinical judgment regarding the presence of risk factors.

## Idiopathic Juvenile Osteoporosis (IJO)

This disorder of unknown etiology presents in pre-pubertal children as bone pain and fragility fractures of spine and long bones; low bone mass is found when densitometry is performed [26, 27]. The diagnosis of IJO is made when other potential causes for bone fragility have been excluded. The etiology of IJO remains elusive. On radiographs, absence of callus at fracture sites and radiolucent bands in metaphyseal regions (i.e., neo-osseus osteoporosis) are characteristic of IJO, whereas callus formation is normal at fracture sites in osteogenesis imperfecta. Many patients with IJO exhibit dramatic "catch-up" bone accrual during puberty. However, for patients who sustain vertebral compression fractures and/or have an extremely low BMD Z-score, pamidronate therapy may be prescribed. This therapy has been shown to be effective in raising lumbar spine BMD and reducing fracture risk over 3 years, and DXA can be a helpful tool to monitor effects of therapy when it is initiated [28].

## Endocrine Disorders

Deficiencies or excesses of certain hormones can limit bone mineral accrual and can contribute to skeletal losses. In Type 1 diabetes mellitus, bone mass is lower in children with this disease compared to healthy controls [29]. With poorly controlled diabetes or associated celiac disease bone mass is notably lower [30, 31]. Of enormous clinical concern is the skeletal effects of long term systemic glucocorticoids prescribed for chronic disease, malignancy, or posttransplantation. The dose, route of administration, specific agent, and duration of glucocorticoid therapy may influence the severity of the skeletal deficits. However, factors such as nutrition, activity, inflammation, and genetic variables appear to modify the skeletal response to chronic glucocorticoid excess, as well [4, 32, 33].

Appropriate treatment to correct endocrine deficits (such as sex steroid replacement therapy for ovarian insufficiency [34]) may be sufficient to prevent or restore deficits in bone mineral density. In other cases, such as with anorexia nervosa, the complexity of the hormonal imbalance that is impairing bone health complicates the therapeutic effort [35, 36].

## Immobilization

Mechanical loading of bone is a key determinant of bone strength. For children who are immobilized due to cerebral palsy, neuromuscular disorders, or congenital or posttraumatic spinal injury, inadequate accrual and increased loss of bone are inevitable [37–40]. In many of these conditions, the adverse effects of immobilization may be compounded by coexisting deficiencies of calories, protein, calcium, or vitamin D intake and by the use of anticonvulsant therapies. Low bone mass and fragility fractures, particularly of the hip and lower extremities, are common in these disorders.

Muscle mass is often impaired in children and adolescents with limited mobility and may also contribute to skeletal losses or inadequate accrual. Research shows that muscle development plays an important role in bone mineral accrual; referred to as the "muscle-bone unit." [41] Modern DXA technology affords reliable assessments of body composition which may inform clinical management in the future, but more research is needed [42].

## Initial DXA Studies

Increased use of DXA for pediatric clinical research has led to an extensive list of conditions associated with low bone mass or fractures in childhood (Table 4.2). However, without systematic screening of large numbers of children with the same diagnosis, the prevalence and severity of low bone density and fractures cannot be established. Little is known about the frequency of fragility fractures in these conditions since cohort sizes are often too small to determine whether fractures exceed the expected incidence for age. Until further research is available, recommendations regarding whom to screen by DXA and how frequently to repeat these studies represent expert opinion rather than evidence-based indications [8].

For a few disorders, subspecialty panels have developed recommendations for DXA examinations based upon analysis of the available literature by assembled experts. For example, in cystic fibrosis the European Cystic Fibrosis Mineralization Guidelines recommended DXA screening no later than at ages 8–10 years and then subsequent DXA measures at designated time intervals depending on the BMD Z-score at baseline [43]. Table 4.3 summarizes the published guidelines for several chronic disorders.

For disorders in which specific recommendations have not been established, the decision to perform DXA assessments should be based upon clinical judgment of risk. Routine DXA screening for the conditions listed in Table 4.2 are not mandated. The decision to perform DXA screening in an individual patient is influenced by disease severity, immobility, bone pain, skeletal deformity, malnutrition, and/or use of medications known to affect bone adversely. As with any test used in clinical practice, bone density testing should be carried out only when it is likely to influence patient management. For example, DXA measures would be indicated if results modify the decision to initiate therapy. If treatment is initiated, DXA screening is appropriate to establish a baseline measurement for monitoring the response to therapy over time.

The potential value of DXA must be weighed against impediments to obtaining useful information from the scans. If the child is too young to remain still or if normative data are not available for the age and gender of the child, the information obtained may not be useful. Given the evolution in DXA technology, whole body measures are reliable in children ≥3 years old and spinal measures are feasible and reproducible even in neonates [44]. Immobilized patients and individuals with skeletal deformities or muscle contractures may be unable to be properly positioned

**Table 4.3** Published recommendations for bone density testing for specific disorders[a]

| Disorder | Recommendations |
|---|---|
| Cystic fibrosis [49] | Baseline DXA scans >8 years if:<br>• <90 % ideal body weight<br>• FEV1 <50 % predicted<br>• Glucocorticoids of ≥5 mg/day for ≥90 days/year<br>• Delayed puberty<br>• History of fractures<br>Baseline DXA at 18 years if no risk factors<br>If normal baseline DXA, repeat every 2–5 years<br>If low baseline DXA (Z-score ≤−2 SD), repeat yearly and consider bisphosphonate therapy |
| Survivor of childhood cancer [50] | DXA at entry into long-term follow-up (typically 2 years following completion of cancer therapy) if:<br>• treated with methotrexate and/or corticosteroids<br>• underwent hematopoietic cell transplant<br>• developed secondary growth hormone deficiency, hypogonadism, delayed puberty, or hyperthyroidism<br>Do not repeat DXA if normal bone density unless ongoing bone health risk factors or mild-moderate impact fractures. |
| Inflammatory bowel disease [51] | DXA scans of the spine and total body less head in children with the diagnosis of IBD or at any point in children with IBD and any of the following risk factors:<br>• Suboptimal growth velocity or height Z-score <−2.0 SD<br>• Weight or BMI Z-score <−2.0 SD or downward crossing percentiles<br>• Primary or secondary amenorrhea<br>• Delayed puberty<br>• Severe inflammatory disease course, especially when associated with decreased albumin level (<3 g/dL)<br>• 6 months or longer of continuous use of systemic glucocorticoids |

[a]These guidelines are primarily based upon the expert opinion of pediatric subspecialists who served on guidelines committees

using standard techniques and skeletal sites. Performing densitometry in young children and in children and adolescents with special considerations is discussed in Chaps. 8 and 9.

The information to be gained from DXA must also be weighed against the risk of misinterpretation. Bone densitometry in children requires specialized skill and attention to avoid errors in acquiring or interpreting densitometry data, as outlined in Chaps. 5 and 6. The most serious errors involve inappropriate reporting of T-scores and use of the WHO criteria for osteoporosis and osteopenia in patients who have not yet reached peak bone mass. These mistakes can cause unwarranted concern and potentially exposing them to inappropriate treatment. Failure to adjust for delayed or advanced maturation or for bone size, and failure to use gender- and ethnic-specific normative data could also contribute to over- or under-diagnosis of low bone mass [45]. To avoid these diagnostic errors, the clinician should arrange for DXA studies to be performed in DXA centers with established expertise in pediatric densitometry. If impossible, DXA results should be reviewed for accuracy by an experienced pediatric DXA consultant.

Selecting the skeletal region to scan will depend upon technical considerations and the clinical indications for the study. Careful positioning and consistent repositioning are required to complete scans for the spine, proximal hip, and total body less head. Skeletal sites with permanent hardware such as a rod or pin should not be scanned. The lumbar spine and total body less head are preferred sites in patients ≤19 years because of the documented high precision and published reference norms [7]. The vertebrae contain considerable trabecular bone, which is selectively lost in response to hypogonadism. By contrast, the total body less head is comprised largely of cortical bone, which is reduced in growth hormone deficiency, hyperthyroidism, and hyperparathyroidism. Thus, the underlying disease process can often dictate the skeletal region that is evaluated.

As in adults, the primary goals of DXA for children and adolescents include monitoring the bone health of high-risk patients, identifying those at greatest risk for fracture, and assessing responses to therapy. Because the relationship between bone density and fracture has not been established in pediatric populations, the diagnosis of osteoporosis should not be made in children and adolescents solely on the basis of densitometric criteria. Per the ISCD [8, 11], as mentioned, the presence of one or more vertebral compression fractures in the absence of local disease or high-energy trauma is indicative of osteoporosis regardless of BMD results obtained by DXA. In the absence of vertebral fractures, the diagnosis of osteoporosis is indicated by the presence of both a clinically significant fracture history and BMD Z-score of ≤2.0 SD. Experts define clinically significant fractures as follows: (1) 2 or more long-bone fractures by the age of 10 year; or (2) 3 or more long-bone fractures at any age up to age 19 years [8, 11]. As discussed earlier, the mechanism of injury is important to take into consideration. It is also important to remember that a normal BMD Z-score does not preclude the potential for underlying skeletal fragility and increased fracture risk in children and adolescents.

## Follow-Up DXA Studies

Bone mass changes slowly, and variability errors for bone densitometry may exceed the rate of change in bone mass [7]. These issues should factor into the decision regarding the timing of repeat DXA studies. Another key factor that dictates the timing of follow-up is the precision or reproducibility of the densitometry measurements, as discussed in detail in Chap. 6 [7]. Variability in repeated measurements can occur in the same individual on the same day. This reflects both the limitations of DXA machinery and software, as well as differences in density due to errors in repositioning the patient. Precision is routinely expressed in terms of the number of standard deviations (SDs) of repeated measurements and how they vary from the mean of multiple measurements. The more precise the measurement, the smaller the change in bone density that can be detected with certainty. Least significant change (LSC), a term used in both pediatric and adult densitometry, describes the minimum increase or decrease between serial DXA measurements that exceeds the variability of the technique itself. The absolute or percent change in bone mineral density meeting the definition of LSC varies both with the precision of the technique and with the level of statistical confidence desired (i.e., 80–95 %). For most sites studied, a true change in bone density will have to be at least 3 % to exceed the error of the technique.

The monitoring time interval (MTI) is an estimate of the minimal time required to be able to detect a meaningful change in bone mineral using a particular densitometric technique [46]. In pediatric populations, yearly rates of bone mineral accrual vary considerably, with the greatest gains occurring several months after peak height velocity [47]. Given the rapid changes in bone size and mineral during the adolescent growth spurt, the MTI would theoretically be shortened. In 1554 healthy children, age 6–16 years, Shepherd et al. showed that MTIs were shortest at the AP spine (MTI 0.2–1.1 years) and longer at the femoral neck and distal third of the radius (0.6–4.3 years) [46]. A complete understanding of precision, LSC and MTI is important for clinicians who order and interpret skeletal assessments by DXA. To repeat a DXA study more frequently than every 12 months is rarely warranted except for clinical research, to monitor response to new drug intervention or rapidly worsening clinical status. Longer intervals between repeat scans may be appropriate if the baseline DXA measures indicates normal bone mineral for age or if the risks for poor bone health wax and wane. Continued threats to bone health such as ongoing glucocorticoid therapy, immobilization, or malnutrition, would prompt a yearly follow-up study to monitor skeletal status more closely and to assess the rate of bone gains or losses.

## Summary Points

- Bone densitometry is performed to determine if deficits in bone mineral are present, to identify those at greatest risk for fracture, to help identify which patients warrant therapy, and to monitor the response to treatment.
- Potential candidates for DXA include children with genetic disorders or chronic diseases associated with low bone mass; children with recurrent fractures, low-impact fractures, or vertebral compression fracture; and those identified as having "osteopenia" on a standard radiograph.
- For some disorders, subspecialty panels have developed guidelines for performing DXAs based upon the available literature and expert opinion.
- For disorders in which specific recommendations have not been established, the decision to perform initial bone densitometry scans is based upon clinical factors such disease severity, bone pain, skeletal deformity, or history of fragility fracture.
- Clinical DXA scans should be performed only if the results will influence patient management.
- The decision to perform a follow-up DXA measurement depends upon initial findings and interval risk factors. To repeat a scan more frequently than every 12 months is rarely warranted except for research, to monitor response to drug intervention or with rapidly worsening clinical status.

- DXA studies should be performed in DXA centers with established expertise in pediatric densitometry to avoid misinterpretation of data.
- Consider potential impediments to obtaining a DXA before ordering the scan. These include a child's inability to remain still without sedation, lack of age- and gender-matched normative data, or skeletal deformities that prevent proper positioning.
- DXA adjustments in analysis and reporting are critically important in those children and adolescents with delayed puberty or short stature.

# References

1. Heaney RP, Abrams S, Dawson-Hughes B, Looker A, Marcus R, Matkovic V, et al. Peak bone mass. Osteoporos Int. 2000;11:985–1009.
2. Golden NH, Abrams SA. Optimizing bone health in children and adolescents. Pediatrics. 2014;134:e1229–43.
3. Mora S, Gilsanz V. Establishment of peak bone mass. Endocrinol Metab Clin N Am. 2003;32:39–63.
4. Rodd C, Lang B, Ramsay T, et al. Incident vertebral fractures among children with rheumatic disorders 12 months after glucocorticoid initiation: a national observational study. Arthritis Care Res. 2012;64:122–31.
5. Huh SY, Gordon CM. Fractures among hospitalized children. Metabolism. 2013;62:315–25.
6. WHO Scientific Group. The assessment of osteoporosis at primary health care level. Geneva: World Health Organization; 2004. Accessed 31 Oct 2014 at http://www.who.int/chp/topics/Osteoporosis.pdf.
7. Crabtree NJ, Arabi A, Bachrach LK, et al. Dual-energy X-ray absorptionmetry interpretation and reporting in children and adolescents: the revised 2013 ISCD pediatric official positions. J Clin Densitom. 2014;17:225–42.
8. Gordon CM, Leonard MB, Zemel BS, International Society for Clinical Densitometry, 2013 Pediatric Position Development Conference: executive summary and reflections. J Clin Densitom. 2014;17:219–24.
9. Bianchi ML, Leonard MB, Bechtold S, et al. Bone health in children and adolescents with chronic disease that may affect the skeleton: the 2013 ISCD pediatric official positions. J Clin Densitom. 2014;17:281–94.
10. Ahmed AI, Ilic D, Blake GM, Rymer JM, Fogelman I. Review of 3530 referrals for bone density measurements of spine and femur: evidence that radiographic osteopenia predicts low bone mass. Radiology. 1998;207:619–24.
11. Bishop N, Arundel P, Clark E, et al. Fracture prediction and the definition of osteoporosis in children and adolescents: the ISCD 2013 pediatric official positions. J Clin Densitom. 2014;17:275–80.
12. Chan GM, Hess M, Hollis J, Book LS. Bone mineral status in childhood accidental fractures. Am J Dis Child. 1984;138:569–70.
13. Goulding A, Jones IE, Taylor RW, Manning PJ, Williams SM. More broken bones: a 4- year double cohort study of young girls with and without distal forearm fractures. J Bone Miner Res. 2000;15:2011–8.
14. Goulding A, Jones IE, Taylor RW, Williams SM, Manning PJ. Bone mineral density and body composition in boys with distal forearm fractures: a dual-energy x-ray absorptiometry study. J Pediatr. 2001;139:509–15.
15. Ma DQ, Jones G. The association between bone mineral density, metacarpal morphometry, and upper limb fractures in children: a population-based case–control study. J Clin Endocrinol Metab. 2003;88:1486–91.

16. Blimkie CJR, Lefevre J, Beunen GP, Renson R, Dequeker J, Van Damme P. Fractures, physical activity and growth velocity in adolescent Belgian boys. Med Sci Sports Exerc. 1992;25:801–8.
17. Cook SD, Harding AF, Morgan EL, Doucet HJ, Bennett JT, O'Brien M, et al. Association of bone mineral density and pediatric fractures. J Pediatr Orthop. 1987;7:424–77.
18. Landin LA. Fracture patterns in children. Analysis of 8682 fractures with special reference to incidence, etiology and secular changes in a Swedish urban population 1950–1979. Acta Orthop Scand Suppl. 1983;202:1–109.
19. DiVasta AD, Feldman HA, Gordon CM. Vertebral fracture assessment in adolescents and young women with anorexia nervosa: a case series. J Clin Densitom. 2014;17(1):207–11.
20. Whyte MP. Osteogenesis imperfecta. In: Favus M, editor. Primer on metabolic diseases and disorders of mineral metabolism. Washington, DC: American Society for Bone and Mineral Research; 2003. p. 470–3.
21. Collins MT, Bianco P. Fibrous dysplasia. In: Favus M, editor. Primer on metabolic diseases and disorders of mineral metabolism. Washington, DC: American Society for Bone and Mineral Research; 2003. p. 466–70.
22. Glorieux FH, Pettifor JM, Juppner H, editors. Pediatric bone biology and diseases. Boston: Academic; 2003.
23. Douros K, Loukou I, Nicolaidou P, et al. Bone mass density and associated factors in cystic fibrosis patients of young age. J Paediatr Child Health. 2008;44:681–5.
24. Sermet-Gaudelus I, Souberbielle JC, Ruiz JC, et al. Low bone mineral density in young children with cystic fibrosis. Am J Respir Crit Care Med. 2007;175:951–7.
25. Rovner AJ, Zemel BS, Leonard MB, Schall JI, Stallings VA. Mild to moderate cystic fibrosis is not associated with increased fracture risk in children and adolescents. J Pediatr. 2005;147:327–31.
26. Bacchetta J, Wesseling-Perry K, Gilsanz V, Gales B, Pereira RC, Salusky IB. Idiopathic juvenile osteoporosis: a cross-sectional single-centre experience with bone histomorphometry and quantitative computed tomography. Pediatr Rheumatol Online J. 2013;11:6. doi:10.1186/1546-0096.
27. Krassas GE. Idiopathic juvenile osteoporosis. Ann N Y Acad Sci. 2000;900:409–12.
28. Baroncelli GI, Vierucci F, Bertelloni S, et al. Pamidronate treatment stimulates the onset of recovery phase reducing fracture rate and skeletal deformities in patients with idiopathic juvenile osteoporosis: comparison with untreated patients. J Bone Miner Metab. 2013;31:533–43.
29. Saha MT, Sievanen H, Salo MK, et al. Bone mass and structure in adolescents with type 1 diabetes compared to healthy peers. Osteoporos Int. 2009;20(8):1401–6.
30. Heilman K, Zilmer M, Zilmer K, Tillmann V. Lower bone mineral density in children with type 1 diabetes is associated with poor glycemic control and higher serum ICAM-1 and urinary isoprostane levels. J Bone Miner Metab. 2009;27:598–604.
31. Diniz-Santos DR, Brandao F, Adan L, et al. 2008 Bone mineralization in young patients with type 1 diabetes mellitus and screening-identified evidence of celiac disease. Dig Dis Sci. 2008;53:1240–5.
32. Rayar MS, Nayiager T, Webber CE, et al. Predictors of bony morbidity in children with acute lymphoblastic leukemia. Pediatr Blood Cancer. 2012;59:77–82.
33. Petryk A, Bergemann TL, Polga KM, et al. Prospective study of changes in bone mineral density and turnover in children after hematopoietic cell transplantation. J Clin Endocrinol Metab. 2006;91:899–905.
34. Khastgir G, Studd JW, Fox SW, et al. A longitudinal study of the effect of subcutaneous estrogen replacement on bone in young women with Turner's syndrome. J Bone Miner Res. 2003;18:925–32.
35. Divasta AD, Feldman HA, Giancaterino C, et al. The effect of gonadal and adrenal steroid therapy on skeletal health in adolescents and young women with anorexia nervosa. Metabolism. 2012;61:1010–20.

36. Misra M, Katzman D, Miller KK, et al. Physiologic estrogen replacement increases bone density in adolescent girls with anorexia nervosa. J Bone Miner Res. 2011;26:2430–8.
37. Fehlings D, Switzer L, Agarwal P, et al. Informing evidence-based clinical practice guidelines for children with cerebral palsy at risk of osteoporosis: a systematic review. Dev Med Child Neurol. 2012;54:106–16.
38. Hough JP, Boyd RN, Keating JL. Systematic review of interventions for low bone mineral density in children with cerebral palsy. Pediatrics. 2010;125:e670–8.
39. Mergler S, Evenhuis HM, Boot AM, et al. Epidemiology of low bone mineral density and fractures in children with severe cerebral palsy: a systematic review. Dev Med Child Neurol. 2009;51:773–8.
40. Bianchi ML, Mazzanti A, Galbiati E, Saraifoger S, Dubini A, Cornelio F, et al. Bone mineral density and bone metabolism in Duchenne muscular dystrophy. Osteoporos Int. 2003;14:761–7.
41. Lee DY, Wetzsteon RJ, Zemel BS, et al. Muscle torque relative to cross-sectional area and the functional muscle-bone unit in children and adolescents with chronic disease. J Bone Miner Res 2015;30:575–83.
42. Pitts S, Blood E, Divasta A, Gordon CM. Percentage body fat by dual-energy x-ray absorptiometry is associated with menstrual recovery in adolescents with anorexia nervosa. J Adolesc Health. 2014;54:739–41.
43. Sermet-Gaudelis I, Bianchi ML, Garabedian M, et al. European cystic fibrosis mineralization guidelines. J Cyst Fibros. 2011;10:S16–23.
44. Kalkwarf HJ, Abrams SA, DiMeglio LA, Koo WWK, Specker BL, Weiler H. Bone densitometry in infants and young children: the 2013 ISCD pediatric official positions. J Clin Densitom. 2014;17:243–57.
45. Leonard MB, Propert KJ, Zemel BS, Stallings VA, Feldman HI. Discrepancies in pediatric bone mineral density reference data: potential for misdiagnosis of osteopenia. J Pediatr. 1999;135:182–8.
46. Shepherd JA, Wang L, Fan B, et al. Optimal monitoring time interval between DXA measures in children. J Bone Miner Res. 2011;26:2745–52.
47. Bailey DA, McKay HA, Mirwald RL, Crocker PRE, Faulkner RA. A six-year longitudinal study of the relationship of physical activity to bone mineral accrual in growing children: the university of Saskatchewan bone mineral accrual study. J Bone Miner Res. 1999;14:1672–9.
48. Pourabbas TB, Erkani MA, Nouraei H, Sadeghian M. Evaluation of bone mineral status in adolescent idiopathic scoliosis. Clin Orthop Surg. 2014;6:180–4.
49. Aris RM, Merkel PA, Bachrach LK, et al. Consensus statement: guide to bone health and disease in cystic fibrosis. J Clin Endocrinol Metab. 2005;90:1888–96.
50. Wasilewski-Masker K, Kaste SC, Hudson MM, LA Esiashvili M, Meacham LR. Bone mineral density deficits in survivors of childhood cancer: long-term follow-up guidelines and review of the literature. Pediatrics. 2008;121:e705–13.
51. Pappa H, Thayu M, Sylvester F, et al. Skeletal health of children and adolescents with inflammatory bowel disease. J Pediatr Gastroenterol Nutr. 2011;53:11–25.

# Chapter 5
# Acquisition of DXA in Children and Adolescents

Nicola J. Crabtree and Kyla Kent

The aim of this chapter is to provide the operator with the basic information required to achieve a high-quality dual-energy x-ray absorptiometry (DXA) scan. Topics such as patient preparation, standard scan acquisition, and common acquisition problems are discussed. This information is intended to supplement instructions provided in operator manuals and individual department protocols.

## Information Prior to Scan

Essential to acquiring a high-quality DXA evaluation is the exchange of information prior to the scan. It is helpful to provide the child and guardian with adequate information about the risks and comfort level of the procedure. It can be helpful to include a picture or diagram of the machine in the appointment letter and also to clarify that no needles or injections are required and that radiation exposure is typically lower than daily exposure from the environment (see Chap. 3). This will help the parent or guardian explains the procedure and hopefully will also allay any fears the child or parent may have about the test.

---

N.J. Crabtree, Ph.D. (✉)
Department of Endocrinology, Birmingham Children's Hospital,
Steelhouse Lane, Birmingham, West Midlands B4 6NH, United Kingdom
e-mail: Nicola.crabtree@bch.nhs.uk

K. Kent, B.A., CBDT
Stanford School of Medicine, 1070 Arastradero Road, Suite 100,
Palo Alto, CA 94304, USA
e-mail: kylaq@stanford.edu

© Springer International Publishing Switzerland 2016                                89
E.B. Fung et al. (eds.), *Bone Health Assessment in Pediatrics*,
DOI 10.1007/978-3-319-30412-0_5

It is equally important for the referring clinician to provide sufficient clinical history to the DXA operator. Specifically, the requisition for densitometry should include the reason for the test, relevant information about diseases or medications, and unusual aspects of the physical exam (e.g., short stature, physical limitations, delayed maturation, or metal implants). The ordering physician should also alert the operator to any potential problems such as mental or physical difficulties that may either prevent the scan being performed or require sedation or modification of standard practice.

## Room Preparation

As with any exam involving children, it is important to ensure the environment is child-friendly. The use of colorful pictures and soft toys will make the scanning room more appealing to a young child and, hence, will make it easier for the child to relax and cooperate during the scan. Maintaining a low noise level and limiting the number of persons in the room also improves cooperation.

## Patient Preparation

Prior to scanning, height and weight should be recorded in light indoor clothes after removal of shoes and any highly attenuating objects that may cause image artifacts such as clothing with metal zippers or buckles or decorations, bras with metal clasps or under-wires, thick elastic waist bands and body jewelry (e.g., umbilical rings) or medical devices (e.g. insulin pumps) that would be in the scanning region. To achieve high-quality results, the child should be scanned in light indoor clothes, scrubs or in a hospital gown. Multiple layers of clothing may lead to a poor-quality scan and may inhibit the operator from noticing possible artifacts underneath clothing layers. In addition, if the whole body scan might be used to assess body composition, it is absolutely necessary that all artifacts that can be removed are and to identify any nonremovable objects (e.g. PICC line, g-tube). The operator should put the child at ease by offering an explanation suitable to his or her level of understanding. The operator should also explain the procedure to the parent or guardian as they are often in the best position to assist and to reassure the child. Throughout the measurements, the operator should keep the child informed of what he or she is doing, of what the scanner will do, of the noises the scanner will make, and of how long each scan and the entire procedure will take.

## Performing the Scan

The goal is to obtain a scan with the child in an ideal scanning position that can be easily reproduced at a follow-up visit. However, this is not always possible. Younger children and those with special needs require adaptations to standard protocols (see

Chap. 9). It is important to assess the child's cooperation prior to starting the scan to avoid any unnecessary radiation exposure caused by having to repeat unusable acquisitions.

## Younger Infants (0–9 Months)

Young infants are among the hardest patients to scan. However, some general guidelines are useful. Before scanning a baby, ask the caregiver to feed and settle the infant and to place him or her on the scanning table in a clean diaper [1]. If necessary, the child can be wrapped in a thin cotton sheet to reduce any small involuntary movements. Room lighting should be subdued to help the baby relax. If it is possible to settle the child, he or she might sleep through the scan, therefore requiring little operator intervention, although some will startle with the movement of the machine. It is important to constantly watch the child for any involuntary movements. If the operator is unable to settle the infant, it is reasonable to reschedule the scan to avoid unnecessary radiation exposure.

## Older Infants (Aged 9–36 Months) and Toddlers

Older infants and toddlers are unlikely to settle easily or to be able to follow instructions. At this age, some children can be quieted by being able to watch television while they are being positioned on the table. Having a parent next to the child is also calming.

However, 9–36-month-olds are difficult to scan since they are often frightened by the equipment and unfamiliar faces. Therefore, the easiest way to scan this group is with light sedation. This must be performed in departments with full resuscitation facilities. Different hospitals will have different sedation procedures, and local protocol should be used at all times. Once the child is sedated, scan acquisition should follow standard scanning procedures, taking extra care that any monitors or lines that are required for the sedation do not overlie the region of interest. Special consideration should be given to this age group to ensure that the benefit of the results from a DXA scan far outweigh the risks of sedation (see Chap. 8 for more details).

## Children (3–12 Years)

Sedation is not usually necessary in children over the age of 3 years; an explanation of the procedure is generally sufficient to reassure the child. The promise of a treat, such as a sticker or certificate, at the end of the scan may also help. Once the child is settled and acquisition has started, it is essential to continually remind him or her to stay still. If it is necessary to gently hold the child, the operator should be aware of where the x-ray tube is located and should keep his or her hands away from the x-ray path.

## Teenagers (13–18 Years)

This age group is theoretically the easiest to scan as they have a greater understanding of the procedure and can usually follow instruction. However, there are some special considerations that should be noted. Teenagers may or may not wish their parent or guardian to be present. They are typically more modest and may be reluctant to undress and put on scrubs or a hospital gown. Some may have body piercings, and if these were obtained recently, teenagers will be particularly reluctant to remove them for the scanning procedure. For females who have attained menarche, the possibility of pregnancy must be considered.

Many of these issues can be addressed with an appropriate information leaflet sent along with the appointment letter or provided just prior to the scan. Teenagers can be advised to wear light indoor clothing without zippers, thick elastic waist bands or metal closures and to remove any jewelry within the region being scanned (such as an umbilical ring, if a spine scan is ordered). Local procedures should be applied regarding the potential for radiation exposure and pregnancy. Some facilities will require a negative serum or urine pregnancy test prior to the scan, whereas others will accept a written or oral statement from the patient that she is not pregnant.

## After the Scan: Communication with the Patient

After successful acquisition of the bone densitometry scan,

- If appropriate, reward the child for cooperating with a sticker or certificate.
- If possible, let the patient and parent see the acquired scan on the screen to help them understand the procedure. Providing a copy of the whole body scan, without analysis, often delights children.
- Inform the parents or guardians how the results of the scan will be transmitted.

## Skeletal Sites to Be Studied

DXA can be used to measure many skeletal sites. In deciding which region or regions of interest to scan, it is important to consider the following:

- Availability of reference data for the acquired region
- Reproducibility and precision of the site to be scanned, and any nonstandard sites or techniques
- Clinical information to be gained
- Radiation exposure
- The clinical or research question to be addressed by the scan

The International Society of Clinical Densitometry (ISCD) guidelines recommend that the posterior –anterior (PA) spine and total body less head (TBLH) are the preferred sites for performing BMC and areal BMD measurements in most pediatric subjects. The guidelines suggest that other sites such as the hip, distal femur, lateral vertebral assessment, and/or forearm, may be useful depending on the clinical need and diagnostic question [2].

All DXA manufactures provide standard procedures for scan acquisition, and these should be followed as closely as possible. However, the operator also should be aware of the points addressed in the following subsections.

## Patient Position

If possible, the child should be positioned according to standard manufacturer's guidelines, ensuring that he or she is comfortable and is able to maintain the position for the duration of the scan. Measurement precision will be affected by poor and nonreproducible positioning. In addition, several of the analysis programs, especially for whole body, require that lines separating the different regions are accurately placed. Incorrect positioning of the patient may result in the inability to correctly place the body part in the correct region for the analysis, thereby influencing the scan results. For example, if the arms are extended above the head for a whole body scan, it is not possible to analyze the arms in the arm regions of interest, thus lowering the whole body bone mineral content (BMC) measurements.

## Scan Area

DXA software will either automatically set the scan area according to the child's height or body size or the area can be adjusted by the operator. Any deviation from the standard protocol should always be noted so that the scan area can be reproduced in a follow-up visit.

## Scan Mode

Bone densitometers have different scan acquisition modes according to the subject's size or desired image resolution. As discussed in Chap. 3, different acquisition modes such as infant mode (GE Lunar & Hologic) or thin mode on the GE Lunar software may be required to differentiate between bone and soft tissue in younger or sicker patients [3–5]. If these programs are used to obtain the initial study, follow-up scans should be performed in these modes to allow for an accurate assessment of change. However, it may be appropriate to scan in the auto low density/pediatric modes and the standard adult mode to allow for flexibility through later growth. The more complex issue may be a child who has lost a large amount of weight between scans. It may not be possible to analyze the new scan if performed in the original scan mode.

Hologic densitometers with software version 12.1 or later have an auto-low density whole body analysis. Use of the actual auto-low density algorithm depends on body weight (it is recommended for children <40 kg) for the whole body scan and poor bone mapping by the standard adult analysis for anterior-posterior (AP) spine and hip scans. The pediatric reference data recently published by Zemel et al were collected with Hologic instruments using the auto-low density algorithms [6].

## Spine Scans

The AP (or posteroanterior [PA]) lumbar spine is one of the preferred sites for measuring pediatric bone mass because of the speed and precision of measurements, the easily identified bony landmarks, and the increasing amount of pediatric normative data [6–19]. The spine is a predominantly trabecular site and is therefore sensitive to metabolic changes in bone turnover. However, the spine may not be indicative of bone changes resulting from low calcium intake or other nutritional deficiencies [20]. It is easily accessible with adequate soft tissue on either side of the vertebrae to allow for bone quantification [21]. However, as with all bones in the child's skeleton, the vertebral bodies will change in size and shape during growth. Factors that may reduce the accuracy of a successful scan include motion, severe scoliosis, vertebral collapse, and interference caused by high-attenuating materials such as metal rods, feeding tubes, umbilical rings, and radiographic contrast material.

## Positioning for the PA Lumbar Spine

In positioning the child for a PA lumbar spine scan, the following steps should be taken:

- Place the child centrally on the scanning table in the supine position, with the spine as straight as possible.
- For follow-up visits, review the scan from the previous visit to ensure consistent positioning.
- Elevate the child's legs using foam pads appropriate for his or her size. Knees should be flexed at a 90° angle to allow the lower back to be pressed flat against the table. This should diminish any lordosis in the lower spine. The knee cushion provided by the manufacturer is generally too large for young children. Smaller cushions can be custom-made to meet the leg dimensions of young children.
- Place the child's arms down by his or her side.
- Check that all removable objects have been moved away from the scan area.

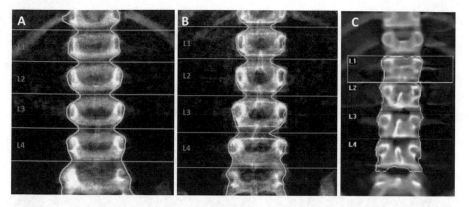

**Fig. 5.1** Correctly acquired spine scans for children of different ages. (**a**) Child, aged 5 years, with hypophosphatasia; (**b**) child, aged 9 years, with osteogenesis imperfecta; (**c**) child, aged 16 years, with multiple stress fractures

- Feel for the patient's iliac crest and umbilicus (or, alternately, lift the shirt to visualize the umbilicus), and position the laser beam approximately 2 cm(1 in.) below this point, ensuring that the beam is centered along the midline of the patient and that the scan area has equal amounts of soft tissue on each side of the spine.
- Start acquisition, reminding the child to stay still and to breathe normally for the duration of the scan.
- Observe the emerging image to ensure that the spine is centrally positioned and is as straight as possible and that L5 and ideally some of the iliac crest is visible. Stop the scan, reposition, and start again if any of these points are incorrect. To minimize radiation exposure, restarting the scan should be kept to a minimum.
- Continue scanning until a rib is seen connected to a vertebral level, usually T12.
- If the scan is started without a bit of the hip showing or stopped without a rib visible on the screen there is a possibility of not correctly labeling the vertebra measured.
- Review the scan for movement, and repeat if necessary.
- The acquired scan should include top of the iliac crest, the top of L5, and the bottom of T12 to aid vertebrae identification; the spine should be centrally located in the scan field, with adequate soft tissue either side of the vertebrae (Fig. 5.1).

## Spine Scan Positioning Problems

It may not always be possible to achieve the ideal scan due to marked scoliosis or vertebral collapse. Figure 5.2 illustrates spine scans from four children with varying degrees of spinal curvature. Both Child (A) and Child (B) have relatively mild deformities, such that scan acquisition and patient positioning are minimally affected; adequate analysis of these patients is possible by rotating or slanting the intervertebral markers. Unfortunately, this is not the case for Child (C) and Child (D). Child (C), a

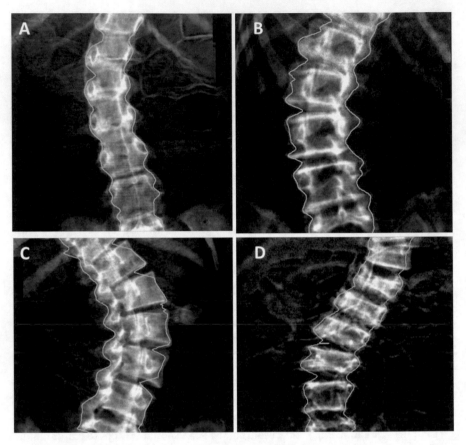

**Fig. 5.2** Spine scans from children with mild to severe scoliosis. (**a**) Child, aged 11 years with spinal cord injury; (**b**) child, aged 17 years with soto syndrome; (**c**) child, aged 15 years, with cerebral palsy; (**d**) child, aged 5 years, with type III osteogenesis imperfecta

young child with cerebral palsy, has a scoliotic and rotated spine, such that the projection of the lower lumbar vertebra appears almost lateral. Although this scan can be analyzed, it is not suitable to compare it to a "normal" reference database since the vertebral areas will not be comparable to normal spine areas. Case (D) also highlights a child with marked scoliosis and vertebral collapse affecting the entire lumbar vertebrae. The degree of collapse and curvature of this child, who has type III osteogenesis imperfecta, makes this scan difficult to analyze and to interpret. In both of these two latter cases, either a whole body and or a radius scan may be more informative.

## Longitudinal Spine Studies

The spine is a useful site to monitor changes in bone mass. However, to achieve successful follow-up scans the operator must:

- Accurately reproduce the patient scan position, using the baseline scan as a guide
- Use the same scan acquisition and analysis parameters (as much as possible)

If there have been significant weight changes between scans, these ideals may not be possible. For weight changes that result in scan mode variation, the mode change should be recorded so that any necessary corrections and other considerations can be made. When weight changes places the child at the borderline between scan modes, scanning in both standard and pediatric modes is recommended. This creates a comparable scan for the previous measure and a new baseline scan for any future follow up. When making these decisions, it is important to consider the additional radiation exposure from repeat scans.

Use of the auto-low density analysis method (Hologic Discovery / Horizon) will allow the results to be compared to a large pediatric reference database collected using this software [6].

Figure 5.3 illustrates a successful series of measurements over a 2-year period beginning at age 16 in a boy being monitored for the effects of three monthly intravenous bisphosphonate treatments.

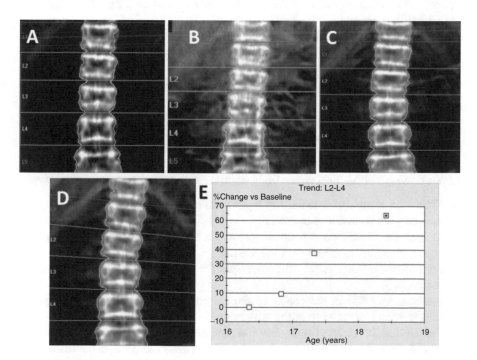

**Fig. 5.3** Serial scans over a 2-year period of a boy from age 16–18 following a bisphosphonate treatment regime

## Whole Body Scans

The whole body is also a preferred site in children. This scan provides measurements of total and regional bone and body composition parameters, making it a useful site for both clinical and research purposes. Growth and disease may affect both bone and body composition values [22].

With older-generation pencil beam densitometers, whole body scan times were as long as 10–20 min. However, with newer fan beam and narrow fan beam machines, scan times have been reduced to a few minutes, thus making it far more feasible to acquire a whole body scan even on a young or fidgety child [23].

Although analysis of specific skeletal regions can be performed from the whole body scan, the precision is relatively poor compared to the good precision for the whole body scan [24].

When acquiring a whole body scan, it is important that the child not wear any high-attenuating objects. Ideally, the child should be scanned in a hospital gown or in light indoor clothing. The operator should be aware that thick elasticized waist bands and plastic buttons may also cause problems with image artifacts. Additionally if body composition is to be calculated, polyvinyl chloride (PVC) sheets or pillows, as well as sand bags used in positioning, will affect the calculations and should therefore be removed from the scanning table. If any cushions or towels etc. are needed for acquisition due to patient comfort, these must be noted and used again for all follow-up scans.

Whole body scanning can be performed in children with internal high-attenuating objects (e.g., metal rods, pins, or plates) if they are likely to remain in situ for follow-up. However, special attention should be given to the analysis and interpretation of such scans, especially when attempting to compare them with normal data.

## Positioning for the Whole Body Scan

In positioning a child for a whole body scan, the following steps should be taken:

- Check the scanning table for any high-attenuating objects, and remove any pillows or pads from the scan area.
- Change the child into a hospital gown or check light indoor clothes for any objects that may interfere with the scan.
- For follow-up visits, review the scan from the previous visit to assure consistent positioning.
- Position the child in the center of the scanning table, with the head approximately 4 cm from the top of the scan region.
- Ensure that the child is lying flat and straight within the scan area, with arms placed alongside the body and the palms flat against the bed. (If the child is too large to place his or her hands in this position, rotate the hands so that they are flat alongside parallel to thighs, thumbs facing the ceiling).

- Ask the child to relax his or her shoulders. Stretch the child's hands toward the foot of the bed.
- Extend the legs on either side of the central line marked on the table, making them as straight as possible, and secure them together with a Velcro strap around the ankles or feet. Alternatively, tape can be used to secure the feet together and to assist the child in keeping hands and arms still while scanning.
- Start the scan, reminding the child to lie still (but to not hold his or her breath). The child should be able to lie comfortably in this position for the duration of the scan. For younger children, it may be necessary to hold either arms or legs to help them maintain this position. If it is necessary to hold the child, be aware of where the x-ray tube is located, keeping your hands away from the x-ray path.
- Once the scan is complete, remind the child to remain still until the scan arm returns to its home position, at which point it will be safe to get down from the scan table.

Figure 5.4 demonstrates acceptable scans of (a) a 5-year-old child with osteogenesis imperfecta, (b) an 11-year-old child with Diamond Blackfan anemia on chronic steroid therapy, and (c) a 16-year-old with Crohn's disease.

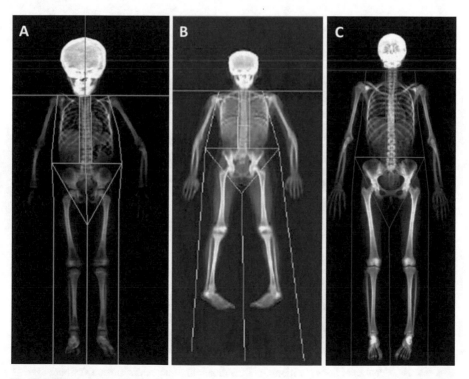

**Fig. 5.4** Correctly acquired total body scans. (**a**) Child, aged 5 years, with Osteogenesis imperfecta; (**b**) child, aged 11 years, with Blackfan Diamond anemia; (**c**) child, aged 16 years, with Crohn's disease

For small children, the length of the scan field may be adjusted to reduce the scan time. However, this may become problematic when comparing scans at follow-up as the child grows larger. For very tall adolescents, it may not be possible to fit the entire body in the scan field; therefore, it is suggested to position the child with his or her head is just below the top of the table and with the feet flexed upward. If the child is still too long for the scan table, the scan should be acquired by excluding the feet from the scan area.

When performing scans on obese adolescents, it can be difficult to position them so that the entire body is in the scan field. Several techniques can be used in this situation, depending on the fat distribution. With centralized obesity, the elbows may be too close to the edge of the scan field. A folded cotton sheet can be wrapped tightly around the middle portion of the body to hold the elbows close to the body. In this case, care should be taken to keep the palms flat on the DXA table.

When these techniques fail, an alternative approach, if the scanner has the software, is to perform a "hemi" scan (Fig. 5.5d). For a hemi scan, position the patient off-center so that the entire right side of the patient and the shoulder and hip of the left side are within the scan area. The measured values for the right side are then used to estimate the bone and body composition parameters for the left side. To estimate total body values the measured and estimated values are combined. In all cases, scans should be monitored for movement and repeated if necessary.

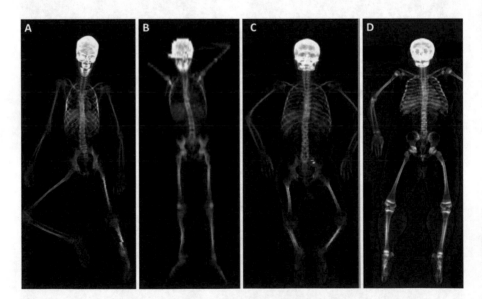

**Fig. 5.5** Non-ideal total body positioning of children with limb contractures. (**a**) Child, aged 11 years, myotubular myopathy; (**b**) child, aged 13 years, with grand mal epilepsy and learning difficulties; (**c**) child, aged 18 years, with Duchenne muscular dystrophy; (**d**) child, aged 16 years, with Duchenne muscular dystrophy, hemi-scan

## Whole Body Scan Positioning Problems

Ideal positioning may not always be possible for children with leg or arm contractures. In these circumstances, research has shown that scanning the child in the semi-lateral position with limbs supported had minimal detrimental effect on whole body scan accuracy and precision [25]. Even children with significant contractures can usually be placed comfortably in the semi-lateral position (see Chap. 9). Figure 5.5 demonstrates suboptimal whole body positioning of four children with limb contractures: (a) a child aged 11 years with myotubular myopathy, (b) a child aged 13 years with grand mal epilepsy and learning difficulties, (c) a child aged 18 years with Duchenne muscular dystrophy, and (d) a hemi-scan of a child aged 16 years with Duchenne muscular dystrophy.

## Hip Scans

The proximal total hip and femoral neck are frequently measured sites in adults. Scanning the proximal hip in children, however, is more difficult because the skeletal landmarks may not be well developed and the femoral neck may be too small for the standard software. These factors contribute to poorer precision in this region. However, there are now more pediatric reference data for this site. The femoral neck region is not recommended in young children since its changing shape makes longitudinal studies difficult and unreliable.

Regardless, if a hip scan is warranted, note that the femoral neck box generated by standard DXA software for this region of interest may be too large for the anatomy of smaller subjects. The operator can customize the width and placement of the neck box for a better fit, but this introduces operator-related variability that can complicate subsequent studies and result in data that is no longer comparable to established reference data sets. The advantage of scanning the proximal hip is that it is a predominately cortical site; therefore, it allows the evaluation of an alternative bone element.

## Positioning for the Proximal Hip Scan

In positioning a child for a proximal hip scan, the following steps should be taken:

- Place the child on the scanning table in the supine position, with the head supported by a small pillow if necessary.
- Rest the arms on the abdomen above the region to be scanned.
- Rotate the whole leg inwards, ensuring that the leg rotates from the hip (to approximately 15–25°) and not from the knee.
- Attach the foot to the hip-positioning aid supplied by the manufacturer. (When performing dual hip measurements, position each hip separately to avoid over-abduction by the adult hip positioner)

- Start the acquisition at the point recommended by the DXA manufacturer, reminding the child to stay still for the duration of the scan.
- Observe the emerging image. The femoral shaft should be parallel to the edge of the bed, the scan should start well below the lesser trochanter, and the image should include the total hip region, with sufficient soft tissue around the greater trochanter (see user manuals for exact machine-specific requirements).
- If the hip is either over- or under-abducted, reposition and restart the scan.
- Stop the acquisition a short distance above the acetabulum.

The acquired scan should include a portion of the femoral shaft, the femoral neck, the whole of the acetabulum, and part of the pelvis. Figure 5.6 illustrates three correctly acquired hip scans. Figure 5.6(a) shows the immature hip of a 6-year-old with osteogenesis imperfecta, Fig. 5.6 (b) shows the hip of a 10-year-old with anorexia nervosa and Fig. 5.6 (c) illustrates the hip of a 17-year-old long distance runner with stress fractures.

Even a developed femur may be problematic to scan and analyze, as illustrated by Fig. 5.7. Figure 5.7(a) shows the shortened femoral neck of a 16-year-old with Charcot-Marie-Tooth disease. The child in Fig. 5.7 (b) is a wheelchair-bound 10-year-old with osteogenesis imperfecta. The unusual load on her femur and femoral neck has resulted in an increased angle between the femoral neck and shaft and, hence, an unusual femoral neck morphometry and an almost absent greater trochanter.

The greatest challenge in the use and interpretation of hip scans in children is in the analysis procedure. Especially in younger and smaller children, the software can fail to properly identify the midline and the border of the greater trochanter. This may require manual placement by the technologist which does introduce error, but if the software does not put regions in the correct place it is not acceptable to just leave them. Comparison to any normative database requires that the regions are correctly placed. Longitudinal comparisons are particularly challenging due to the changes in bone size as children grow. Guidelines for longitudinal analysis of scans are provided by McKay et al [26] and are discussed in detail in Chap. 6.

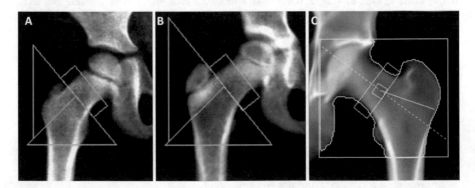

**Fig. 5.6** Correctly acquired hip scans. (**a**) Child, aged 6 years, with osteogenesis imperfecta; (**b**) child, aged 10 years, with anorexia nervosa; (**c**) child, aged 17 years, with multiple stress fractures due to long distance running

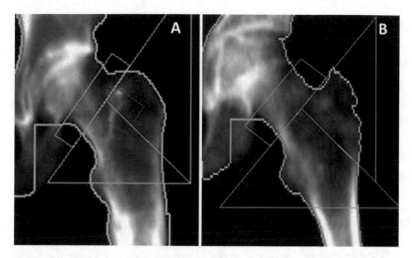

**Fig. 5.7** Problems associated with hip morphometry of under-loaded bones. (**a**) Child, aged 16 years, with Charcot-Marie-Tooth disease (walks with crutches); (**b**) child, aged 10 years, with osteogenesis imperfecta (mostly wheelchair-bound)

## Vertebral Fracture Assessment (VFA)

The importance of identifying vertebral fractures has been highlighted with the most recent definition of osteoporosis; suggesting that osteoporosis can be defined by the identification of one or more vertebral compression fractures, in the absence of local disease or high-energy trauma [27]. Until recently the gold standard technique for identifying these fractures was lateral x-rays. However, VFA by DXA using newer generation bone densitometers has been shown to have excellent sensitivity for vertebral fracture identification, especially for clinically relevant moderate (Grade 2) to severe (Grade 3) vertebral fractures [28, 29].

Although image resolution from a DXA scanner is lower than that of conventional spinal radiographs, VFA has several advantages. DXA systems are capable of acquiring the whole spine in a single projection in both the posterior-anterior and lateral projections; whereas with conventional radiographs the thoracic and lumbar spine requires two separate exposures/films. VFA with parallel beam geometry results in images without image magnification and artifactual concave vertebral endplates ("bean" can affect) due to the parallax effect of the divergent X-ray beam of conventional spinal radiographs. Most significantly for children, the radiation dose from a DXA VFA scan is approximately 10–100 times lower than the radiation dose from lumbar and thoracic spine radiography [28]. Moreover, the vertebral fracture assessment by DXA can be performed at the same time as the routine DXA assessment and negate the need for additional visits to the hospital for further spine imaging. However, the current use of VFA is still machine-dependent. For older DXA scanners such as the GE Lunar Prodigy and the Hologic QDR series, the image resolution is not sufficient to reliably diagnose vertebral fractures in children and as such VFA scanning on such devices is not recommended [30].

## Positioning for the Vertebral Fracture Assessment Scan

In positioning a child for a VFA scan, the following steps should be taken:

### *In the Decubitus Position*

- Unfold the spine positioner board and set it against the back rail of the scanner table.
- Place the child on the scanning table in decubitus position, with the head supported by a small pillow if necessary.
- Place the arms 90° from the chest, away from the region to be scanned to be scanned.
- Position the patient's knees towards the chest until the lower back and both shoulders are flat against the lateral positioner.
- Make sure the patient's spine is parallel to the scanner table, using small foam pads where necessary.
- Place a foam wedge below the bottom knee and between the knees to help straighten the pelvis and improve patient comfort.
- Start the acquisition at the point recommended by the DXA manufacturer (just below L5), reminding the child to stay still for the duration of the scan.
- Observe the emerging image. Ensure all of the posterior elements are in the scan filed with sufficient soft tissue visible to identify the anterior edge of the vertebrae.
- Stop the acquisition in the upper thoracic region insuring all visible vertebrae are in the field of view.
- Check for movement.

### *In the Supine Position*

- Place the child on the scanning table in supine position, with the head supported by the VFA positioning aid.
- Place their arms over their head resting on the VFA positioning aid (if available).
- Make sure the patient's spine is straight and positioned exactly in the center of the scan field and parallel to the edge of the scan table.
- Raise the knees using foam pads to flatten out the base of the spine (see PA spine positioning).
- Start the acquisition at the point recommended by the DXA manufacturer (just below L5), reminding the child to stay still for the duration of the scan.

- Observe the emerging image. Ensure all of the posterior elements are in the scan filed with sufficient soft tissue visible to identify the anterior edge of the vertebrae.
- Stop the acquisition in the upper thoracic region insuring all visible vertebrae are in the field of view.
- Check for movement.

Figure 5.8 highlights three correctly acquired VFA scan; Fig. 5.8(a) is a 8-year-old child with congenital nemaline myophathy and vertebral fracture; Fig. 5.8 (b) is a 14-year-old child with multiple low-trauma fractures, Fig. 5.8 (c) is a 17-year-old child with Duchenne muscular dystrophy and vertebral fractures and Fig. 5.8 (d) is a 23-year-old young adult with thalassemia.

The greatest challenge when performing VFA scans is to get the spine as straight as possible, with no vertebral rotation, no air in the field of view and no movement. It is often helpful to ask the child to hold their breath for the "Fast" 10 s scan to avoid breathing artifacts on the emerging image. Additionally, when scanning in the decubitus position, it is necessary to place some padding between the trunk and the table to maintain a parallel projection of the spine with the scanning table. This is

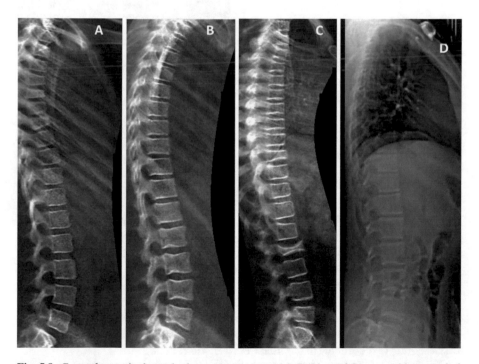

**Fig. 5.8** Correctly acquired vertebral assessment scans. (**a**) Child, aged 8 years, with congenital nemaline myopathy and vertebral fractures; (**b**) child, aged 14, with multiple low-trauma fractures; (**c**) child, aged 17 years with Duchenne muscular dystrophy and vertebral fractures; (**d**) young adult, aged 23 with thalassemia

**Fig. 5.9** Example of a
VFA scan acquired in the
decubitus position (**a**)
without padding and (**b**)
with padding between the
patient's waist and the scan
table

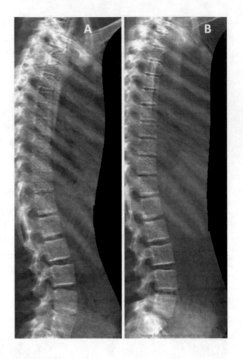

illustrated in Fig. 5.9. Figure 5.9 (a) is a 16-year-old child scanned without under
trunk padding and Fig. 5.9 (b) highlights how the projection of the spine can be
improved with the addition of small pads between the patient's waist and table.

## Other Sites

### *Radius and Lateral Distal Femur*

The radius and lateral distal femur are scanned less commonly in children, although
they can provide useful information, particularly for those unable to lie still or who
are too contracted for a whole body exam, those who exceed the weight limitations
for the table or are too thick to fit under the arm of the table.

The radius can be scanned using either axial or peripheral devices although axial
devices are preferred if the site is being used for serial scans. It is usual to measure
the nondominant arm at the ultradistal and distal third section. Within these two
regions, it is possible to measure sections of predominantly trabecular (in the ultradistal radius) and cortical (in the distal third section) bone.

The forearm-positioning device should be used if the child is large enough to reach it
while keeping the elbow at shoulder level and flexed at a 90° angle. For smaller children,
cushions may be needed to achieve the proper position. When these positioning techniques fail, the child can be positioned on the table and scanned in the supine position.

In patients with joint contractures, it may be possible to perform a lateral distal femoral scan. This scan is achieved by placing the child on his or her side on the scanning table, with the femur to be imaged parallel to the edge of the bed (see Chap. 9). The leg is scanned using forearm software and is analyzed using the forearm subregional analysis software with an adapted technique [31].

# Interference

## *Artifacts*

Unfortunately, a frequent problem when scanning children is interference caused by metal artifacts and motion. Problems caused by artifacts should be limited to only those resulting from immovable objects such as pins, plates, rods, and feeding tubes. External highly attenuating objects such as leg braces, plaster casts, or monitors should be removed prior to scanning, or the scan should be rescheduled when these devices are no longer required.

Figure 5.10 illustrates examples of both removable and immovable internal and external artifacts. Child A has a subclavian portocatheter in situ which could not be removed and child B has had spinal rod included in the scan field. Artifacts such as these cause minimal interference for longitudinal scanning if they remain in place for the follow-up period, but they will affect the ability to compare the results to

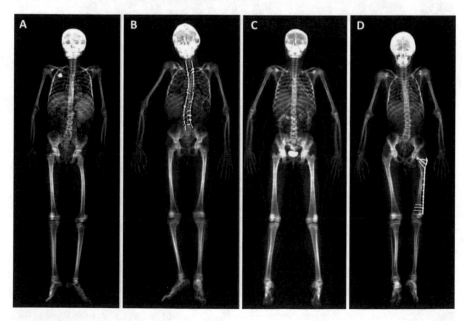

**Fig. 5.10** Whole body artifacts. (**a**) Subclavian portocatheter; (**b**) spinal rodding; (**c**) IV contrast for computed tomography scan; (**d**) internal femur fixation

reference data (Chap. 6). Child C IV contrast from a computed tomography scan performed earlier in the day; the scan should have been delayed until contract media had passed though the bowel. Finally, child D has had orthopedic rods placed in his femur following a fracture. The rod was subsequently removed which made comparison with prior results difficult. When it is not possible to remove the interfering object or to postpone the scan, data from the whole body scan can be used by estimating the values for the affected side based upon results from the unaffected side.

Not all artifacts are limited to the whole body scan. Figure 5.11 illustrates a selection of spine scans affected by internal artifacts. Excluding a specific region of interest during analysis may reduce the effect of such artifacts, but the exclusion makes comparison to a reference range difficult.

Unavoidable interferences may also occur as result of the child's clinical condition or treatment. Figure 5.12 (a) illustrates a common pattern of high-density endplates associ-

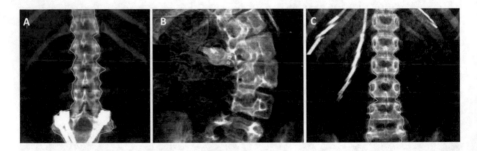

**Fig. 5.11** Lumbar spine artifacts. (**a**) Spinal rod; (**b**) percutaneous endoscopic gastroscopy feeding tube; (**c**) nasogastric tube and central line

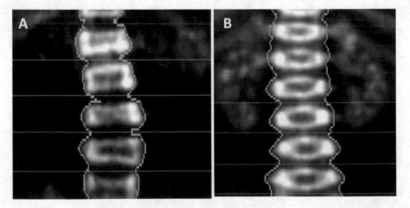

**Fig. 5.12** Artifacts resulting from treatment or clinical conditions. (**a**) Child, aged 3 years, with osteogenesis imperfecta, after bisphosphonate treatment; (**b**) child, aged 4 years, with primary oxalosis type I and calcium deposits in his kidneys

ated with bisphosphonate treatment. Figure 5.12 (b) illustrates a child with primary oxalosis type I, in whom kidney calcium deposits may affect soft tissue estimation.

## Poor Edge Detection

Poor edge detection may be a result of photon starvation (when not enough x-rays can pass through the body) at the detectors or poor tissue differentiation observed with extremely low-density bone. Figure 5.13 illustrates three examples in which poor edge detection has occurred. Figure 5.13 (a) is of a 13-year-old with Crohn's disease who has extremely low spine density. The 16-year-old in Fig. 5.13(b) has a brain tumor and associated obesity: the child has more than 60 % body fat. The 6-year-old child in Fig. 5.13 (c) has marked lymphedema and fluid overload due to severe liver disease.

In all of these examples, the densitometer had difficulty distinguishing between bone and soft tissue, which resulted in erroneous values being generated during the analysis. With densitometers that allow for modifications in the acquisition parameters, photon starvation can be overcome by rescanning the child in a different scan mode using an increased sample time e.g. array mode for Hologic scanners will increase the scan time from fast array mode by approximately 30 s. Poor tissue differentiation may be overcome at the analysis stage by analyzing the acquired image with a specific low-density analysis package.

The most recent version of the Hologic (Waltham, MA) software for the QDR Discovery and Horizon models includes an auto-low density analysis. BMD values for this mode do not differ as much from standard analysis mode results as did older low-density software versions. However, it is uncertain as to whether there is a significant bias associated with this analysis mode [32]. Use of the "auto-low density" software will ensure that the scan results obtained are comparable to the pediatric reference data provided by the manufacturer which were obtained from healthy children using this software [6].

Similar changes have occurred in the pediatric whole body analysis mode. Since the edge detection algorithm can have a significant impact on the results for bone area, BMC, and BMD, it is of critical importance that the reference data used to interpret the results have been obtained using the same scan analysis procedures.

## Movement

The most common problem when scanning young children is movement, resulting in significant variations in BMD and poor reproducibility. Although most analysis techniques can cope with a small amount of movement (Fig. 5.14), any movement in the scan field will reduce the measurement precision and may produce unreliable results. If the child is unable to stay still for the duration of the scan, the following points need to be considered.

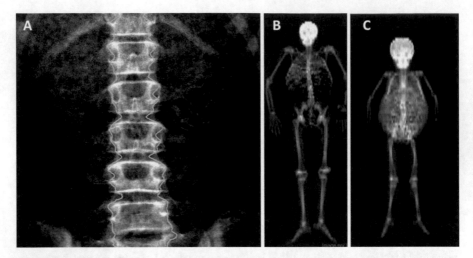

**Fig. 5.13** Poor edge detection. (**a**) Under-mineralized spine; (**b**) obese child scanned in incorrect mode resulting in photon starvation; (**c**), poor tissue differentiation in a young child with liver disease

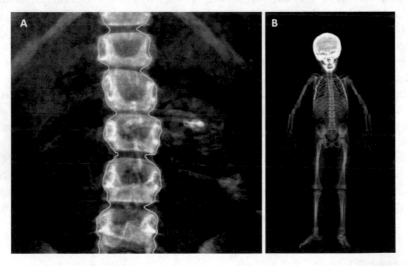

**Fig. 5.14** Effects of movement; (**a**) Lumbar spine with small lateral movement; (**b**) total body scan with small lateral movements

- How urgent is the scan? Can it be delayed until the child is older and able to understand and cooperate better?

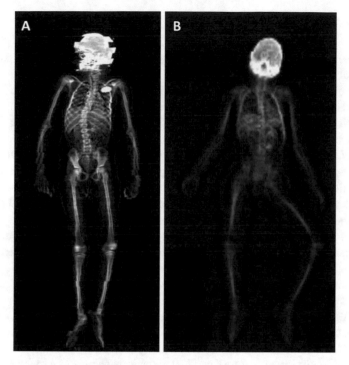

**Fig. 5.15** Effects of sedation. (**a**) Unsedated 12-year-old child with microcephaly; (**b**) sedated 5-year-old child with cerebral palsy

- Would practicing remaining still be helpful? Sometimes this can be done at home prior to scanning.
- Is sedation necessary? It is not always young children who require sedation; sometimes older children with learning difficulties may require sedation to achieve an analyzable scan (Fig. 5.15).

The aim of this chapter has been to give general guidelines for scan acquisitions that are appropriate to most children scanned on most DXA machines. Obviously, each center will have different scan protocols, and these should be followed as closely as possible. The operator should always minimize radiation exposure by only performing clinically useful scans. By explaining the procedure to the child, the operator is likely to reduce fear, to maximize cooperation, and to obtain scans of the highest possible quality.

## Summary Points

- Different age groups require unique considerations with regard to obtaining the optimal scan.
- Every effort should be made to prepare the child and family prior to the procedure to avoid having to repeat scans.
- Specific details are provided for positioning patients for the two most frequently used scans; spine and total body, as well as for alternative scans of the proximal femur (i.e., hip) and the lateral spine for vertebral fracture assessment (VFA).
- Spine scans can be performed on most pediatric patients. Spine reference data for children ages 3–5 (machine specific) are currently available for all major DXA scanners. For younger aged children the technician would need to refer to published data for the calculation of a spine Z-Score.
- Total body scans can be performed on all pediatric patients who are able to remain still during the procedure without sedation. Gender-specific pediatric reference ranges, for patients age 3 or older are available.
- Hip scans can be performed on older children, in whom the hip is more developed. Pediatric reference ranges for children ages 5 and older are available. However, this site is only recommended for older children e.g. 11years and above, when the software is better able to detect the typical regions of interest.
- Vertebral fracture assessment by DXA using newer densitometers is a sensitive tool for identifying moderate (grade 2) and severe (grade 3) vertebral fractures.
- Other scans such as the distal radius and the lateral distal femur are currently used primarily for research purposes or in special populations
- Scan interference such as movement, attenuating artifacts, and excess fluid should be reduced as much as possible. This may require postponing scans if there are non-removable artifacts or the child is unable to cooperate. If the scan is required urgently, selective skeletal sites may be analyzed or sedation may be needed (to avoid motion).

## References

1. Koo WWK, Massom LR, Walters J. Validation of accuracy and precision of dual energy X-ray absorptiometry for infants. J Bone Miner Res. 1995;10(7):1111–5.
2. Crabtree NJ, Arabi A, Bachrach LK, Fewtrell M, El-Hajj Fuleihan G, Kecskemethy HH, et al. Dual-energy X-ray absorptiometry interpretation and reporting in children and adolescents: the revised 2013 ISCD Pediatric Official Positions. J Clin Densitom. 2014;17(2):225–42.
3. Wang J, Thorton J, Horlick M, Formica C, Wang W, Rahn M, et al. Dual-energy X-ray absorptiometry in pediatric studies. J Clin Densitom. 1999;2(2):135–41.
4. Picaud J-C, Duboeuf F, Vey-Marty B, Delmas P, Claris O, Salle BL, et al. First all-solid pediatric phantom for dual-X-ray absorptiometry measurements in infants. J Clin Densitom. 2003;6(1):17–23.
5. Laskey MA. The influence of tissue depth and composition on the performance of the Lunar dual-energy X-ray absorptiometer whole-body scanning mode. Eur J Clin Nutr. 1992;46:39–45.
6. Zemel BS, Kalkwarf HJ, Gilsanz V, Lappe JM, Oberfield S, Shepherd JA, et al. Revised reference curves for bone mineral content and areal bone mineral density according to age and sex

for black and non-black children: results of the bone mineral density in childhood study. J Clin Endocrinol Metab. 2011;96(10):3160–9.

7. Arabi A, Nabulsi M, Maalouf J, Choucair M, Khalife H, Vieth R, et al. Bone mineral density by age, gender, pubertal stages and socioeconomic status in healthy Lebanese children and adolescents. Bone. 2004;35:1169–79.

8. Binkley TL, Specker BL, Wittig TA. Centile curves for bone densitometry measurements in healthy males and females aged 5–22 years. J Clin Densitom. 2002;5(4):343–53.

9. Crabtree N, Machin M, Bebbington N, Adams J, Ahmed F, Arundel P et al. The Amalgamated Paediatric Bone Density Study (The ALPHABET Study): the collection and generation of UK based reference data fro paediatric bone density. Bone Abstracts. 2013;2.

10. Kalkwarf HJ, Zemel BS, Yolton K, Heubi JE. Bone mineral content and density of the lumbar spine of infants and toddlers: influence of age, sex, race, growth, and human milk feeding. J Bone Miner Res. 2013;28(1):206–12.

11. Khadilkar AV, Sanwalka NJ, Chiplonkar SA, Khadilkar VV, Mughal MZ. Normative data and percentile curves for Dual Energy X-ray Absorptiometry in healthy Indian girls and boys aged 5–17 years. Bone. 2011;48(4):810–9.

12. Min JY, Min KB, Paek D, Kang D, Cho SI. Age curves of bone mineral density at the distal radius and calcaneus in Koreans. J Bone Miner Metab. 2010;28(1):94–100.

13. Sala A, Webber CE, Morrison J, Beaumont LF, Barr RD. Whole-body bone mineral content, lean body mass, and fat mass measured by dual-energy X-ray absorptiometry in a population of normal Canadian children and adolescents. Can Assoc Radiol J. 2007;58(1):46–52.

14. Tan LJ, Lei SF, Chen XD, Liu MY, Guo YF, Xu H, et al. Establishment of peak bone mineral density in Southern Chinese males and its comparisons with other males from different regions of China. J Bone Miner Metab. 2007;25(2):114–21.

15. Ward KA, Ashby RL, Roberts SA, Adams JE, Zulf Mughal M. United Kingdom reference data for the hologic QDR discovery dual energy X-ray absorptiometry scanner in healthy children aged 6–17 years. Arch Dis Child. 2007;92(1):53–9.

16. Xu II, Chen JX, Gong J, Zhang TM, Wu QL, Yuan ZM, et al. Normal reference for bone density in healthy Chinese children. J Clin Densitom. 2007;10(3):266–75.

17. Zanchetta JR, Plotkin H, Alvarez-Filgueira ML. Bone mass in children: normative values for the 2–20 year old population. Bone. 1995;16(4):393S–9.

18. Zhou W, Langsetmo L, Berger C, Adachi JD, Papaioannou A, Ioannidis G, et al. Normative bone mineral density z-scores for Canadians aged 16 to 24 years: the Canadian Multicenter Osteoporosis Study. J Clin Densitom. 2010;13(3):267–76.

19. Kelly TL, Wilson KE, Heymsfield SB. Dual energy X-Ray absorptiometry body composition reference values from NHANES. PLoS One. 2009;4(9):e7038.

20. Specker BL. The significance of high bone density in children. J Pediatr. 2001;139(4):473–5.

21. Carrascosa A, Gussinye M, Yeste D, del Rio L, Audi L. Bone mass acquisition during infancy, childhood and adolescence. Acta Paediatr. 1995;411:18–23.

22. Bianchi ML, Leonard MB, Bechtold S, Hogler W, Mughal MZ, Schonau E, et al. Bone health in children and adolescents with chronic diseases that may affect the skeleton: the 2013 ISCD Pediatric Official Positions. J Clin Densitom. 2014;17(2):281–94.

23. Mazess RB, Hanson JA, Payne R, Nord RH, Wilson M. Axial and total body bone densitometry using a narrow-angle fan-beam. Osteoporos Int. 2000;11:158–66.

24. Shepherd JA, Wang L, Fan B, Gilsanz V, Kalkwarf HJ, Lappe J, et al. Optimal monitoring interval between DXA measures in children. J Bone Miner Res. 2011;26(11):2745–52.

25. Henderson RC, Lark RK, Renner JB, Fung EB, Stallings VA, Conaway M, et al. Dual X-ray absorptiometry assessment of body composition in children with altered body posture. J Clin Densitom. 2001;4(4):325–35.

26. McKay HA, Petit MA. Analysis of proximal femur DXA scans in growing children: comparison of different protocols for cross-sectional 8-month and 7-year longitudinal data. J Bone Miner Res. 2000;15(6):1181–8.

27. Bishop N, Arundel P, Clark E, Dimitri P, Farr J, Jones G, et al. Fracture prediction and the defi-
    nition of osteoporosis in children and adolescents: the ISCD 2013 Pediatric Official Positions.
    J Clin Densitom. 2014;17(2):275–80.
28. Adiotomre E, Summers L, Broadley P, Lang I, Morrison G, Offiah A. Replacing conventional
    spine radiographs with dual energy x-ray absorptiometry in children with suspected reduction
    in bone density. Bone Abstracts. 2013.
29. Crabtree N, Chapman S, Hogler W, Shaw N. Is vertebral fracture assessment by DXA more use-
    ful in a high fracture risk paediatric population than in a low-risk screening population? Bone
    Abstracts. 2013;2.
30. Makitie O, Doria AS, Henriques F, Cole WG, Compeyrot S, Silverman E, et al. Radiographic ver-
    tebral morphology: a diagnostic tool in pediatric osteoporosis. J Pediatr. 2005;146(3):395–401.
31. Kecskemethy HH, Harcke HT. Assessment of bone health in children with disabilities.
    J Pediatr Rehabil Med. 2014;7(2):111–24.
32. Simpson DE, Dontu VS, Stephens SE, Archbold LJ, Lowe V, O'Doherty MJ, et al. Large
    variations occur in bone density measurements of children when using different software. Nucl
    Med Commun. 2005;26(6):483–7.

# Chapter 6
# Analysis and Evaluation of DXA in Children and Adolescents

Babette S. Zemel and Heidi J. Kalkwarf

## Introduction

Optimal bone accretion during childhood is critical for the development of a healthy adult skeleton. In children, a variety of health conditions and medical treatments can threaten skeletal development. Bone fragility at any point in the life cycle is largely determined by bone mass and density. Other factors, such as bone size and geometry, micro-repair mechanisms, and bone turnover, also contribute to bone fragility but are less easily measured in a clinical setting. One of the major steps in assessing bone health is to conduct a bone density test using dual energy x-ray absorptiometry (DXA). DXA scans acquired from children are unique from those acquired on adults because of smaller bone size, the presence of growth plates, and the need to accommodate the growing skeleton when monitoring changes over time. Once acquired, DXA measurements need to be compared to appropriate reference ranges in order to interpret the results. In this chapter, we will address (1) the fundamentals of scan analysis in children; (2) selection of reference data; and (3) other considerations in the evaluation of DXA scan results.

B.S. Zemel, Ph.D. (✉)
Department of Pediatrics, The Children's Hospital of Philadelphia,
34th St. and Civic Center Blvd, Philadelphia, PA 19027, USA
e-mail: zemel@email.chop.edu

H.J. Kalkwarf, Ph.D.
Gastroenterology, Hepatology and Nutrition, Cincinnati Children's Hospital,
3333 Burnet Avenue, MLC 2010, Cincinnati, OH 45229, USA
e-mail: Heidi.Kalkwarf@cchmc.org

© Springer International Publishing Switzerland 2016                                         115
E.B. Fung et al. (eds.), *Bone Health Assessment in Pediatrics*,
DOI 10.1007/978-3-319-30412-0_6

# Fundamentals of Scan Analysis

Over the past decade, significant advancements in DXA software have improved and standardized the ability to analyze scans on pediatric patients, primarily through improved edge detection algorithms that are better able to identify the shape of smaller, less dense bones. The precision of DXA scans in children is close to that of adults [1], providing confidence that DXA results in children are reproducible under optimal circumstances. The accuracy of analysis is dependent upon the quality of the scans obtained. Correct patient positioning during scan acquisition is critical for appropriate scan analysis. With poor patient positioning, the assumptions of scan analysis algorithms may be violated. The direction and magnitude of poor positioning on bone density results are unknown making it difficult to interpret the results. In situations of gross movement, it might not be possible to analyze the scan. (Details regarding correct positioning for pediatric patients are provided in Chap. 5: Acquisition of Bone Scans)

With high-quality scans, analysis is routine given the current auto-analysis software for most DXA models. Analysis of spine, whole body, forearm, and proximal femur scans is typically a four-step process: (1) identifying and choosing among the available software for the DXA machine, (2) confirming or correcting the global region of interest (ROI), (3) confirming or modifying subregional landmarks and (4) confirming or editing the bone map.

## *Spine Analysis*

Analysis of spine scans should follow manufacturer's guidelines. The child should be positioned so that their spine is straight and centered in the scan field. Scans should be carefully inspected for motion artifact. Lateral motion appears as abnormally or implausibly shaped vertebral bodies. Lateral motion invalidates scan results. In very young children, breathing can produce unavoidable motion in the anterior-posterior direction, as opposed to lateral motion. Breathing motion appears as regularly spaced horizontal white lines (or streaks) throughout the scan image and is unlikely to affect results. Figure 6.1 illustrates scans with motion artifact, with breathing artifact and without motion.

Contemporary software versions have edge detection algorithms that function well for young children with much lower bone density than adults. The global ROI may be adjusted to the left or right so that it can be centered around the vertebral column; however, the box width is not adjustable. The top line for ROI must be positioned within the intervertebral space between T12 and L1. The bottom line of the ROI must be positioned within the intervertebral space between L4 and L5. These lines may be angled slightly if necessary to account for alterations in spine anatomy such as scoliosis.

Once the global ROI is adjusted, the bone map is either confirmed or edited. Editing should only be done when the bone map is grossly erroneous. The placement of the three horizontal intervertebral lines between L1 and L2, L2 and L3, and

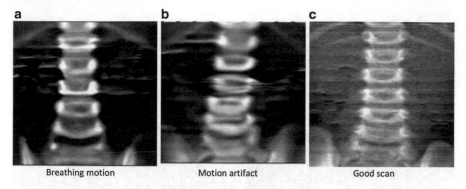

Fig. 6.1 Lumbar spine scans in infants showing (**a**) anterior-posterior "breathing" movement, (**b**) lateral movement, and (**c**) no movement

L3 and L4 should be confirmed or adjusted as necessary. Interfering factors within the global ROI such as belly button rings can invalidate the results of the spine scan; unlike adults, there are no reference data at this time to determine the Z-scores for individual vertebrae or combinations of vertebrae. Under these circumstances, alternative scans are recommended. Like adults, a deviation in the increasing progression of bone area and bone mineral density from L1 to L4 suggests a possible vertebral deformity or compression fracture, requiring further investigation. There are no major differences in the final assessment of spine scans for children as compared to adults.

## *Whole Body Scan Analysis*

Specifics of whole body scan acquisition are described in Chap. 5. Prior to analyzing, scan images should be carefully inspected for motion and other artifacts such as snaps, buttons, pocketed cell phones, etc. The quality of the scan is important as poor patient positioning or movement will affect the accuracy of the results. Children should be scanned with their head at the end of the table to achieve uniform positioning for follow-up scans as the child grows. The scan length may be shortened to decrease the scan time. However, care should be taken to make the scan length sufficiently long that the entire child will fit within the scan window. It is helpful to mark the table top at 130, 140, and 150 cm so the operator can determine the appropriate scan length when the child is lying on the table. Figure 6.2 shows whole body scan images with and without motion or other artifacts.

Manufacturer's guidelines should be followed for analysis of whole body scans, including defining standard, manufacturer-specified subregions. The technologist must adjust the lines defining the subregions for appropriate scan analysis. There are ten subregions: head, left and right arms, left and right ribs, thoracic and lumbar spine, pelvis, and right and left legs. The bone map is not visible on whole body

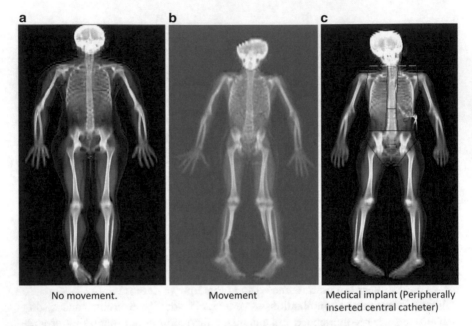

No movement.                    Movement                    Medical implant (Peripherally
                                                             inserted central catheter)

**Fig. 6.2** Whole body scans in children illustrating (**a**) a good scan with no movement, (**b**) a scan with movement in the head and legs, and (**c**) a scan of a child with a medical artifact (PICC line)

scans. Therefore, the technologist should examine the BMC and aBMD results within each subregion to confirm that bone is detected. This is particularly important for very young children because of their smaller bone size and lower bone density. Presently, Hologic does not recommend the use of standard whole body scans in children less than 3 years of age (Thomas Kelly, personal communication) because the bone map is likely to be incomplete. The infant whole body scan mode is an alternative, but currently is a tool for research applications only. GE Lunar devices presently do not provide technical support for infant scans.

Of note, Hologic software performs an automatic weight-based adjustment to the edge detection algorithm of whole body scans for children under 40 kg (i.e., 88 lb).

## Forearm Analysis

Young children may be too small to sit in a chair and achieve the optimal position for a forearm scan. It is often more feasible to position the child on the table. They can be placed in a supine position with their elbow bent at 90 degrees and forearm parallel to the edge of the table, or they can be placed prone on the table with their arm above their head with the forearm parallel to the edge of the table as shown in Fig. 6.3. Regardless of the postural method used, the position of the forearm in the scan field should meet the manufacturer recommendation and the analysis of the forearm scan is the same.

In growing children, the growth plate and epiphysis of the radius and ulna will be visible in the image and the ulnar styloid might not be present. In very young children, the ulnar epiphysis might not be visible. Generally, the manufacturer's guidelines for scan analysis should be followed, but the ROI should be placed so that the ultradistal region excludes the dense bone tissue at the proximal edge of the growth plate as shown in Fig. 6.4.

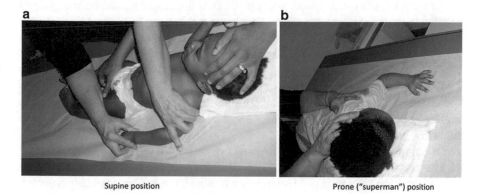

**Fig. 6.3** Forearm scan positions in young children showing (**a**) the supine position, and (**b**) the prone "superman" position. The superman position should be used only when the supine position is not possible. The arm can be held in position during the scan provided the "helper's" hands are not in the scan field

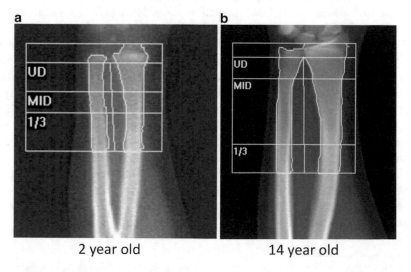

**Fig. 6.4** Placement of regions of interest in forearm scans of children. The distal border of the ultradistal region of interest should be proximal to the growth plate

## *Proximal Femur Analysis*

Acquisition of proximal femur scans is described in Chap. 5. The scans should be inspected for proper positioning. The femur should be rotated 10°–15° and the lesser trochanter is just barely visible. If the lesser trochanter is too prominent, then the leg is not internally rotated sufficiently. In young children, it may be difficult to visualize the lesser trochanter, but in older children, especially adolescent boys, the lesser trochanter is quite prominent. The shaft of the femur should be straight and parallel to the edge of the scan field. The lower edge of the ROI should encompass the lesser trochanter. As with all scans, inspection for motion or other artifacts is important, and the bone map should be inspected to be sure that it is correct.

Once the bone map is complete, the next step is to let the software determine the midline, Ward's triangle,[1] the base of the greater trochanter, and the neck box placement. The midline should be perpendicular to the narrowest part of the neck region. A misplaced midline can be caused by very low density bone or by unusual proportions in a growing child.

In Hologic systems, increasing the border of the global ROI to include additional soft tissue near the head of the femur may allow the software to find the midline more accurately. If the midline is still incorrectly positioned, it should be manually adjusted. However, manual adjustments should be made with caution because it can be difficult to reproduce the analysis; it is best to use auto-analysis for the midline when possible.

The next step is to inspect the position of the neck box. The default width should not be changed unless the top of the box is in the head of the femur or the bottom is overlapping the ischium. If either of these is the case, the box should be moved or, possibly, narrowed the smallest amount possible. Any changes in the size or location of the neck box should be noted on the report. Additionally, if the neck box width is changed, BMC Z-scores and bone mineral apparent density (BMAD) results cannot be used because the calculations assume this region is at the default box size.

The femoral neck ROI should be positioned so that the lower outer corner is just touching the bone in the neck region at the point where the curve of the greater trochanter meets the curve of the neck region. The other three corners must be in soft tissue. If the patient is very small or has a very short hip axis length, it may not be possible to place the neck box without overlapping the ischium region. In this case, go back to the mapping step and manually delete bone away from the neck region. Once this region is deleted, place the neck box appropriately. Figure 6.5 illustrates good quality proximal femur scans for an older and younger child.

GE Lunar models have a slightly different ROI, which uses the midline placement and triangulation to place the lower edge of the global ROI. The neck region for GE Lunar models is also perpendicular to the midline but is located in the center of the whole neck region.

---

[1] We do not recommend using Ward's triangle region in children. This region is defined as the region of least density within the femoral neck. Therefore, the region is in a different location for each child and may change location over time, making interpretation meaningless.

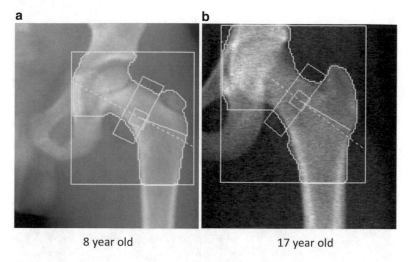

**Fig. 6.5**   Placement of regions of interest in proximal femur scans in children

## *Lateral Distal Femur*

The lateral distal femur scan is frequently used to assess bone health in children with chronic diseases who are immobilized as described in Chap. 9. Details of scan procedures are also published [2, 3]. The scan should be acquired with the femur parallel to the long edge of the table using the forearm scan mode. Subregional forearm analysis is used to analyze these scans rather than the auto-analysis function, which requires bone length. The scan is analyzed by placing contiguous ROI boxes around three regions: (1) the anterior distal region of the femur placed proximally to the growth plate, a region that is primarily trabecular bone; (2) the metadiaphysis, which includes both trabecular and cortical bone; and (3) the diaphysis, which is entirely cortical bone (Fig. 6.6). The height of the ROI is determined by the width of the diaphysis, and calculated as twice the diaphyseal width times the aspect ratio. For the first region, only the anterior portion of the bone is included in the ROI. The posterior edge of the ROI is positioned at the midpoint of the bone width at the growth plate. The anterior portion of the first ROI should extend beyond the soft tissue. For regions 2 and 3, the width of the box should be large enough to extend over soft tissue and centered across the bone.

   The scan should be inspected for movement artifact. With modest movement in one region, it is possible to use the other regions for interpretation. However, with excessive movement, it may be impossible to properly size and align the ROI boxes because of the interdependency of their positions.

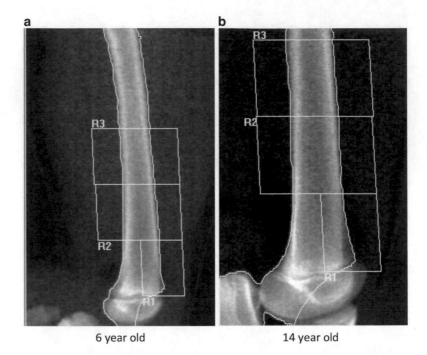

6 year old                              14 year old

**Fig. 6.6** Analysis of lateral distal femur scans in children


## *Manufacturer, Model, and Software Differences*

Bone mineral density (BMD) results for the same person measured on different instruments may differ, especially if the instruments are from different manufacturers [4]. These differences may be due machine calibration differences, or unique manufacturer software and acquisition methods. Due to these discrepancies, it is recommended that, whenever possible, the same instrument, model, and software version be used to assess an individual patient over time.

It is not always feasible to conduct serial measurements on identical instruments, as would be the case for a patient who receives care at multiple clinics or for clinics that have upgraded their DXA technology over time. In an attempt to allow comparisons among manufacturers, the three most common instrument manufacturers (Hologic, GE Lunar, and Norland) established cross-calibration factors [5], which permitted calculation of the standardized BMD (sBMD). The sBMD is expressed in $mg/cm^2$ to avoid confusion with manufacturer-specific areal BMDs, which are expressed in $g/cm^2$ [5–7]. The equations to convert measurements of spine and hip aBMD were established using scans obtained on adult women and phantoms [5], with further adjustments published for the spine [8] and femur [9]. A comparison of sBMD values for 30 postmenopausal women measured on Hologic Delphi and GE-Lunar Prodigy devices showed differences of 0.5 % for the right total hip and

4.1 % for lumbar spine L1 to L4 [10]. The equations for the spine do not apply well to men [11]. Most conversion equations are based on adults, were developed on older generation DXA scanners, and have not been validated for children. Only one study has established a standardization formula based on a sample that included children, but their results are restricted to whole body scans [12].

If equipment is upgraded or replaced, the differences between devices must be considered. If only software analysis versions are upgraded, it is possible to reanalyze prior scans using the new software so that follow-up values will be less divergent. If the instrument is replaced, it is recommended that cross-calibration be performed by scanning a set of 30 individuals with a range in age, size, and aBMD that reflects the clinical population on both the old and new instruments. Guidelines for performing the cross-calibration can be found at http://www.iscd.org/resources/calculators/. If this is not possible, the change in instrument manufacturer, model, or software should be noted on the clinical report.

## Follow-Up Scan Analysis

Analysis of longitudinal changes in growing children can prove to be difficult. Although no one approach has been shown to be best, some practices can minimize error. Prior scan images should be carefully examined during positioning and scan acquisition to optimize comparability of repeated measurements. Good practice should be used in positioning and analysis at all time points. If there is deviation from good practice in the prior or current scan, this should be noted on the report. Documentation of manufacturer, model, and software should be noted on all clinical reports, and specific comments should be included on serial reports when there are changes in the machine model or software used.

Manufacturers recommend that all follow-up scans be analyzed using the compare mode. In rapidly growing children, it is often necessary to make adjustments to the global ROI and subregions, especially if follow-up scans occur over a large period of time. The compare mode can and should be used to ensure similar positioning of the ROI between time points. Regardless of whether or not the compare function is used, it is important that technologists in the same clinic follow a consistent protocol for all children and that researchers report details of scan analyses in manuscripts.

## Fundamentals of Evaluation

Age-related increases in BMC and aBMD are complex. BMC and aBMD undergo nonlinear increases relative to age, and the variability in these measures also increases as shown in Fig. 6.7. Like growth in height and weight, DXA results need to be evaluated relative to reference ranges (similar to growth charts) that account

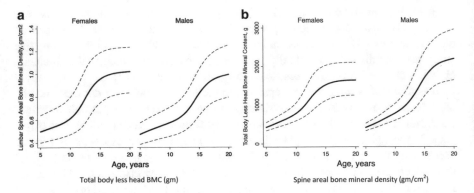

**Fig. 6.7** Age related increases in BMC and aBMD during growth

for the expected age- and sex-specific changes in growing children. The selection of reference ranges is central to the evaluation process because DXA results for children are expressed as Z-scores, the number of standard deviations above or below the median for age and sex. In older adults, the T-score is used. The T-score compares a DXA result to the mean and standard deviation for young adults when bone mass is at its peak. A T-score should never be used in children as they have not yet reached peak bone mass. For children, Z-scores are used as an indicator of "bone mineral status," i.e., how an individual's measurement compares to those of peers with the same age and sex. Use of inappropriate reference ranges can yield Z-scores that misrepresent "bone mineral status" (e.g., low bone density for age). The points below highlight the important considerations in selecting reference data.

Children whose BMC or BMD is close to the median for their age and sex will have a Z-score of approximately zero. A Z-score of 2 corresponds to the 97.7th percentile, and a Z-score of −2 corresponds to the 2.3rd percentile. An advantage of Z-scores over percentile values is that very low or very high values that are outside the reference population distribution (i.e., greater than the 100th percentile or less than the 0th percentile) can be quantified. This is especially important for longitudinal follow-up of children with low BMD as it allows for quantifying the changes in BMD relative to the expected values for age and sex.

## Normative Data

### Ideal Characteristics of Reference Data

The first step in the interpretation of DXA measurements in pediatric patients is appropriate selection of reference data. Reference data should have several characteristics. The data should be derived from a sample of healthy children who are representative of the overall population. Healthy children can be defined as those who are free of chronic diseases, medication use, and physical limitations that might affect bone mineral accrual. They should also be of normal nutritional, growth, and developmental status because these are known to affect bone health. Because of the possibility of regional differences in lifestyle, ethnic composition, sunlight exposure, and so forth, a multiregional sample is optimal to capture normal variability. The sample needs to be of sufficient size to adequately characterize the variability in bone measures for both boys and girls. Because the variability in bone measures increases with age, it is important to assure sufficient sample sizes at all ages so that the age-dependent differences in variability can be well characterized.

## Calculation of the Z-Score

The purpose of reference data is to gather the necessary information for calculating Z-scores (standard deviation scores). Expression of DXA outcomes in children as Z-scores requires knowing age- and sex-specific characteristics of the BMC or aBMD distributions so that a child's measurement is compared to those of the same age and sex in the reference population.

The simplest approach to calculate Z-scores involves use of age and sex-specific means and standard deviations from reference data as shown in Eq. (1).

$$Z - \text{score} = (\text{observed} - \text{mean}) / \text{standard deviation} \qquad (1)$$

This approach assumes that the age- and sex-specific values are normally distributed, and that the sample sizes for each age and sex group are large enough to characterize the distribution. It also assumes that annual age increments are an appropriate grouping; during periods of rapid bone accrual, smaller age groupings may be needed. A limitation of this approach is that random sampling fluctuations can result in erratic differences between adjacent age groups.

The distribution of bone measures is sometimes skewed, so more sophisticated biostatistical techniques have been used, including parametric regression modeling [13, 14], multivariate semi-metric smoothing [15] and the LMS method [16]. These techniques provide "smoothed" values over the age range to avoid random sampling fluctuations. Bone outcomes become increasingly variable with advancing age and are often skewed owing to variation in timing of puberty (i.e., early and later maturing children), and the increasing influence of environmental, genetic, and behavioral factors on bone outcomes. The LMS method of characterizing reference values addresses these concerns and provides a method for smoothing across age ranges, accounting for changes in variation with age, and skewness in the distribution [16]. The LMS method uses a power transformation to normalize data. The optimal power to obtain normality is calculated for a series of age groups, and the trend is summarized by a smooth (L) curve. Smoothed curves for the median (M) and coefficient of variation (S) are also calculated, and these three measures, L, M, and S, are used to describe the data distribution. When the LMS method is applied, the distribution and exact percentiles can be described using Eq. (2) as follows:

$$\text{percentile curve} = M \times \left[ \left(1+\left(L \times S \times Z\right)\right)^{(1/L)} \right] \qquad (2)$$

using the $L$ (skewness), $M$ (median), and $S$ (coefficient of variation) values, and $Z$ corresponding to the Z-score equivalent of standard percentiles (e.g., the 50th percentile is a Z-score of zero; the 2.3rd percentile is equivalent to a Z-score of −2.0).

For an individual, the exact Z-score can be calculated as:

$$Z - \text{score} = \left( \left[ \left(\text{Observed value} / M\right)L \right] - 1 \right) / \left(L \times S\right) \qquad (3)$$

## Selection of Reference Data

Most DXA software includes pediatric reference data and provides the calculated Z-score in the DXA report, but good documentation regarding the source of the reference data is sometimes lacking. Clinicians and researchers should be aware of the reference data used to generate Z-scores and the impact that this may have on interpretation of results. Options for selecting pediatric reference data include: (1) using the database incorporated into the manufacturer's software; (2) comparing your data to published data; or (3) using locally collected normative values. Each approach has its benefits and limitations. The database incorporated into the manufacturer's software may derive from a single published study, a blending of several published studies, or other adjustments that are not explicitly described. For example, the U.S. reference data from the Bone Mineral Density in Childhood Study (see below) were acquired on Hologic DXA devices. These data have been blended into Hologic pediatric databases. Likewise, GE Lunar incorporated these reference data into the enCore 2011 software, presumably with adjustments because the reference data were collected using Hologic DXA devices. As with all decisions related to acquiring, analyzing, and interpreting DXA scans, the most important point is to be aware of the sources used to calculate Z-scores, the limitations involved and providing documentation to ease interpretation of changes at follow-up.

The ideal approach is to have reference data that meet the criteria described above for each DXA model, unless it is well-established that the results of different DXA models (different models of the same manufacturer and among different manufacturers) are interchangeable. DXA results obtained with machines from different manufacturers and, in some instances, different software versions by the same manufacturer are not always comparable. For example, the differences between Hologic version software 11.2 and 12.1 in the analysis of whole body scans results in changes of up to 25% in total body aBMD in the smallest subjects, but no differences in aBMD in subjects weighing more than 40 kg [17]. A comparison of GE Lunar models showed that the Prodigy model measured total body BMC was 9.4% lower in small children and 3.1% higher for larger children compared to the DPX-L model [18]. These examples underscore the need to be familiar with the software version in use, and the reference data selected for calculating Z-scores.

The advantage of using published reference data is that details of the population are described in the manuscript. A listing of published reference ranges can be found in Crabtree et al. [19]. The youngest age for most reference data bases is 5 years, although there are some that go to age 3 years. Information about reference ranges for children less than 5 years of age can be found in Kalkwarf et al. [20].

Presently, the most robust published pediatric reference data acquired on Hologic systems come from the Bone Mineral Density In Childhood Study (BMDCS). In 2001, the U.S. National Institutes of Health initiated the multicenter, prospective, longitudinal BMDCS to develop reference data in a multiethnic sample [21, 22]. Reference ranges for ages 5–20 years were developed using over 10,000 measurements on ~2000 healthy youth. Standardized eligibility criteria, equipment, and procedures for data collection were used. Whole body, lumbar spine, proximal femur, and forearm scans were acquired using Hologic Delphi/Discovery systems, and analyzed centrally. Preliminary [21] and final [22] age and sex-specific reference ranges, established using the LMS method (described above) have been published based on this large cohort, with separate reference ranges for African American and non-African American children. These reference data can be used to calculate Z-scores for pediatric subjects in Hologic software version 12.3 or higher. A website calculator is available at https://bmdcs.nichd.nih.gov/. Both Hologic and GE Lunar systems have adopted these reference ranges in their software.

Another large reference data set that is anticipated comes from the Amalgamated Paediatric Bone Density Study (Alphabet) study [23]. The data set is a collation of bone density measurements on over 3000 healthy children, ages 5–20 years, measured in seven centers the UK on GE Lunar (DPX-L, Prodigy, and iDXA) or Hologic Discovery DXA devices. Using in vivo and in vitro cross calibration among devices, standardization across devices was achieved using transformation equations. Sex-, age-, and size-specific reference curves have been generated, but are not yet published.

## Population Ancestry

A final consideration in the selection of reference data is the occurrence of differences in bone mineral accrual according to population ancestry [22, 24–28]. In particular, African Americans have significantly greater BMD and lower fracture rates than other ethnic groups. For other ethnic or ancestry groups, differences in bone mineral accrual are usually attributable to body size, so size-adjusted Z-scores (see below) obviate the need for ethnic-specific reference data. For African Americans vs. others, differences in growth, body composition, skeletal maturation, and the timing of puberty only partly explain group differences. The International Society of Clinical Densitometry (ISCD) Pediatric Positions Statement recommends the use of race-specific reference data when possible [19]. As noted above, the BMDCS has published reference ranges for African American and Non-African American youth [21, 22].

DXA reports should explicitly state whether race-specific reference data are used because choice of reference data affects the Z-score and clinical interpretation. It is not known, however, if race-specific reference data allow better identification of fracture risk as compared to non-race-specific reference data. Nevertheless, the use of race-specific reference curves provides an indication of an individual's "bone mineral status" relative to their genetic potential as defined by their ancestry group. This is more of a theoretically based consideration than an evidence-based one. In the absence of evidence-based guidelines for the use of ethnic-specific reference data, the rationale chosen by the ISCD may reasonably be applied to children.

### Size Adjustments

DXA is a two dimensional imaging modality that systematically results in lower aBMD in smaller individuals because it is an areal ($g/cm^2$), not a volumetric ($g/cm^3$) measure. This limitation of DXA is of particular concern in pediatric evaluations because of the age-related changes in bone size that occur with growth, and the variability in growth among children of similar age. Many children in need of a DXA evaluation have chronic diseases that place them at risk for poor bone mineral accrual because of malabsorption, poor dietary intake, inflammation, reduced physical activity, or medications. These same factors also contribute to faltering growth and delayed maturation relative to same-age peers. Under these circumstances, estimating the effect of size-related artifacts on DXA measurements is important for the clinical interpretation because it provides an indication of the degree to which a low BMC or aBMD Z-score is due to small body size vs. an abnormality in bone accretion.

The ISCD Pediatric Positions [19] state "In children with short stature or growth delay, spine and total body less head (TBLH) BMC and aBMD results should be adjusted. For the spine, adjust using either bone mineral apparent density (BMAD) or the height Z-score. For TBLH, adjust using the height Z-score." In a study of low trauma fracture cases, lumbar spine BMAD performed best in identifying children with fracture [29] (odds ratio 9.3, 95 % confidence interval (CI) 5.8–14.9). Spine BMAD is calculated using the formula in Eq. 4 below.

$$\text{Spine BMAD}_{L1\text{-}L4} = \sum \left( BMC / Ap^{3/2} \right) \tag{4}$$

where Ap is the projected bone area from the DXA measurement. A limitation of this approach is that reference ranges for spine BMAD are not yet available.

The height Z-score adjustment method was developed because the relationship between stature and BMC/aBMD changes as a function of age [22, 30]. The steps are more complex, requiring the initial calculation of BMC or aBMD Z-score and height-for-age Z-score, which are then used to calculate an adjusted Z-score. The calculations can be performed by the website calculator at https://bmdcs.nichd.nih.gov/. An important caveat of this approach is that it has not been used in fracture studies to determine whether it improves fracture prediction.

# Interpreting Scans

*The importance of the Z-score*: The BMC or aBMD Z-score, the central element in interpreting DXA results, provides information about how an individual's BMC or aBMD compares to peers of similar age, sex, population ancestry (if ancestry-specific reference ranges are used) and size (if a size adjustment applies). Statistically, the normal range is defined as ±2 standard deviations (Z-scores). Accordingly, the ISCD Pediatric Positions define a Z-score <−2 as low BMC or aBMD [19]. By definition, 2.3 % of the reference population will have a Z-score less than −2. The threshold of <−2 has not been directly linked to fracture risk or other bone health outcomes.

*Fracture prediction*: Ultimately, the goal of obtaining a DXA scan is to assess bone health and prevent future fractures. Fractures are common in otherwise healthy children: 30–50 % of children will experience at least one fracture before they reach adulthood [31, 32]. Epidemiologically, fracture patterns in children are different from adults in several key characteristics. Childhood fractures peak around ages 11–14 in boys and 8–11 years in girls, and then decline as young adulthood is attained [33]. Fractures are more common in boys than in girls, and the most common site of fractures is the upper extremity. Most studies of the association of DXA outcomes and fractures in children have been conducted using samples of healthy children. One population cohort study determined that the risk of fracture increased by 89 % for every 1 SD decrease in size adjusted bone Z-score [34]. A case-controlled study of forearm fracture among children who experienced forearm injuries reported a 28–41 % increase in fracture risk for every 1 SD decrease in bone Z-score [35]. However, despite these associations, the sensitivity of DXA to identify fracture risk is poor in healthy children.

Among children with health conditions detrimental to bone accretion, bone density Z-scores are also predictive of fracture. In a study of children referred for clinical bone health assessment (osteogenesis imperfecta, long-term corticosteroid treatment, immobility, thalassemia, anorexia nervosa, etc.), the diagnostic odds ratio for a vertebral fracture for children with lumbar spine BMAD Z-score <−2 was 9.3 (95% CI: 5.8–14.9) [29]. The odds ratio for a fracture for children with total body less head BMC (adjusted for lean body mass and height) Z-score of <−2 was 6.5 (95 % CI: 4.1–10.2). The abilities of the models to discriminate children at risk of fracture, assessed by area under the curve in ROC analyses, were 0.73 and 0.74, respectively, indicating acceptable discrimination. Among immobilized children, risk of fracture increased by 6–15 % for every 1.0 decrease in lateral distal femur Z-score [36]. In a prospective study of children diagnosed with acute lymphoblastic leukemia, risk of vertebral fracture over the following 12 months increased by 80 % for every one standard deviation decrease in spine aBMD Z-score at diagnosis [37]. The ability of the model to discriminate children at risk of fracture was 0.81, indicating acceptable discrimination. These studies underscore the utility of DXA in bone health assessment and future fracture risk. No studies to date have established a threshold above which fracture risk escalates, and the relationship between BMC or aBMD Z-score and fracture risk appears to be continuous.

*Other considerations*: Other factors that are often considered in interpreting BMC or aBMD Z-scores are bone age, pubertal maturation, and body composition [19]. Both bone age and puberty stage are affected by the timing of physical maturation. The timing of puberty has a long lasting effect on bone accretion. Early maturing children have greater bone density at the end of puberty or in early adulthood [38, 39]. Likewise, boys with delayed maturation have lower bone density relative to age [40]. Males with later age at peak height velocity, an indicator of pubertal timing, had lower bone density at age 18 but not at age 25 years [41]. However, there are no specific evidence-based guidelines on how to incorporate pubertal maturation or bone age into the interpretation of DXA results at this time. Body composition, especially lean body mass, has very strong positive associations with BMC and aBMD at all ages [42]. The extremes of the nutritional status continuum (undernutrition and obesity) are expected to impact bone Z-scores in children. However, for all of these considerations, there are no evidence-based guidelines on how to incorporate such information into the interpretation of the BMC or aBMD Z-score. Additional considerations when interpreting DXA bone results include the history, the clinical exam (including growth status, bone age, and pubertal status), the presence of other risk factors (including bone pain and fracture history), and laboratory values.

*Discrepant Z-scores*: BMC/aBMD Z-scores from different skeletal sites (e.g., lumbar spine, total body) are positively correlated, but the correlation is far from perfect, ranging from 0.4 to 0.7 (Zemel unpublished data). This means that not all individuals who have a high bone Z-score at one skeletal site will have a similarly high Z-score at another skeletal site. Discrepancies in bone Z-scores at different skeletal sites may be due to the composition of bone at those sites. The spine and femoral neck have a high percentage of trabecular bone, whereas the total body and forearm have a high percentage of cortical bone. Differences in disease processes or medication exposures may differentially target specific bone compartments. Similarly, bone loading physical activity stimulates bone accretion. Excessively high bone loading physical activity or non-ambulatory status can account for discrepancies in bone Z-scores between different skeletal sites. Generally, the lowest Z-score should be of greatest clinical concern.

*Definition of osteoporosis in children*: The bone density test is an important component of skeletal health assessment. However, unlike adults, the definition of osteoporosis in children cannot be made on densitometric criteria alone. The 2013 ISCD Pediatric Positions defined osteoporosis in childhood as follows [43]:

"One or more vertebral compression (crush) fractures, in the absence of local disease or high-energy trauma.

In the absence of vertebral compression (crush) fractures, the diagnosis of osteoporosis is indicated by the presence of both a clinically significant fracture history and BMD Z-score <−2.0.

A clinically significant fracture history is one or more of the following:

- Two or more long bone fractures by age 10 years
- Three or more long bone fractures at any age up to 19 years

A BMD/BMC Z-score greater than −2.0 does not preclude the possibility of skeletal fragility and increased fracture risk."

*Longitudinal Follow-Up*: Follow-up DXA scans should only be obtained if results will influence therapeutic decision-making. The timing of follow-up scans should be carefully considered for each individual patient as there is very little evidence to support the optimal interval for follow-up in children. Important considerations may include the initial indication for the DXA scan, the disease processes and treatments that occur following the initial DXA scan, and the child's age. The time interval needs to be long enough that a "meaningful change" (i.e. beyond measurement error) in BMC or aBMD is likely to occur. The monitoring time interval can be calculated based on the precision of DXA scans and the age and sex-specific annual rate of change. This has been estimated in healthy children participating in the BMDC study [1]. They found the monitoring time interval was as low as 3 months for some skeletal sites and age groups because of the rapid rate of change in children less than 15–16 years. In practice, DXA exams are rarely repeated more frequently than every 12 months, and longer intervals (i.e., >12 months) may also be appropriate. Occasionally, evaluations made at time intervals <12 months are warranted to monitor response to new drug intervention or to monitor rapidly worsening clinical status.

Changes in DXA results should be evaluated in the context of the growth that has occurred in that interval. Height increases result in larger skeletal size and greater BMC, but not necessarily greater aBMD because BMC and bone area may not increase proportionately. Since aBMD is the ratio of BMC to bone area, the disproportionate changes in BMC and bone area can make it appear as if aBMD is declining when, in fact, BMC and bone area are both increasing. Presently, there is no way to determine whether the gain in BMC or aBMD for a given amount of height growth is appropriate. At best, one should evaluate size adjusted Z-scores at baseline and follow-up to serve as an indicator of BMC/aBMD relative to growth.

In adults, bone loss is the main cause for a decline in *T*-score and is often expressed as a percentage change in aBMD. In children, failure to gain bone at the rate expected for age and sex is the more likely cause of a declining Z-score. Therefore, a percentage change in aBMD is difficult to interpret. Under some rare conditions, bone loss may occur in childhood, for example, in the case of a child with hematologic malignancies who begin therapy [44].

# Conclusions

Bone measurements by DXA are an essential component of a bone health evaluation in children at risk for poor bone mineral accrual, fractures, and osteoporosis later in life. DXA imaging is widely available, of relatively low cost, and has minimal radiation exposure. Children have smaller bones and are not always able to remain motionless during scans. Consequently, scan analysis requires attention to these concerns. Nevertheless the DXA precision in children is close to that in adults. Studies of healthy children and of children with chronic medical conditions show that DXA BMC and aBMD are predictive of future fractures; the risk of fracture increases as aBMD and BMC Z-scores decline. Substantial efforts have been made to develop appropriate DXA reference data for children ≥5 years of age and to identify the best approaches to account for delayed growth and altered body composition. Reference data for children <5 years of age and further advancements in ways to incorporate skeletal and sexual maturation in to interpretation of DXA results are needed. Great care should be taken in the selection of appropriate reference data that most closely match the device and software version used in the evaluation. Additional considerations when interpreting DXA bone results include medical history, the clinical exam (including growth status, bone age, and pubertal status), presence of other risk factors (including bone pain and fracture history), and laboratory values.

## Summary Points

- Analysis and evaluation of DXA scans are contingent upon acquisition of high-quality scans, devoid of movement and other artifacts that may affect BMC or aBMD results.
- Analysis of follow-up scans should use the "compare mode" to optimize the comparability of aBMD results. In addition, accurate placement of the ROI according to manufacturer's guidelines and examination of the "bone map" are important to ensure the scan is analyzed appropriately.
- To account for age-related increases in BMC and aBMD in growing children, age, sex, and race-specific reference values should be used to calculate a Z- score. The T-score should never be used for children.
- Reference data used to calculate Z-scores should be selected based on (1) data collected from the same instrument manufacturer and a similar software version as the clinical scan of interest, (2) provision of sex and race-specific reference curves, and (3) a large sample size used to generate the curves.
- In children with growth delay, it is important to estimate the effect of size-related artifact on aBMD Z-scores. This may be achieved by use of adjustments that incorporate the child's height for age Z-score or by use of BMAD.
- BMD or BMC Z-scores alone cannot be used to diagnose osteoporosis, but they are an indicator of how a child's DXA result compares to his or her peers. Low or very low Z-scores should trigger additional evaluations; however, even children without low Z-scores may not be achieving their genetic potential for bone mass.
- Interpretation of DXA scan results should be done within the context of other relevant clinical information such as patient history, growth assessment, clinical exam, and presence of other risk factors.

# References

1. Shepherd JA, Wang L, Fan B, et al. Optimal monitoring time interval between DXA measures in children. J Bone Miner Res. 2011;26:2745–52.
2. Zemel BS, Stallings VA, Leonard MB, et al. Revised pediatric reference data for the lateral distal femur measured by Hologic Discovery/Delphi dual-energy X-ray absorptiometry. J Clin Densitom. 2009;12:207–18.
3. Henderson RC, Lark RK, Newman JE, et al. Pediatric reference data for dual X-ray absorptiometric measures of normal bone density in the distal femur. AJR Am J Roentgenol. 2002;178:439–43.
4. Wang J, Thornton JC, Ioannidou E, et al. Four commonly used dual-energy X-ray absorptiometry scanners do not identically classify subjects for osteopenia or osteoporosis by T-score in four bone regions BIz11.5. J Clin Densitom. 2005;8:191–8.
5. Genant HK, Grampp S, Gluer CC, et al. Universal Standardization for dual X-ray absorptiometry: patient and phantom cross-calibration results. J Bone Miner Res. 1994;9:1503–10.
6. Hanson J. Standardization of femur BMD. J Bone Miner Res. 1997;12:1316–7.
7. Steiger P. Standardization of measurements for assessing BMD by DXA. Calcif Tissue Int. 1995;57:469.
8. Hui SL, Gao S, Zhou XH, et al. Universal standardization of bone density emasurements: a method with optimal properties for calibration among several instruments. J Bone Miner Res. 1997;12:1463–70.
9. Lu Y, Fuerst T, Hui S, Genant HK. Standardization of bone mineral density at femoral neck, trochanter and Ward's triangle. Osteoporos Int. 2001;12:438–44.
10. Fan B, Lu Y, Genant H, Fuerst T, Shepherd J. Does standardized BMD still remove differences between Hologic and GE-Lunar state-of-the-art DXA systems? Osteoporos Int. 2010;21:1227–36.
11. Ganda K, Nguyen TV, Pocock N. Gender disparity in BMD conversion: a comparison between Lunar and Hologic densitometers. Arch Osteoporos. 2014;9:180.
12. Shepherd JA, Fan B, Lu Y, et al. A multinational study to develop universal standardization of whole-body bone density and composition using GE Healthcare Lunar and Hologic DXA systems. J Bone Miner Res. 2012;27:2208–16.
13. Hastie T, Tibshirani R. Generalized additive models. New York: Chapman and Hall; 1990.
14. Horlick M, Wang J, Pierson Jr RN, Thornton JC. Prediction models for evaluation of total-body bone mass with dual-energy X-ray absorptiometry among children and adolescents. Pediatrics. 2004;114:e337–45.
15. Short DF, Zemel BS, Gilsanz V, et al. Fitting of bone mineral density with consideration of anthropometric parameters. Osteoporos Int. 2011;22:1047–57.
16. Cole TJ, Green PJ. Smoothing reference centile curves: the LMS method and penalized likelihood. Stat Med. 1992;11:1305–19.
17. Shypailo RJ, Ellis KJ. Bone assessment in children: comparison of fan-beam DXA analysis. J Clin Densitom. 2005;8:445–53.
18. Crabtree NJ, Shaw NJ, Boivin CM, Oldroyd B, Truscott JG. Pediatric in vivo cross-calibration between the GE Lunar Prodigy and DPX-L bone densitometers. Osteoporos Int. 2005;16:2157–67.
19. Crabtree NJ, Arabi A, Bachrach LK, et al. Dual-energy X-ray absorptiometry interpretation and reporting in children and adolescents: the revised 2013 ISCD Pediatric Official Positions. J Clin Densitom. 2014;17:225–42.
20. Kalkwarf HJ, Zemel BS, Yolton K, Heubi JE. Bone mineral content and density of the lumbar spine of infants and toddlers: influence of age, sex, race, growth, and human milk feeding. J Bone Miner Res. 2013;28:206–12.
21. Kalkwarf HJ, Zemel BS, Gilsanz V, et al. The bone mineral density in childhood study: bone mineral content and density according to age, sex, and race. J Clin Endocrinol Metab. 2007;92:2087–99.
22. Zemel BS, Kalkwarf HJ, Gilsanz V, et al. Revised reference curves for bone mineral content and areal bone mineral density according to age and sex for black and non-black children: results of the bone mineral density in childhood study. J Clin Endocrinol Metab. 2011;96:3160–9.

23. Crabtree N, Machin M, Bebbington N, et al. The Amalgamated Paediatric Bone Density Study (The ALPHABET Study): the collation and generation of UK based reference data for paediatric bone densitometry. In: International Conference on Children's Bone Health; 2013 June, 2013; Rotterdam, The Netherlands: bioscientifica; 2013. p. OC1.
24. Bachrach LK, Hastie T, Wang MC, Narasimhan B, Marcus R. Bone mineral acquisition in healthy Asian, Hispanic, black, and Caucasian youth: a longitudinal study. J Clin Endocrinol Metab. 1999;84:4702–12.
25. Ellis KJ. Body composition of a young, multiethnic, male population. Am J Clin Nutr. 1997;66:1323–31.
26. Ellis KJ, Abrams SA, Wong WW. Body composition of a young, multiethnic female population. Am J Clin Nutr. 1997;65:724–31.
27. Nelson DA, Simpson PM, Johnson CC, Barondess DA, Kleerekoper M. The accumulation of whole body skeletal mass in third- and fourth-grade children: effects of age, gender, ethnicity, and body composition. Bone. 1997;20:73–8.
28. Wang MC, Aguirre M, Bhudhikanok GS, et al. Bone mass and hip axis length in healthy Asian, black, Hispanic, and white American youths. J Bone Miner Res. 1997;12:1922–35.
29. Crabtree NJ, Hogler W, Cooper MS, Shaw NJ. Diagnostic evaluation of bone densitometric size adjustment techniques in children with and without low trauma fractures. Osteoporos Int. 2013;24:2015–24.
30. Zemel BS, Leonard MB, Kelly A, et al. Height adjustment in assessing dual energy x-ray absorptiometry measurements of bone mass and density in children. J Clin Endocrinol Metab. 2010;95:1265–73.
31. Cooper C, Dennison EM, Leufkens HG, Bishop N, van Staa TP. Epidemiology of childhood fractures in Britain: a study using the general practice research database. J Bone Miner Res. 2004;19:1976–81.
32. Landin LA. Epidemiology of children's fractures. J Pediatr Orthop. 1997;6:79–83.
33. Khosla S, Melton 3rd LJ, Dekutoski MB, Achenbach SJ, Oberg AL, Riggs BL. Incidence of childhood distal forearm fractures over 30 years: a population-based study. JAMA. 2003;290:1479–85.
34. Clark EM, Ness AR, Bishop NJ, Tobias JH. Association between bone mass and fractures in children: a prospective cohort study. J Bone Miner Res. 2006;21:1489–95.
35. Kalkwarf HJ, Laor T, Bean JA. Fracture risk in children with a forearm injury is associated with volumetric bone density and cortical area (by peripheral QCT) and areal bone density (by DXA). Osteoporos Int. 2011;22:607–16.
36. Henderson RC, Berglund LM, May R, et al. The relationship between fractures and DXA measures of BMD in the distal femur of children and adolescents with cerebral palsy or muscular dystrophy. J Bone Miner Res. 2010;25:520–6.
37. Alos N, Grant RM, Ramsay T, et al. High incidence of vertebral fractures in children with acute lymphoblastic leukemia 12 months after the initiation of therapy. J Clin Oncol. 2012;30:2760–7.
38. Gilsanz V, Chalfant J, Kalkwarf H, et al. Age at onset of puberty predicts bone mass in young adulthood. J Pediatr. 2011;158:100–5 (5 e1-2).
39. Chevalley T, Bonjour JP, Ferrari S, Rizzoli R. The influence of pubertal timing on bone mass acquisition: a predetermined trajectory detectable five years before menarche. J Clin Endocrinol Metab. 2009;94:3424–31.
40. Finkelstein JS, Neer RM, Biller BM, Crawford JD, Klibanski A. Osteopenia in men with a history of delayed puberty. N Engl J Med. 1992;326:600–4.
41. Darelid A, Ohlsson C, Nilsson M, Kindblom JM, Mellstrom D, Lorentzon M. Catch up in bone acquisition in young adult men with late normal puberty. J Bone Miner Res. 2012;27:2198–207.
42. Hogler W, Briody J, Woodhead HJ, Chan A, Cowell CT. Importance of lean mass in the interpretation of total body densitometry in children and adolescents. J Pediatr. 2003;143:81–8.
43. Bishop N, Arundel P, Clark E, et al. Fracture prediction and the definition of osteoporosis in children and adolescents: the ISCD 2013 Pediatric Official Positions. J Clin Densitom. 2014;17:275–80.
44. El-Hajj Fuleihan G, Muwakkit S, Arabi A, et al. Predictors of bone loss in childhood hematologic malignancies: a prospective study. Osteoporos Int. 2012;23:665–74.

# Chapter 7
# Reporting DXA Results for Children and Adolescents

Ellen B. Fung

## Abbreviations

| | |
|---|---|
| BMAD | Bone mineral apparent density |
| BMC | Bone mineral content g |
| aBMD | Areal bone mineral density g/cm$^2$ |
| vBMD | Volumetric bone mineral density g/cm$^3$ |
| DXA | Dual energy X-ray absorptiometry |
| ISCD | International Society of Clinical Densitometry |
| HAZ | Height for age Z-score |
| NOF | National Osteoporosis Foundation |
| VFA | Vertebral fracture assessment |
| WHO | World Health Organization |

## Introduction

Accurate acquisition and interpretation of bone densitometry scans in the pediatric patient are necessary first steps toward any clinical assessment process. The dual-energy X-ray absorptiometry (DXA) report fulfills the role of transmitting data clearly to the referring clinician. A timely, concise, and informative report is essential to relay the DXA findings and to avoid costly and potentially dangerous misinterpretations by physicians unfamiliar with pediatric densitometry data.

E.B. Fung, Ph.D., R.D., C.C.D. (✉)
UCSF Benioff Children's Hospital Oakland,
Children's Hospital Oakland Research Institute,
Oakland, CA, USA
e-mail: efung@mail.cho.org

© Springer International Publishing Switzerland 2016
E.B. Fung et al. (eds.), *Bone Health Assessment in Pediatrics*,
DOI 10.1007/978-3-319-30412-0_7

Reports generated using the DXA manufacturer's proprietary software have advanced significantly since X-ray-based bone densitometers were widely marketed in the late 1980s. Typically, these reports provide basic patient demographic data and a graphical image of the skeletal scan, as well as numeric data for bone area, bone mineral content (BMC), and areal bone mineral density (aBMD) for each region of interest (and sub-region of the spine or whole body). Additionally, the patient's aBMD data are compared with reference data derived from healthy controls to generate standard deviation scores: Z-scores represent comparisons with age-matched norms, and T-scores, comparisons with young adults.

Until recently, regardless of the age of the subject, most of the standard software provided by the manufacturer automatically reported both Z- and T-scores (e.g. Hologic software version earlier than 12.5) including the resulting diagnoses of osteopenia or osteoporosis, as established by the World Health Organization for older adults [1]. For the inexperienced operator, the software-generated reports appear to provide a comprehensive clinical evaluation of the results sufficient to estimate risk for osteoporosis in a young child. However, interpretation based solely on these computer-generated reports is inappropriate and often misleading when interpreting the DXA results of children and adolescents. Quite clearly, T-scores should not be used in children. Furthermore, the terms osteopenia and osteoporosis are not to be used in pediatric densitometry in isolation of clinically pertinent information. It is crucial that the software-generated report be modified and supplemented by a formal written report provided by an expert experienced with interpreting pediatric densitometry.

DXA software programs allow creation of customized reports that eliminate the appearance of T-scores in patients less than 50 years of age, and remove mention of "osteopenia" or "osteoporosis" in an individual <21 years of age. Both of these revisions are in accordance with current International Society for Clinical Densitometry guidelines position statements [2, 3].

Since the first edition of this text, guidelines for the reporting of DXA results from both adult and pediatric patients have become more common. The International Society for Clinical Densitometry (ISCD) has now published two guidelines for the standardization of DXA scanning, interpretation and reporting in pediatrics; the first was published in 2008 [3] and most recently in 2013 [2]. There have also been position papers by the ISCD on unifying the reporting of body composition measures in adults [4] as well as how to document vertebral fractures observed on Vertebral Fracture Assessment (VFA) scans [5]. VFA is a full lateral spine scan, an option on newer DXA devices, used in some pediatric practices. An entire chapter in this textbook is devoted to the topic of vertebral fracture and its assessment (Chap. 10). Body composition measures are routinely acquired as part of the whole body scan, but often not reported. This chapter offers guidelines specifically tailored to the pediatric patient, primarily for the reporting of bone densitometry but also includes suggestions for how to report body composition and VFA results. Examples of reporting formats used at pediatric imaging centers are provided in the Appendix D.

# The DXA Report: Purpose and Audience

The clinical DXA report has three main purposes: (1) to present the numeric data in a concise, organized, and easily understood fashion to the referring physician; (2) to provide enough technical information to allow for comparison to subsequent DXA studies or to those studies performed at other densitometry centers; and (3) to provide a preliminary interpretation of the findings in a clinical context. The report may also include recommendations to the patient or physician based on the findings.

Pediatric bone densitometry reports are sent only to the referring physician in most cases. However, some families may also request a copy of the report; therefore it is important to both define all technical and clinical terminology used and to provide an objective, nonjudgmental review.

Failure to communicate results effectively to the referring physician or patient/parent may be due simply to letters being lost or misunderstood. Health literacy is a factor in the understanding of health-related communication and is a problem for most people in the US [6]. As part of a study to improve knowledge of osteoporosis in adult patients, researchers from Iowa developed a generic DXA results letter intended for patients [7]. The letter was sent to women recently diagnosed with osteoporosis [7], and was used also a motivational tool. As the field of pediatric densitometry develops, this study could serve as a model for the importance of communication of information with patients.

The technical DXA report ideally contains five elements: (1) patient demographics, (2) a brief medical history, (3) test results, (4) technical comments, and (5) interpretation and occasionally recommendations. Each element will be described in detail below, and data that are typically included in each section are elucidated. At some imaging centers, the manufacturer generated copy of the scan image with numeric results is provided with a copy of the report.

The formal report may be written by any qualified, expert in densitometry. However, in several regions of the United States, the report must be signed or cosigned by a board-certified physician in order to receive insurance reimbursement (for the physician's co-pay portion of the DXA service). In other regions, there is not a separate billing (e.g. CPT code) for a physicians' review of the exam and any experienced, qualified operator may report the results. For details regarding training and educational courses available for both technologists and physicians seeking training in bone densitometry acquisition and reporting procedures, please see Appendix A, Table 4.

# Report Components

In recent years there has been consensus as to the components that should be provided in every pediatric clinical DXA report [2, 3]. Tables 7.1 and 7.2 list the relevant recommended content for pediatric patient reports suggested by the ISCD and the NOF. These components are provided as guidelines and need not be considered standard for all institutions. A more abbreviated version of the DXA report could be

**Table 7.1** Components of the Baseline DXA Report

| |
|---|
| **I. Patient & provider information** |
| Patient name |
| Medical record number |
| Date of birth |
| Gender |
| Ethnicity/race |
| Referring physician/provider |
| Measured weight, height (specify units: kg/Ib; cm/in) |
| Calculated BMI, height, weight %, or Z-scores |
| Primary diagnosis, indications for DXA test |
| *List of current relevant medications* |
| *Bone age or pubertal stage* |
| *Inclusion of possible risk factors, including documentation of nontraumatic fractures, sports participation* |
| *Calcium intake or use of calcium supplements* |
| *Use of vitamin D supplements* |
| *25OH vitamin D laboratory value* |
| **II. Test results** |
| Skeletal sites scanned |
| aBMD, BMC, bone area for each site |
| aBMD Z-scores for each site by chronological age |
| *BMD Z-scores for each site by bone age (if available)* |
| *BMD Z-scores for each site adjusted for HAZ (as needed)* |
| **III. Technical comments** |
| Manufacturer, model of instrument used |
| Software version *(e.g. Hologic Apex 5.3.1)* |
| Technical quality of the scans obtained |
| *Limitations of the study* (e.g., *artifacts, scoliosis*) |
| Pediatric reference source(s) used for Z-score calculation |
| **IV. Interpretation & recommendations** |
| Qualitative assessment of aBMD Z-score results |
| *Assessment of calcium intake in reference to DRI* |
| *Adjustments made for body size, bone age, pubertal delay* |
| *Recommendations for necessity and timing of follow-up DXA scan studies* |
| V. Body composition components[a] |
| *Body mass index, $kg/m^2$* |
| *Total mass, with head, g* |
| *Total lean mass, g* |
| *Total fat mass, g* |
| *Percentage fat mass (%)* |
| VI. VFA vertebral fracture assessment components[b] |
| *Visual evaluation documentation of vertebral height abnormalities* |
| *Fracture diagnosis including type (wedge, biconcave, crush)* |
| *Severity (mild, moderate, severe) and grade (1, 2 or 3) of abnormality* |

(continued)

**Table 7.1**  (continued)

The components in plain font are considered standard at most densitometry centers. Those in *italics* are provided as suggestions
**What should NOT be included:** *aBMD T-scores, and terms "Osteopenia" & "Osteoporosis" based on the results from the DXA examination alone*
Semi-quantitative VFA criteria by Genant- *Ref.* [24] *Genant H, et al. JBMR 1993:1137–1148*
*Modified from*
*Reference* [2]: *Crabtree NJ et al. J Clin Densitom 2014;17:2:225–242*
[a]*Reference* [4]: *Petak S et al. J Clin Densitom 2013 16;4:508*
[b]*Reference* [5]: *Vokes T et al. J Clin Densitom 2006;9:1:37*

**Table 7.2**  Additional Components of the Follow-Up DXA Report

| |
|---|
| **I. Patient & provider information** |
| Indication for follow-up DXA scan |
| *Interval fractures, change in clinical status, medications* |
| **II. Test results** |
| Skeletal sites scanned |
| BMD, BMC, bone area for each site |
| *Annualized change in BMC, BMD* |
| *Change in BMD Z-scores* |
| **III. Technical comments** |
| Which previous scans are being used for comparison? |
| Statement regarding what denotes statistical significance for change in BMD at the center, or LSC |
| *Recommendation for necessity and timing of follow-up DXA scan* |

The elements in plain font are considered standard at most densitometry centers. Those in *italics* are provided as suggestions
*Modified from*
*Reference* [2], *Crabtree NJ, et al. J Clin Densitom 2014;17:2:225–242*

used, particularly when the referring physician is familiar with the procedure and the resulting data obtained. However, one must also consider that technical consistency in the report is important as it allows for comparison amongst patients within a clinic, as well as critical information necessary for follow-up scans.

## Patient Demographics

The optimal report includes basic patient demographics (i.e., age, gender, and ethnicity or race) and anthropometrics. Weight and height taken at the time of the DXA scan should always be included in the report, along with their respective units (kg/lb or cm/in). It is very important to document patient height and weight since DXA measures areal, and not true volumetric, bone mineral density. As discussed previously in Chap. 6, bone density is underestimated in small patients as a result of the two-dimensional nature of the instrumentation [8, 9]. Documentation of patient size will be important for interpretation of the scans during the evaluation phase.

Body mass index (kg/m$^2$), growth percentiles, and standard deviation Z-scores should be calculated using current growth charts. The WHO (between 1997 and 2003) completed the Multi-Center Growth Reference Study in 8500 children measured in six countries (Brazil, Ghana, India, Norway, Oman, USA). The new international growth charts (children 0–5 years) have now been adopted for use in many countries in that they represent optimal growth with no nutritional failure. In the United States and Australia, growth charts for older children include those developed by the Centers for Disease Control in 2002 [10], whereas in the United Kingdom, growth charts were recently updated (January, 2013) to combine both UK-WHO data and UK90 now simply: UK Growth Chart [11]. Examples of these growth charts are provided in Appendix B.

The demographic and anthropometric data are helpful in determining if body size is sufficiently above or below the expected range to warrant adjustment of DXA results. For those with short stature or growth delay, the ISCD recommends the use of either Bone Mineral Apparent Density (BMAD), an estimate of volumetric BMD, or Height for age Z-score (HAZ) calculations to adjust the spine aBMD; HAZ is recommended to adjust the whole body scans [2]. Unfortunately, there are no published pediatric norms to calculate Z-scores from BMAD adjustments. Therefore, aBMD Z-scores are available only for HAZ adjustments [12]. Explanation of the modifications being made should be part of the interpretation section of the DXA report.

## Medical History

The report should include a brief summary of the relevant clinical history. This might include the primary medical diagnosis, the use of medications known to affect aBMD (e.g., growth hormone, certain anti-convulsants, glucocorticoids, proton pump inhibitors), fracture history, mobility status, endocrine abnormalities, pubertal status, bone age, and family history of osteoporosis. Physical activity level, dietary history, and use of vitamin or mineral supplements may also be useful.

As discussed in Chap. 5, clinical information prior to the scan improves both the acquisition and the interpretation of bone densitometry. Ideally, the patient's medical history should be obtained directly from the referring physician. This type of information is typically gathered with a Referral or Request for Procedure form. However, some patients will be referred for bone densitometry assessment without a complete medical history.

If the referring physician has not relayed the indications for the scan and the relevant medical history, it is possible to ask the patient, parent, or both for relevant medical information. At most imaging centers, patients are asked to complete a brief registration questionnaire at the time of the DXA procedure. Examples of pediatric DXA registration questionnaires and request for procedure forms are provided in Appendix D (see also Figure 7.1).

The DXA technologist should review the questionnaire with the parent, giving particular attention to details surrounding fracture history, endocrine or growth abnormalities, orthopedic surgeries, medication and supplement usage, and family history of osteoporosis. If, for some reason, the questionnaire cannot be adequately

**Bone Densitometry Clinic – Children's Registration Questionnaire**

Patient's Name (Last, First):__A.B_____        Today's Date:  3/24/2015

Gender:  o Male      X Female                           Date of Birth:  XX/XX/XXXX

Ethnicity: **White**

Referring Doctor: ___Dr. D_____    Department:____Gastroenterology____
             (who you would like to receive report)

Have you had this type of examination before?          o Yes   **X** No
    If yes, where did you have this done?_____

Have you ever been told you have scoliosis or a curvature of the spine? o Yes    **X** No

Why have you been referred for a bone density scan? _____possible low bone density_____

Have you ever had surgery on your hip?        o Yes   X No
    If yes, which hip was it performed on?        o Right  o Left   o Both

Do you participate in at least 60 min of physical activity every day?      o Yes   X No

Have you ever broken (fractured) a bone?                        o Yes    X No
    If yes, when was your last fracture? _____

Have you had any exams within the last 7 days where a contrast material was used (e.g. barium, MRI)? NO
    If so, which exam? _____When was this done?_____

Does your family have a history of osteoporosis?                X Yes    o No
  If yes, please describe relation to patient (e.g. mother, grandmother, aunt etc.)__grandmother_____
  If yes, was this a hip fracture?__arm fx_____  Is this person taking medication for osteoporosis?___yes, fosamax_

Have you ever taken corticosteroids (e.g. steroids/prednisone)?        X Yes   o No

Do you currently take any prescribed medications?                X Yes   o No
    If so, please list them here:___Remicade, and Delzicol _____

Do you take **calcium supplements** on a regular basis?        o Yes   X No
    If yes, how much?_____500_____mg   and how frequently? _ 2x/day_____

Do you take **vitamin D supplements** on a regular basis?      o Yes   X No
    If yes, how much?_____IU    and how frequently? _____

**For FEMALE patients only:**  Have you begun to menstruate?                    o Yes    X No
          If yes, Do you have a regular menstrual period?      o Yes    o No
          Is there any chance that you may be pregnant?       o Yes    X No

**Calcium Intake:**   For each food listed below, please indicate the number of servings you (the patient) consumes of these calcium rich foods <u>in a typical week</u>. If you consume 1/2 cup of milk on your cereal each morning you can respond:       Milk = 0.5 servings per day **OR**  3.5 servings per week

|  | Serving Size | # servings / week |
|---|---|---|
| Milk any type (including fortified soy milk) alone or in co | 1 cup | 7 |
| Calcium fortified orange juice | 1 cup | 0 |
| Yogurt | 1 cup | 0 |
| Cheese (alone or in sandwiches, casseroles etc) | 1 slice | 0 |
| Ice Cream, frozen yogurt, pudding or custards | ½ cup | 0 |
| Macaroni & cheese, quesadillas, tacos/burritos | 1 cup or item | 0 |
| Pizza (any type) | 1 slice | 0 |
| Tofu | ½ cup | 0 |
| Beans (white, navy, pinto, baked) | ½ cup | 0 |
| Almonds or Pistachios | 1 oz (about 24) | 2.5 |
| Cooked green vegetables | ½ cup | 3 |
| Breakfast Cereal: specify cereal type:_____ | 1 cup | 0 |

**Fig. 7.1** Example Registration Questionnaire for 'Patient AB'

completed at the time of examination (e.g., because of a language barrier or because the child is not accompanied by a parent), the form can be faxed to the referring clinic for completion after the DXA procedure is completed.

## Test Results

For each skeletal site that is assessed, aBMD, BMC, and bone area should be included, as should the corresponding aBMD Z-score, to allow the clinician to determine if the measured values are within the expected range for age. BMC and bone areas are used to calculate estimates of volumetric BMD at the spine [BMAD] and should be included in the report. Reporting BMC and bone area also allows the clinician to examine subsequent changes due to bone growth.

Calculating changes in aBMD over time requires thoughtful consideration in pediatric patients. Although no one approach has been shown to be best, some practices can minimize error. Prior to any calculations or interpretations, scan images should be carefully examined during scan acquisition to optimize comparability of repeated measurements. Many experts believe that it is more informative to examine changes in BMC, rather than aBMD, in pediatric patients because of the variable of growth (see more detail in Chap. 6: Evaluation) [13]. In adult patients, the size of the skeleton remains relatively constant, making longitudinal comparisons of aBMD appropriate. In pediatric patients, bone growth leads to changes in bone area as well as BMC. These parameters may not increase in parallel. In fact, Bailey et al. [14] have shown that peak height velocity precedes the periods of peak bone mineral accrual by several months in teens. In recent years, there are more robust pediatric-specific reference data. However, BMC Z-scores are infrequently reported because they have yet to be incorporated into the manufacturer software. For this reason, the aBMD Z-score is typically reported and, as needed, adjusted for bone and body size.

Calculating the pediatric aBMD Z-score, however, can be challenging because there is still no universal pediatric reference data set for all DXA manufacturers. Some centers have chosen to utilize the normative data in the manufacturer's most recent software program, whereas others use published or locally collected reference values. The source of the reference data used to calculate the aBMD Z-score should always be cited in the report because the Z-score will vary if a different reference data set is used [15]. Now that race-specific reference data are more readily available for pediatric populations, and are known to significantly affect Z-score generation and clinical interpretation, it is crucial to identify when race-specific reference data are used in the DXA analysis [12].

Within the results table itself, the units for reporting DXA results are now standardized. The International Society for Clinical Densitometry has published guidelines for nomenclature for both bone densitometry and body composition, and has standardized decimal places for numeric data frequently reported (see Table 7.3).

**Table 7.3** ISCD Guidelines for DXA Reporting Nomenclature for a Pediatric Report

| Measure | Decimal places | Example |
|---|---|---|
| BMD (g/cm²) | 3 | 0.655 |
| Z-score | 1 | −1.5 |
| BMC, spine or hip scan (g) | 2 | 28.52 |
| BMC, whole body scan (g) | 0 | 1652 |
| Area, spine or hip scan (cm²) | 2 | 44.66 |
| Area, whole body scan (cm²) | 0 | 1850 |

## Technical Comments

The report should include sufficient detail regarding how the DXA was performed and interpreted to allow comparisons with previous and future densitometry studies. Given the intrinsic differences between densitometers and the software used for bone densitometry assessment, the manufacturer and model of the instrument should be specified (e.g., Hologic Discovery A) (see Table 7.1 and further discussion in Chap. 3). Similarly, the software mode used to acquire and analyze the scan should also be provided (e.g., auto-low density software). If reference data are used in the calculation of Z-scores that are different from the manufacturer's normative data, the source for the normative data should be cited.

Prior to the preparation of the report, careful visual review of each scan must be made to ensure that artifacts do not affect data obtained. The report should outline any technical difficulties encountered with obtaining the scan (see example DXA report Fig. 7.2). Documentation is important, both for the initial interpretation of the DXA scan and to alert the DXA technologist to these effects when acquiring future scans. These might include scoliosis, degenerative disease, vertebral compression fractures, or nonremovable metal artifacts (see Table 7.4). Nonremovable artifacts in the scan field region of interest can cause significant errors in spine BMD measurements when the artifact is near or lying-over lumbar spine vertebrae [16, 17]. When these types of artifacts are present, BMD measurements should be questioned. Scans with motion artifacts or removable metal objects (e.g., metal from the underwire or clasp of a bra, a belt buckle, a pant zipper, or a belly button ring) should not be reported. These scans should be repeated before the patient leaves the clinic. Additionally, if the default position of neck box is changed in the analysis of the proximal femur scan this must be clearly documented in the report as neither the BMC Z-score nor BMAD calculations are valid (see Chap. 6). Analysis of longitudinal changes in growing children can prove to be difficult. As was highlighted in Chaps. 5 and 6, good practice should be used in positioning and analysis for all DXA scans. If there is deviation from good practice in the baseline or current scan, this should be noted on the report.

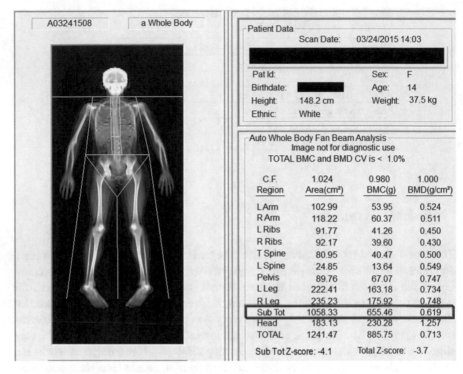

**Fig. 7.2** Example Whole Body Scan Image from Hologic Scanner for 'Patient AB'

**Table 7.4** Examples of Technical Problems Noted on Reports

| I. Representative Technical Comments | |
|---|---|
| Spine scan | Scoliosis noted in lumbar region |
| | Compression fracture in L1, L2-4 used for analysis |
| | Osteoarthritis noted in L1, L2-4 used for analysis<br>Surgical clip noted near L2, did not interfere with scan<br>G-tube noted proximal to L1, L2-4 used in analysis |
| Proximal femur scan | Left hip replacement, right proximal femur scanned |
| | Incomplete hip rotation, prominent lesser trochanter |
| Whole body scan | Permanent pins in right wrist secondary to fracture |
| | Gold crowns on molar teeth<br>Indwelling Port-a-cath in upper right quadrant |
| **II. Avoidable artifacts** | |
| Spine scan | Pant zipper artifact in L3, L4 |
| Proximal femur scan | Metal coin artifact in pocket, interferes with femoral neck |
| Whole body scan | Bracelet on left forearm<br>Necklace |
| | Underwire bra in upper left and right quadrants |

## *Interpretation and Recommendations*

The most challenging and controversial elements of the pediatric DXA report are "Interpretation" and "Recommendations." For postmenopausal women, the interpretation of DXA results are fairly straightforward, based upon WHO criteria for osteoporosis [1] and the Fracture Risk Assessment Tool (FRAX®), released in 2008 [18], these tools assist in determining which patients are most suitable for pharmacological therapy. Though diagnostic categories for low bone mass in pediatrics have been clarified, there is still no established algorithm to calculate the 10-year probability of fracture in a pediatric patient, similarly there is no consensus as to how bone density results alone should guide decisions regarding treatment.

The aBMD Z-score is presented in numeric terms within the results table of the DXA report; additionally, these results can be reported in qualitative terms. As the term "low BMD for chronological age" is appropriate to use for pediatric patients with aBMD Z-scores less than or equal to −2.0 [2]. In patients with delayed growth or puberty, it may also be appropriate to adjust for bone size and maturation. These adjustments should be explained in this section of the report (see example DXA report Figs. 7.2 and 7.3). For example, the report for an 18-year-old female with a height-for-age Z-score of −2.8 might include both the Z-score based upon reference data for healthy 18-year-old females, as well as a HAZ adjusted Z-score that takes into account the short stature [12]. Of note, there is no single adjustment that will be appropriate for every clinical situation. The limitations of these possible adjustment factors are described in detail in Chap. 6 (Fig. 7.2).

An assessment of fracture risk in children should not be reported based on DXA data alone. In addition, the terms "osteopenia" and "osteoporosis" should not be used in pediatric DXA reports since they refer specifically to WHO fracture risk criteria developed for postmenopausal women [2]. The term osteoporosis may be used for the pediatric patient with low bone mass (≤−2.0) combined with a significant fracture history. Significant fracture history in a pediatric patient in the absence of a vertebral compression fracture is defined as at least two or more long bone fractures by age 10 or three or more long bone fractures by age 19 [2, 19]. There is a relationship between low aBMD Z-score by DXA and fracture risk in pediatric patients, but it is far less developed [20, 21].

Interpretation of follow-up scans should include a discussion of changes in BMC, aBMD, and aBMD Z-scores. In follow-up scans, most pediatric patients would be expected to have an increase in BMC, bone area, and aBMD. It is important not to confuse an increase in aBMD or BMC with an improvement in bone mineral status. In order for the change to be an improvement, the aBMD Z-score of the follow-up scan should be greater than the previous aBMD Z-score. If aBMD has decreased overtime, examination of changes in BMC and bone area may help explain the reason for the change in aBMD (i.e., the loss of mineral or an increase in bone area). Given the current paucity of robust pediatric reference data for BMC by chronological age, the aBMD Z-score for each scan is typically reported (Fig. 7.3).

Interpretation of repeat scans also requires attention to physical changes that have occurred in the growing patient as well as any new pertinent medical findings

## Bone Densitometry Report

Report Date: 03/25/2015                          Date of Birth: XX/XX/XXXX
Scan Date: 03/24/2015                            Technologist: L.C.
Previous Scan Date: None at CHRCO                Referring Physician: Dr. D.

Patient History: A.B. is a 14 y.o. 2 mo old premenarchial female patient referred for initial bone mineral density assessment. She has a past medical history of Crohn's disease, diagnosed in January, 2014. Family history is notable for a twin sister also recently diagnosed with Crohn's disease and low bone mass as well as a grandmother with a fracture history, currently being treated with alendronate. Current prescribed medications include infliximab infusions every 8 weeks and daily mesalamine. Calcium intake is estimated to be 350 mg/day (diet only + 1000 mg calcium supplementation). She does not take additional vitamin D supplementation.

Lab Results:    25OH Vit D:    19 ng/mL       10/24/2014
History of corticosteroid use:    Yes
Fracture history:                 None reported

Anthropometrics:
Height: 148.2 cm (Z = -2.0)       Weight: 37.5 kg (Z = -1.8)       Body mass index: 17.1 kg/m$^2$ (Z= -0.9)

| | Spine, L1-L4 | Total Hip | Whole Body* |
|---|---|---|---|
| Type of Analysis | Fast Array | Fast Array | Auto Whole Body |
| Area, cm2 | 35.84 | 24.37 | 1058 |
| BMC, g | 19.53 | 13.34 | 655 |
| aBMD, g/cm2 | 0.545 | 0.548 | 0.619 |
| BMD Z-score | -3.7 | -3.6 | -4.1 |
| HAZ Adjusted Z-score | -2.6 | | -3.2 |
| | | | |
| Body Composition | Lean, g | Fat, g | Fat, % |
| | 25102 | 12227 | 32.0 |

Instrument Hardware / Software: Hologic Discovery A Bone Densitometer (v 12.6.1)
Anthropometric Z-scores based on CDC 2-20 Years.
*Whole body scan less head reported in accordance with ISCD recommendations
HAZ Adjusted Z-scores according to Zemel BS, et al. J Clin Endo Metab. 2010;95(3):1265-73.
Notable interfering factors: None

Interpretation & Recommendations: A.B. BMD Z-scores are considered below the normal range for chronological age, as defined by the ISCD guidelines for pediatric patients as a BMD Z-score less than -2.0. Given BMD can be underestimated in patients who are small for age, A.B.'s results were adjusted for her height for age Z-score (-2.0). When this is done, her height adjusted spine BMD Z-score is -2.6, her adjusted whole body BMC Z-score: -2.9, and whole body BMD Z-score: -3.2. Therefore, some of the deficits observed may be considered instrument artifact, but low bone mass remains even after height adjustment. A.B.'s calcium intake is consistent with recommendations for age of 1300 mg/day, whereas her circulating vitamin D level is in the deficient range (<20 ng/mL). Recommend continued focus on calcium intake and monitoring of 25OH vitamin D to maintain a level >30 ng/ml for optimum bone mineralization. Repeat DXA scans as clinically indicated, typically in one year.

Summary of Key Terms:
BMC: bone mineral content (g); aBMD: areal bone mineral density (g/cm2)
Z-score: number of SD's above or below the mean of a healthy population matched for age and gender.
ISCD: International Society for Clinical Densitometry. HAZ: height for age Z-score
Least significant change (LSC) for a spine scan in serial DXA for our center: 0.026g/cm$^2$

**Fig. 7.3** Example DXA Report for 'Patient AB'

when possible. Specifically, observations of delay in growth or pubertal development of the child should be acknowledged because these alterations may also affect bone growth. Significant dietary changes (e.g., the resolution of anorexia nervosa or the initiation of calcium supplementation) might influence bone health and may be noted. If physical activity has increased or decreased significantly since the last examination or if the patient was confined to bedrest due to illness for a significant time period, this too may be noted. Detailing fractures that have occurred is critical, as is documentation of pertinent medical findings since the last examination, for example, bone age assessments or initiation or cessation of corticosteroid therapy.

Typically, repeat DXA scans are performed every 1–2 years, but may be repeated as often as every 6 months if a patient has a significant change in therapy or has had a worsening in clinical status. The optimal time interval between DXA measures in children has been addressed using data from the Bone Mineral Density in Childhood Study (BMDCS) [22]. The study found that the optimal interval differs by pubertal stage and skeletal site. On average, spine and total body less head were the most reproducible skeletal sites with the shortest calculated interval between scans in children <14 years (~6 months). Otherwise, scans were to be repeated annually.

In order to determine if changes in BMD exceed the variability or "noise" of repeated scans, calculations must be made a priori for what is commonly referred to as the least-significant change (LSC). The LSC takes into account both the instrument's and the technologist's precision estimates, as well as the level of statistical confidence that is thought to be clinically relevant. Details for performing these precision studies and guidelines for how to calculate the LSC have been provided elsewhere [23] (see Chap. 3). The LSC for the DXA center should be included in any densitometry report of longitudinal data. Only changes in the region of interest that are equal to or greater than the LSC can be considered significant.

## Other Components

A formal DXA report should include a header identifying the name of the clinic and the location at which the scan studies were performed, a signature line for the author of the report, and a footer that defines all key terminology.

There are advantages and disadvantages to including a copy of the DXA proprietary software report. These reports provide the raw data upon which the report is based and the scan images in which acquisition errors may be observed. Unfortunately, in early software versions (Hologic < version 12.5) these reports may also contain the $T$-scores and the WHO classification guidelines, which are inappropriate for use in pediatric subjects. Therefore, if included, the finalized report from the DXA center must caution against the use of the $T$-score. When the DXA software proprietary reports are provided to the referring physician, the summary report should still include BMC, bone area, and aBMD, and also the complete information on the DXA equipment used, in case the propriety and summary reports get separated in the medical record. For clinics that transmit reports by fax, be aware that color images do not reproduce well in facsimile.

Optional maxims to include at the end of the report might include suggestions on the timing of the next DXA examination, recommendations for calcium and vitamin D dietary intake or supplementation, and encouragements for cessation of smoking and participation in non-impact weight bearing physical activity to improve bone mineralization.

In conclusion, the DXA report for the pediatric patient is an important part of the imaging exam. Without the report, manufacturer proprietary images and numerical data could be mis-interpreted by referring physicians unfamiliar with $T$-scores, $Z$-scores, software and reference data in the field of pediatric densitometry. Careful review of patient scans prior to reporting, and review of patient medical history will improve the accuracy and utility of the pediatric DXA report. A timely, concise, and informative report which relays the DXA findings will avoid costly and potentially dangerous mis-interpretations by physicians unfamiliar with pediatric densitometry data.

## Summary Points

- A timely, concise, and informative DXA report is essential to relay densitometry findings and to avoid costly and potentially dangerous misinterpretations by referring physicians unfamiliar with interpreting pediatric densitometry data.
- Enough information should be provided in the report to allow for comparison to previous and subsequent DXA studies.
- The technical DXA report ideally has five basic elements: (1) patient demographics, (2) a brief medical history, (3) test results, (4) technical comments, and (5) interpretation and often recommendations.
- Medical history information to include in the report: primary medical diagnosis, use of medications known to affect bone health, fracture history, anthropometric data and when available, pubertal status, bone age, as well as focused dietary and physical activity history.
- Careful review of the DXA scan images must be made prior to reporting of results to avoid misinterpretation of the findings based on artifacts in the scan field.
- Reporting densitometry data in pediatrics is unique and different than for adult patients—the most challenging and controversial elements are interpretation and recommendations.
- Inclusion of the model and software used for scan acquisition, as well as the reference data used in the interpretation of the data, is crucial to the pediatric report.
- $T$-scores should never used, and the terms "osteopenia" and "osteoporosis" should not be included in pediatric DXA reports without documentation of significant fracture history.
- For pediatric patients with significant growth delays, spine aBMD Z-score should be adjusted for using either BMAD or HAZ calculations; whole body aBMD Z-score should be adjusted for height for age Z-score.

## References

1. World Health Organization. Assessment of fracture risk and its application to screening for post-menopausal osteoporosis WHO technical report series. World Health Organ Tech Rep Ser. 1994;843:1–129.
2. Crabtree NJ, Arabi A, Bachrach LK, Fewtrell M, El-Hajj Fuleihan G, Kecskemethy HH, Jaworski M, Gordon CM. Dual-energy X-Ray absorptiometry interpretation and reporting in children and adolescents: the revised 2013 ISCD pediatric official positions. J Clin Densitom. 2014;17(2):225–42.
3. Gordon CM, Bachrach LK, Carpenter TO, Crabtree N, El-Hajj Fuleihan G, Kutilek S, Lorenc RS, Tosi LL, Ward KA, Ward LM, Kalkwarf HJ. Dual energy X-ray absorptiometry interpretation and reporting in children and adolescents: the 2007 ISCD pediatric official positions. J Clin Densitom. 2008;11(1):43–58.

4. Petak S, Barbu CG, Yu EW, Fielding R, Mulligan K, Sabowitz B, Wu CH, Shepherd JA. The official positions of the International Society for Clinical Densitometry: body composition analysis reporting. J Clin Densitom. 2013;16(4):508–19.
5. Vokes T, Bachman D, Baim S, Binkley N, Broy S, Ferrar L, Lewiecki ME, Richmond B, Schousboe J. Vertebral fracture assessment: The 2005 ISCD official positions. J Clin Densitom. 2006;9(1):37–46.
6. Berkman ND, Sheridan SL, Donahue KE, Halpern DJ, Crotty K. Low health literacy and health outcomes: an updated systematic review. Ann Intern Med. 2011;155(2):97–107.
7. Edmonds SW, Solimeo SL, Lu X, Roblin DW, Saag KG, Cram P. Developing a bone mineral density test result letter to send to patients: a mixed-methods study. Patient Prefer Adherence. 2014;8:827–41.
8. Fewtrell MS, British Paediatric Adolescent Bone Group. Bone densitometry in children assessed by dual x-ray absorptiometry: uses and pitfalls. Arch Dis Child. 2003;88:795–8.
9. Fewtrell MS, Gordon I, Biassoni L, Cole TJ. Dual x-ray absorptiometry (DXA) of the lumbar spine in a clinical pediatric setting: does the method of size adjustment matter? Bone. 2005;37:413–9.
10. Kuczmarski RJ, Ogden CL, Guo SS, Grummer-Strawn LM, Flegal KM, Mei Z, Wei R, Curtin LR, Roche AF, Johnson CL. 2000 CDC growth charts for the United States: methods and development. Vital Health Stat. 2002;11:1–190.
11. Freeman JV, Cole TJ, Chinn S, Jones PRM, White EM, Preece MA. Cross sectional stature and weight reference curves for the UK, 1990. Arch Dis Child. 1995;73:17–24.
12. Zemel BS, Leonard MB, Kelly A, Lappe JM, Gilsanz V, Oberfield S, Mahboubi S, Shepherd JA, Hangartner TN, Frederick MM, Winer KK, Kalkwarf HJ. Height adjustment in assessing dual energy x-ray absorptiometry measurements of bone mass and density in children. J Clin Endocrinol Metab. 2010;95(3):1265–73.
13. Heaney RP. BMD: the problem. Osteoporos Int. 2005;16:1013–5.
14. Bailey DA, McKay HA, Mirwald RL, Crocker PRE, Faulkner RA. A six-year longitudinal study of the relationship of physical activity to bone mineral accrual in growing children: The University of Saskatchewan Bone Mineral Accrual Study. J Bone Miner Res. 1999;14:1672–9.
15. Leonard MB, Propert KJ, Zemel BS, Stallings VA, Feldman HI. Discrepancies in pediatric bone mineral density reference data: potential for misdiagnosis of osteopenia. J Pediatr. 1999;135:182–8.
16. Sherman ME, Shepard J, Frassetto L, Genant HK. Discrepancy in results between spine and hip scans of a woman with end stage renal disease. J Clin Densitom. 2002;5(1):95–8.
17. Morgan SL, Lopez-Ben R, Nunnally N, Burroughs L, Fineberg N, Tubbs RS, Yester MV. "Black hole artifacts"—a new potential pitfall for DXA accuracy? J Clin Densitom. 2008;11(2):266–75.
18. Watts NB, Lewiecki EM, Miller PD, Baim S. National Osteoporosis Foundation 2008 clinician's guide to prevention and treatment of osteoporosis and the World Health Organization Fracture Risk Assessment Tool (FRAX): what they mean to the bone densitometrist and bone technologist. J Clin Densitom. 2008;11(4):473–7.
19. Bishop N, Arundel P, Clark E, Dimitri P, Farr J, Jones G, Makitie O, Munns CF, Shaw N. Fracture prediction and the definition of osteoporosis in children and adolescents: the ISCD 2013 pediatric official positions. J Clin Densitom. 2014;17(2):275–80.
20. Clark EM, Tobias JH, Ness AR. Association between bone density and fractures in children: a systematic review and meta-analysis. Pediatrics. 2006;117(2):e291–7.
21. Clark EM, Ness AR, Tobias JH. Bone fragility contributes to the risk of fracture in children, even after moderate and severe trauma. J Bone Miner Res. 2008;23(2):173–9.
22. Shepherd JA, Wang L, Fan B, et al. Optimal monitoring time interval between DXA measures in children. J Bone Min Res. 2011;26(11):2745–52.
23. Bonnick SL. Bone densitometry in clinical practice: application and interpretation. 2nd ed. Totowa, NJ: Humana Press; 2004. p. 287–300.
24. Genant HK, Wu CY, van Kuijk C, Nevitt MC. Vertebral fracture assessment using a semiquantitative technique. J Bone Miner Res. 1993;8(9):1137–48.

# Chapter 8
# DXA Evaluation of Infants and Toddlers

Bonny L. Specker and Teresa L. Binkley

## Introduction

The clinical assessment of bone health or bone fragility of infants and toddlers has typically relied on standard radiography to assess density and specific disease conditions (e.g., rickets, fracture). Radiography is subjective, is not quantitative, and large changes must occur before low bone density can be detected [1]. This lack of sensitivity led to a significant interest in objective, quantitative measurements in the clinical evaluation and monitoring of changes in bone mineral content (BMC) and bone mineral density (BMD) of infants and toddlers. Methods such as dual energy X-ray absorptiometry (DXA) allow for quantitative measurements that have good precision and can reliably assess and monitor changes in BMC and BMD. Preterm infants are known to have significant osteopenia and were one of the first populations to be studied using DXA [2]. Despite this interest in the preterm infant, research in this age group lagged behind that of older children and adolescents. However, given the extensive amount of literature on DXA bone measures in preterm and term infants that now exists [3–11], and the interest in utilizing quantitative measurements to evaluate and monitor changes in BMC and BMD, the International Society of Clinical Densitometry (ISCD) recently developed guidelines for infants and children less than 5 years of age [12].

The purpose of this review is to briefly discuss the use of quantitative ultrasound (QUS) and peripheral quantitative computed tomography (pQCT) for assessing bone parameters, and provide greater details on the use of DXA in infants and toddlers. Evidence for a relationship between bone density and fractures will be discussed, as well as the appropriate skeletal sites to measure, issues that are relevant

B.L. Specker, Ph.D. (✉) • T.L. Binkley, Ph.D.
EA Martin Program, South Dakota State University,
SWC, Box 506, 1021 Medary Avenue, North Brookings, SD 57006, USA
e-mail: bonny.specker@sdstate.edu; teresa.binkley@sdstate.edu

© Springer International Publishing Switzerland 2016                                   151
E.B. Fung et al. (eds.), *Bone Health Assessment in Pediatrics*,
DOI 10.1007/978-3-319-30412-0_8

to infants and toddlers, factors that are associated with bone measurements, and a summary of the current recommendations on who should be scanned and how results should be presented.

## Methods for Quantifying Bone

QUS, pQCT, and DXA have been used to assess bone in adults and techniques are covered in more detail in Chap. 2. These methods have been modified to accommodate measurement of small bones with lower density.

### *Ultrasound and pQCT*

The velocity and attenuation of the ultrasound waves are measured and expressed as speed of sound (SOS) and broadband attenuation (BUA). SOS through bone is defined by the ratio of the traversed distance to the transit time (m/s) and is dependent on the density, the micro- and macrostructure, and the elastic modulus, which reflects the stiffness of a material. Energy is lost when the ultrasound wave travels through the material and this phenomenon is known as attenuation. Although not discussed in detail here, there are normative pediatric reference data sets for several of the available ultrasound devices [13–17]. Infant and toddler QUS measurements are typically made at the mid-tibia, distal third of the radius, or at the phalanges. The main advantage of QUS is that it is easily transportable to the bedside for use in infants and toddlers for whom DXA measurements are not feasible (e.g., preterm infants in the neonatal intensive care unit, studies where measurements need to be in the field). QUS is technically simpler and more economical compared with DXA and pQCT. Some investigators have found that QUS measures are correlated with areal BMD (aBMD) [18, 19], although others suggest that since QUS measures more than just density there should not be a correlation [13, 20]. Pluskiewica and coworkers found that DXA and phalangeal QUS measurements do not identify the same patients with reduced bone mineral status and speculated that this was because these two techniques are measuring different bone properties [20]. The disadvantages of QUS include the influence of probe size [21] and subcutaneous fat thickness [22] on speed of sound measurements.

Peripheral quantitative computed tomography (pQCT) is used to measure volumetric BMD (vBMD) in the peripheral skeleton. This technology has the ability to separate and measure both trabecular bone tissue, generally found at the end of the long bones, and cortical bone tissue found in the shaft. By the mid to late 1990s, pQCT was being used to investigate geometric and biomechanical bone properties [23, 24], establish reference data [25, 26], correlate muscle and bone strength [27–29] and obtain measurements in older children [30, 31]. Utilization of pQCT to measure bone characteristics of infants and toddlers has been limited, though some studies have been published [32–36]. General advantages of pQCT are that it yields volumetric measures of bone density (vBMD, mg/cm³), as well as geometric measures and biomechanical strength indices. These measurements may inform why DXA measures are affected among children with specific diseases or conditions [37, 38]. For example, aBMD by DXA may be low due to a thin cortical shell leading to decreased BMC rather than an actual reduction in vBMD. Disadvantages of pQCT include lack of standard scan sites, standard acquisition parameters (voxel sizes and scan speeds are set by the operator and vary among studies) and analysis algorithms, which have limited its clinical utility. Additional considerations for use in infants and toddlers include difficulty in positioning an arm or leg in the measurement gantry. Pediatric positioning devices were developed in the late 1990s and have reduced movement and increased the percent of valid scans, but these devices were developed for older children and not infants and toddlers. In addition, infants and toddlers have smaller bones with thinner cortices, and cortical vBMD cannot be accurately measured at cortical thicknesses <2 mm [32]. Binkley et al. found that mean cortical thickness at the distal 20 % tibia site in 3–4 year old children was 1.2 mm thereby excluding the measurement of cortical vBMD [32]. Despite the inability to obtain cortical vBMD measurements, total cross-sectional bone area, cortical area, and cortical thickness can be accurately measured in these children and provide important information. An additional consideration of pQCT is the inability to obtain repeated measurements at the same bone site in longitudinal studies due to variations in longitudinal bone growth rates. Movement also can cause errors in locating the measurement site, especially if the movement occurs between the scout view and slice imaging. pQCT measures of healthy older children have been used to establish reference ranges for bone growth patterns that can be used as a comparison when studying the bone of diseased children [26, 39, 40]. pQCT measurements in healthy children have been done to test the effects of activity, bone loading, diet, pubertal stage, and hormonal status on bone [7, 33, 41–46]. Despite the increasing number of studies reporting pQCT results in older children and the establishment of normative reference ranges, reference data for infants and toddlers are limited.

## *DXA*

DXA was introduced in the late 1980s for use in postmenopausal women; scan acquisition and analysis applications for infants and young children using pencil beam technology began in the early 1990s. Pencil beam technology was replaced by fan-beam technology leading to a significantly faster scan acquisition time. Although there were numerous studies validating bone and body composition measurements against small animal carcass data for pencil beam devices, only a few studies have validated the Hologic fan-beam scanners [47, 48]. No validation of the GE/Lunar current generation fan-beam devices has been carried out for small subjects.

The speed of a DXA scan and the minimal radiation exposure allow it to be easily used in pediatric populations. Effective doses of radiation exposure for the whole body scan and pediatric spine scans are all less than 5 μSv [49, 50], well below the annual radiation exposure limits recommended by the National Council for Radiation Protection [51] for public infrequent exposures of 5000 μSv and approximately the same as the annual negligible individual dose of 10 μSv.

Since DXA images are two-dimensional, a true measure of vBMD cannot be obtained. BMD obtained from DXA is referred to as areal BMD (aBMD) and is a function of both the amount of bone mineral and the projected bone area (aBMD = BMC/bone area (g/cm$^2$). It is important to consider bone size when assessing bone measures in only two dimensions since a larger bone size may artificially inflate aBMD measurements [52]. This is illustrated in studies that show that aBMD increases with age, despite vBMD remaining relatively constant until the time of puberty when there is a large increase [53, 54]. Mathematical methods have been proposed to adjust aBMD to more closely reflect vBMD [30, 55]. These methods include the calculation of bone mineral apparent density (BMAD), which for the spine divides BMC by the projected bone area to the power of 1.5 [56], or inclusion of bone and body size parameters in a regression approach (size-adjusted bone mineral content (SA-BMC)) [55, 57]. BMAD has only been used in a few infant studies [58, 59]. Expressing BMC-for-bone area or BMC-for-height [55] or correcting for bone size by using length or height-for-age Z-scores [60] have been suggested as alternatives to correct for the influence of size on aBMD measures.

## Relationships Between Bone Measurements and Fracture

Although bone density in adults has been shown to be associated with fracture risk, the association between bone measures and fracture risk in children has only recently been confirmed in longitudinal studies. Several older case control studies were completed that showed decreased aBMD in children with a fracture [61–63]. However, the BMD measurements in these studies took place a significant time after the fracture when BMD could be decreased due to immobilization or decreased activity levels. However, findings from longitudinal studies [64, 65], or a recent case-control study where bone measurements were obtained soon after fracture [66], also found associations between fracture risk and low BMC or BMD. Although these studies found that low BMC or BMD is associated with increased fracture risk in older children, there are few data on the relationship between BMC or BMD and fracture risk in infants and toddlers.

It has been hypothesized that poor bone accrual during growth in humans affects lifelong bone strength [67, 68]. BMC, aBMD, and bone area have all been shown to be directly related to bone strength in growing animals, with BMC being the best overall predictor [69]. Although fractures in healthy infants are not common due to their non-ambulatory state and low risk of accidental trauma, the increase in mobility during the second and third years of life places toddlers at greater risk of sustaining a trauma that may result in a fracture. Fracture rates increase steadily in childhood from about 2 years of age until their peak in early adolescence [70].

DXA is the preferred method for assessment of bone health in older children and adolescence as outlined in the 2007 ISCD Position Statements owing to its widespread availability, low cost, ease of use, good precision and safety [71]. These advantages hold true for use in infants and toddlers as well, as outlined by the 2013 ISCD Position Statement [12].

## Commonly Measured Skeletal Sites

Whole body and regional scans (lumbar spine, proximal femur, forearm) are available on most DXA devices. The whole body and lumbar spine are the most common DXA measurement sites in infants and toddlers and are the preferred sites recommended in the 2013 ISCD statement [12].

### Whole Body

Analysis of the whole body provides information on BMC, bone area, and lean and fat mass. The rapid growth rate and bone accrual that occurs during infancy makes it likely to observe changes in whole body BMC over a short period.

Some investigators have recommended that whole body BMC, not aBMD, is the correct bone measure in growth studies [55, 72], but because whole body BMC is so dependent on body size it is important to view measurements in terms of length or height of the infant or toddler. It also has been proposed that the head BMC be omitted from whole body scan results due to the large contribution of the head to total bone mass in this age group and the significant changes in the proportion of the head to whole body BMC that occur early in life [73]. The 2007 ISCD recommendations for children older than 5 years was to exclude the head from whole body scan results and report the results as total body less head (TBLH). The rationale was that because the skull contains such a large percent of the overall BMC that TBLH results might be more sensitive to observing changes in BMC if the disease or condition being studied does not affect the skull. However, there is a possibility that bone is redistributed during loading and unloading: head BMC is lower, while BMC of the remaining skeleton is higher, in young gymnasts compared to non-gymnasts [74], and the skull has a significant increase in BMC, while BMC of the remaining skeleton has a decrease, during prolonged bed rest studies of older individuals [75, 76].

Another reason for using TBLH for infants is that the head is difficult to position and movement artifacts are often a problem in this area of the scan when measuring infants and toddlers. The 2013 ISCD guidelines made no recommendation for inclusion or exclusion of the head region from whole body DXA results since there are no data regarding fracture prediction or how specific disease affect whole body bone distribution. Due to the difficulties in obtaining a movement-free whole body scan (see below) and the lack of appropriate normative data bases, the 2013 ISCD guidelines for infants and young children stated that DXA whole body BMC measurements for children <3 years are of limited clinical utility [12].

## Regional Scans

Region-specific scans can be completed at numerous bone sites on DXA. In addition, regional measurements can be obtained from the whole body scan, although the two types are not comparable with regional measurements from the whole body scan having a poorer resolution [77]. Regional scans of the spine, femur, and forearm are feasible since movement is minimized due to short scan times (<30 s) and it is possible to hold the infant or toddler without interfering with the scan image.

The spine scan is the most commonly reported regional scan in infants and has been successfully used in newborns as early as 27 weeks of gestation and weighing as little as 1.2 kg [78]. The scan speed for the current fan-beam devices is about 30 s and precision estimates in 307 infants and toddlers aged 1–36 months for spine BMC and aBMD are 2.2 and 1.8 % respectively, with better precision at older ages [79]. Normative spine BMD curves for infants aged 0–364 days and spine BMC and aBMD curves for 1–36 month olds using the Hologic Discovery A fan-beam densitometer [58, 79] are shown in Figs. 8.1 and 8.2, respectively.

Hazell and coworkers compared forearm DXA data from 57 children aged 2–5 years obtained on a Hologic 4500 Discovery and found these data to agree with a

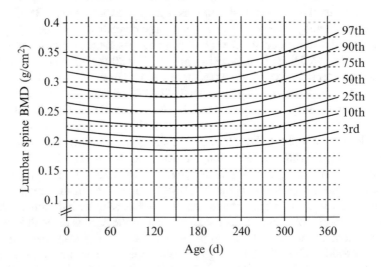

**Fig. 8.1** Spine BMD-for-age reference curve for infants, birth to 12 months. Taken from Gallo et al. [58]. Data were obtained on a Hologic QDR 4500A ($n=59$)

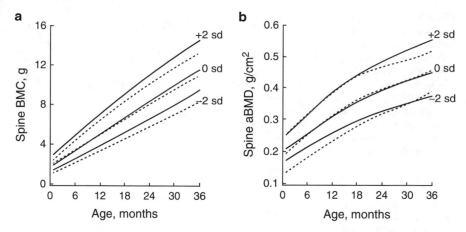

**Fig. 8.2** Median and ±2 standard deviation curves for lumbar spine BMC (**a**) and aBMD (**b**) for age for boys (*solid lines*) and girls (*dashed lines*). Taken from Kalkwarf et al. [79]. Data were obtained on a Hologic Discovery A fan-beam (*n* = 307)

portable DXA (pDXA) [80]. Precision estimates of forearm bone measurements using the current generation of DXA devices in infants and toddlers are not currently available in the literature.

Proximal femur scans have been performed on children as young as 2–3 years of age [81–84] and the whole femur in infants up to 12 months of age [58, 85]. The analysis of these scans is difficult due to the short femoral neck, low bone density, and the shape of the trochanter, leading the ISCD to recommend that the proximal femur scan not be obtained for clinical purposes in children <5 years of age.

## Bone Measurement Issues

### Equipment and Software Differences

Despite the extensive use of DXA in infants, discrepancies exist among studies in the reported normative values for BMC, aBMD, and body composition. In a large part these discrepancies are due to differences in the acquisition and analysis software among DXA manufacturers and the various software versions. Whole body BMC values vary significantly between pencil- and fan-beam devices as well as between adult and pediatric software analyses [86]. Hammami and coworkers compared the differences among adult, pediatric, and infant software analyses on a Hologic QDR4500A (Fig. 8.3) [87]. They found that the adult software significantly underestimated BMC, and overestimated aBMD, compared to the infant software while there was some improvement using the pediatric software [87].

**Fig. 8.3** Relationships between adult, pediatric, and infant whole body software for fan-beam DXA. Measurements using adult software (*dashed line*) are more than twice the measurements obtained using infant software. Results using pediatric software (*dotted line*) also are greater than infant software results, but not to the same extent as use of adult software. The solid line is the line of identity. Modified from Hammami et al. [87]

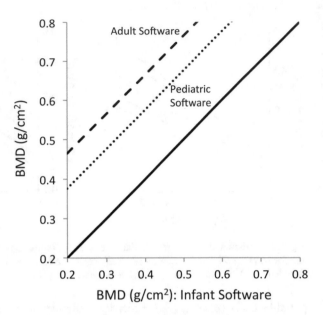

The Hologic QDR-1000W and QDR-1500 were the original pencil beam devices that had an infant whole body application and are now obsolete. These original pencil beam devices were replaced by the QDR-2000 that could operate in both the single beam and fan-beam modes. Eventually the QDR-4500 replaced the QDR-2000. The different DXA devices, models, and software versions are summarized in Table 8.1 and reference data for different devices are given in Table 8.2.

**Whole Body Scans**

There have been several types of software that have been used to obtain whole body scans, including infant, pediatric, and adult whole body scan software; the infant whole body scan software that does not come standard with the purchase of the device. The infant whole body scan takes about 3 min and bone edge detection algorithms are optimized to detect very low density bone. The pediatric software algorithm, which is now obsolete, was a default analysis used at body weights of less than 40 pounds. The acquisition and analysis algorithms for the infant, pediatric, and adult whole body scans differ and are not comparable [87].

Whole body scans of newborn infants with GE/Lunar Prodigy devices also have been reported [88, 89], with a scan time of about 6 min. It is unclear if the infant and regular whole body scan results converge at some body weight or are comparable. There are currently no studies that have performed head-to-head comparisons of devices from different manufactures and software versions for their impact on infant whole body bone measurements. GE/Lunar Prodigy normative values are about 30 % lower than data obtained on Hologic devices in infants 6 months of age.

**Table 8.1** DXA densitometers using pediatric or infant software

| Manufacturer | Model[a] (production years) | | Software versions | Published data by software version |
|---|---|---|---|---|
| Hologic Quantitative Digital Radiography (QDR) | QDR-1000 & 1000 W (1987–1994) | Pencil-beam | Various | v5.35 (PWB)—Brunton et al. [123]<br>v5.47 (PWB)—Picaud et al. [124]<br>v5.56—Brunton et al. [123]<br>v5.56—(PWB) Specker et al. [7]<br>v5.64P (IWB)—Zia-Ullah et al. [77]<br>v4.57Q (infant spine)—Zia-Ullah et al. [77]<br>v5.71p (IWB)—Koo et al. [125]<br>Infant spine—Koo et al. [78] |
| | QDR-1500R (1987–1994) | Pencil-beam | Various | v5.67P (IWB)—Avila-Diaz et al. [126] |
| | QDR-2000 (1987–1994) | Pencil-/fan-beam | Various | IWB v5.64—Picaud et al. [124]<br>IWB v5.73p—Koo et al. [127] |
| | QDR-2000+ (1992–1994) | Pencil-/fan-beam | Various | IWB v5.73P—Zia-Ullah et al. [77]<br>Infant spine v4.76Q—Zia-Ullah et al. [77]<br>v5.71p—Koo [125, 127] |
| | QDR-4000 (1997–2003) | | Various | Cannot do infant whole body |
| | QDR-4500 series (1995–2004) | Fan-beam | V9.x-Apex 4.x (if upgraded) | IWB—Koo et al. [127, 128]<br>IWB vKH6—Hammami et al. [87, 104] |
| | Delphi series (2000–2004) | Fan-beam | V11.2-Apex 4.x (if upgraded) | IWB Elite v11.2—Gallo et al. [58] |
| | Discovery series (2003-pres) | Fan-beam | V12.0-v12.7 Apex 2.x Apex 3.x (aka V13.x) Apex 4.x (aka V14.x) Apex 5.x (aka V15.x) | Infant spine fast array v12.7—Kalkwarf et al. [79]<br>IWB APEX 13.2.1—Gallo et al. [85] |

(continued)

**Table 8.1** (continued)

| Manufacturer | Model[a] (production years) | | Software versions | Published data by software version |
|---|---|---|---|---|
| GE/Lunar | DPX | Pencil-beam | | |
| | Prodigy | Fan-beam | | IWB v12.10—Godang et al. [88] IWB v12.10– Ay et al. [89] |
| | iDXA | Fan-beam | | IWB v11-30.062 enCore2007 [129] |

*C* compact system, *SL* supine lateral feature added (C-arm rotates around patient), *W* whole body feature added, *A* research system with all features, *IWB* infant whole body

Software versions for Hologic QDR that affected pediatric measurements

V12.1 & V12.3—Auto Whole Body analysis added for subjects less than 40 kg. This replaced the former pediatric whole body analysis. Auto Whole Body analysis can be turned off to be identical to V12.01

V12.5—ISCD compatible reports with ISCD Pediatric reference data for <20 years added

V12.4, V2.5, V12.6—No changes in data collection during scan or analysis: BMD, BMC, and Area results are identical

APEX 2.2—Reference curves for children updated with Bone Mineral Density Childhood Study (BMDCS) data. Analysis method for <20 years changed for AP spine and hip to match BMDCS methods

APEX 3.0.1—Does not support "pediatric whole body" and does not provide legacy "Low Density Spine." Auto Whole Body and Auto Low Density are used instead

APEX 3.1—Supports AP spine analysis for infants and toddlers birth to 3 years of age. Depends on the scan date set in the computer and date of birth entered

APEX 3.3—Added NHANES whole body bone and composition reference data for children

APEX 3.4—Reference data for whole body BMD versus age extended down to age 3 using Hologic Pediatric reference data for ages 3–6 and BMDCS references data at age 7. Report provides whole body subtotal BMD (excluding head) for ages <20 years

APEX 4.0—Infant Whole Body acquisition mode for infants aged birth to 1 year

Calibration of Infant Whole Body fat and lean changed on Discovery W, Wi, and Explorer models resulting in greater fat mass. Calibration for A models did not change

NHANES White Whole Body BMD versus age reference data is extended down to age 3 using the Hologic Pediatric reference data for ages 3–6 years and the BMD Children Study reference data at age 7 years

Whole body pediatric curves for lean vs. height and lean vs. subtotal BMC included (lean does not include BMC)

APEX 4.5.2 & 5.5.2—new "Infant Whole Body" analysis added. Excluded more bone pixels from body composition resulting in higher percent fat in most infants. The existing "Infant Whole Body" is still available but manufacturer recommends a transition

[a]Hologic models

**Table 8.2** Publications providing normative data on healthy infants and toddlers

| Reference | Device | Population N (male) age | | |
|---|---|---|---|---|
| Location | Model software | | Bone site | Mean ± SD |
| *Whole body* | | | | |
| Venkataraman et al. [130] Oklahoma City, OK Oklahoma Memorial Hospital | DXA — not specified | 28 Newborns 1.46 ± 0.12 d | WB BMC (g) WB bone area (cm²) | 80.5 ± 6.63 241 ± 13 |
| Atkinson et al. [131] Hamilton, Ontario, Canada McMaster University | Hologic QDR 1000 W Pediatric WB v5.56 | 46 Neonates Age <1 m | WB BMC (g) | 74 ± 13 |
| Specker et al. [7] Cincinnati, Ohio University of Cincinnati | Hologic QDR 1000 W Pediatric WB v5.56 | Infants Phase 1: 92 infants (39 M) Age 1, 3, 6 m Phase 2: 87 infants (37 M) Age 6, 9, 12 m | WB BMC (g) 1 m 3 m 6 m 9 m 12 m | 91.9 ± 14.1 123.1 ± 16.9 161.8 ± 24.1 198.6 ± 28.7 236.2 ± 35.8 |
| Koo et al. [132] Memphis, Tennessee University of Memphis | Hologic QDR 1000 W Pediatric WB v5.64P | 130 Newborn and infant Age N 1–8 d 65 (37 M) 9–390 d 65 (34 M) 9–90 d 16 91–150 d 17 151–270 d 12 271–390 d 20 | WB BMC (g) 1–8 d 9–90 d 91–150 d 151–270 d 271–390 d WB bone area (cm²) 1–8 d 9–90 d 91–150 d 151–270 d 271–390 d | 68.2 ± 10.2 103.4 ± 21.4 137.1 ± 20.0 196.4 ± 26.6 253.2 ± 41.3 308 ± 26 431 ± 58 527 ± 45 650 ± 64 754 ± 88 |
| Butte et al. [133] Houston, Texas Baylor College of Medicine | Hologic QDR 2000 Infant WB v5.56–5.71P | Newborns and infants Age N 0.5 m 76 (33 M) 12 m 74 (32 M) 24 m 72 (29 M) | WB BMC (g) 0.5 m Girls 0.5 m Boys 12 m Girls 12 m Boys 24 m Girls 24 m Boys | 68 ± 12 68 ± 13 208 ± 31 221 ± 33 298 ± 48 321 ± 38 |

(continued)

**Table 8.2** (continued)

| Reference<br>Location | Device<br>Model software | Population<br>N (male) age | Bone site | Mean ± SD |
|---|---|---|---|---|
| Avila-Diaz et al. [126]<br>Mexico City, Mexico | Hologic<br>QDR 1500<br>Infant WB<br>v5.67P | 48 Infants<br>(26 M)<br>1–5 m<br>Age N<br>33±4 d 37<br>63±4 d 35<br>94±11 d 29<br>126±10 d 18<br>147±6 d 16 | WB BMC<br>(g)<br>1 m<br>2 m<br>3 m<br>4 m<br>5 m<br>WB bone<br>area (cm²)<br>1 m<br>2 m<br>3 m<br>4 m<br>5 m | 82.6±11.9<br>103.8±16.0<br>111.0±15.1<br>129.3±17.7<br>134.0±20.0<br>377.7±36.6<br>437.2±61.8<br>467.7±39.3<br>499.3±43.5<br>521.0±46.0 |
| Hammami et al. [104]<br>Detroit, Michigan<br>Wayne State University | Hologic<br>QDR 4500A<br>vKH6 | 73 Newborns<br>(32 M)<br>3.0±2.1 d | WB BMC<br>(g)<br>Bone area<br>(cm²) | 89.3±14.1<br>371±33 |
| Ay 2011 et al. [89]<br>Rotterdam, The Netherlands<br>Erasmus Medical Center | GE lunar<br>prodigy<br>IWB v12.10 | 252 Infants<br>(145 M)<br>Boys:<br>6.4±0.8 m<br>Girls:<br>6.3±0.7 m | WB BMC<br>(g)<br>Boys<br>Girls | 120.9±23.5<br>110.5±20.4 |
| Gallo 2012 [58]<br>Winnipeg, MB, Canada<br>University of Manitoba | Hologic<br>QDR 4500A<br>Elite<br>IWB v11.2 | 52 Infants<br>(36 M)<br>Age N<br>2–4 w 62<br>6 m 35<br>12 m 11 | WB BMC<br>(g)<br>2–4 w<br>6 m<br>12 m<br>WB BMC<br>less head<br>(g)<br>2–4 w<br>6 m<br>12 m | 76.0±14.2<br>169.5±29.0<br>227.0±29.7<br>45.6±8.1<br>87.7±16.3<br>114.8±21.9 |
| *Lumbar spine* | | | | |
| Brallion et al. [134]<br>Lyon, France<br>Eduard Herriot Hospital | Hologic<br>QDR 1000<br>UHR v4.10 | 10 Newborns<br>1 d | L1-L5<br>LS BMC<br>(g)<br>LS BMD<br>(g/cm²) | 2.34±0.42<br>0.268±0.030 |
| Salle et al. [135]<br>Lyon, France<br>Eduard Herriot Hospital | Hologic<br>QDR 1000<br>UHR v4.20 | 57 Newborns<br>(29 M)<br>Age ≤48 h | L1-L5<br>BMC (g)<br>L1-L5<br>BMD (g/cm²) | Data presented<br>graphically with normal<br>range by weight (kg)<br>and length (cm) |

(continued)

**Table 8.2** (continued)

| Reference<br>Location | Device<br>Model software | Population<br>N (male) age | Bone site | Mean±SD |
|---|---|---|---|---|
| Kurl et al. [136]<br>Kuopio, Finland<br>Kuopio University<br>Hospital | Lunar DPX<br>Pediatric AP<br>spine<br>V3.8E | 41 Infants<br>(19 M)<br>Age 2–6 m | L2-L4<br>BMC (g)<br>Boys<br>Girls<br>L2-L4<br>Bone Area<br>(cm²)<br>Boys<br>Girls<br>L2-L4<br>BMD (g/<br>cm²)<br>Boys<br>Girls | 2.26±0.58<br>1.93±0.57<br>8.74±1.20<br>8.27±1.10<br>0.25±0.04<br>0.23±0.05 |
| Zia-Ullah 2002 [77]<br>Memphis, Tennessee<br>University of<br>Tennessee | Hologic<br>QDR 1000 W<br>IS v4.57Q | 99 Infants<br>(58 M)<br>Age 1–391 d | L1-L4<br>BMC (g)<br>Bone area<br>(cm²)<br>BMD (g/<br>cm²) | 2.2±1.5<br>8.8±4.2<br>0.231±0.049 |
| Ay 2011 [89]<br>Rotterdam, The<br>Netherlands<br>Erasmus Medical<br>Center | GE lunar<br>prodigy<br>IS v12.10 | 252 Infants<br>(145 M)<br>Boys:<br>6.4±0.8 m<br>Girls:<br>6.3±0.7 m | LS BMC<br>(g)<br>Boys<br>Girls<br>LS BMD<br>(g/cm²)<br>Boys<br>Girls | 2.7±0.5<br>2.6±0.4<br>0.31±0.04<br>0.33±0.04 |
| Gallo 2012 [58]<br>Winnipeg, MB,<br>Canada<br>University of<br>Manitoba | Hologic<br>QDR 4500A<br>Elite<br>Auto low<br>density spine<br>v11.2 | 62 Infants<br>(36 M)<br>Age N<br>2–4 w 62<br>6 m 62<br>12 m 57 | L1-L4<br>BMC (g)<br>2–4 w<br>6 m<br>12 m<br>L1-L4<br>Bone area<br>(cm²)<br>2–4 w<br>6 m<br>12 m<br>L1-L4<br>BMD (g/<br>cm²)<br>2–4 w<br>6 m<br>12 m | 2.35±0.42<br>3.59±0.63<br>5.37±1.02<br>8.86±1.10<br>14.28±2.01<br>17.67±2.52<br>0.266±0.044<br>0.252±0.031<br>0.304±0.044 |

(continued)

**Table 8.2** (continued)

| Reference | Device | Population N (male) age | | |
|-----------|--------|------------------------|---|---|
| Location | Model software | | Bone site | Mean ± SD |
| Kalkwarf [79] | Hologic | 307 (158 M) | | L1-L4 BMC (g) |
| Cincinnati, Ohio | Discovery A | Age N | | L1-L4 BMD (g/cm²) |
| Children's Hospital | Infant spine | 1–6 m 37 | | Data presented |
| Medical Center | v12.7 | 6.1–12 m 50 | | graphically by age and |
| | | 12.1–18 m 51 | | in table as Z-score |
| | | 18.1–24 m 59 | | |
| | | 24.1–30 m 56 | | |
| | | 30.1–36 m 54 | | |

*d* day, *m* month, *h* hour, *w* week, *WB* whole body, *BMC* bone mineral content, *BMD* bone mineral density; *IWB* infant whole body

*IS* infant spine, *LS* lumbar spine

**Spine Scans**

Scan acquisition is performed using the standard posterior-anterior (PA) spine scan. Hologic Apex software provides the ability to analyze spine scans for infants and toddlers by automatically determining the specific algorithm and bone edge detection thresholds. Bone edge detection thresholds are set based on age for children 36 months and younger, and by bone map evaluation for children older than 36 months. The algorithms were developed so that the same software can be used and scans compared across all ages. There are multiple scan modes (array, fast array, turbo) for acquisition of spine scans on the Hologic devices, but data comparing the various modes for infants and toddlers are lacking. Since it is not known whether these modes are comparable, it would be prudent to use the same scan mode on repeated measurements of the same child and when identifying appropriate normative data sets. The GE/Lunar densitometers also have the capability to perform spine measurements in infants and toddlers. Means ±1 standard deviation of spine BMC obtained from different publications are shown in Fig. 8.4 and illustrate differences in normal ranges that are observed among the different devices for various ages.

## *Performing a Scan in Infants or Toddlers*

Infants are among the most challenging subjects to measure using DXA. Before measuring an infant it is helpful to feed and calm them and to place the infant on the scanning table in a clean diaper. If necessary, the child could be swaddled in a thin cotton sheet or blanket to reduce small involuntary movements. Subdued room lighting also may also help. Very young infants (i.e., <3 months of age) will usually sleep through the measurement and will require limited operator intervention (Fig. 8.5).

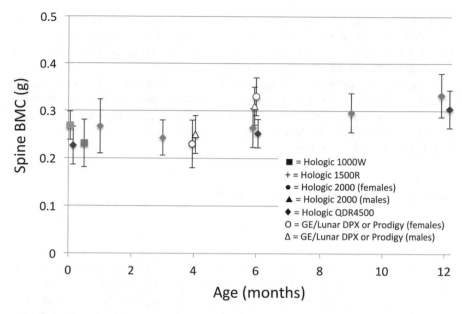

**Fig. 8.4** Published normative data (means ±1 SD) for spine BMC in infants. *Filled square* = Hologic 1000 W; *Plus Sign* = Hologic 1500R; *filled circle* = Hologic 2000 (females); *filled triangle* = Hologic 2000 (males); *filled diamond* = Hologic QDR4500; *open circle* = GE/Lunar Prodigy (females); *open triangle* = GE/Lunar Prodigy (males). Different colors represent different studies

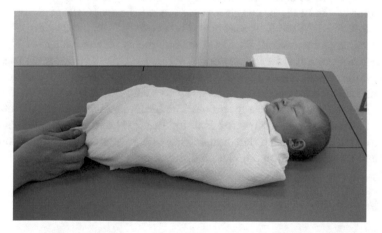

**Fig. 8.5** Swaddling and positioning of an infant prior to whole body DXA measurement

Swaddling becomes ineffective for keeping infants motionless for the required 3–6 min as the infants become older and stronger. Stranger anxiety in infants around 8–9 months of age also makes this age especially difficult to scan. In the event of movement, DXA scans can be repeated with the hope of obtaining a movement-free image. Gallo et al. reported that when making up to two attempts, they obtained movement free whole body scans on 99 % of infants at 1 month of age compared to 81 % at 12 months of age [85]. Few studies report success rates obtaining movement free scans or the number of attempts to obtain one.

Some investigators have used restraints on 6- and 12-month old infants scanned with fan-beam densitometers [89], but it is important the make sure that the restraints are radiolucent or scan results may be affected. Some studies have found an effect of multiple layers of cloth on bone measurements, which seems to be more of a problem with the fan-beam devices [87, 90].

## Normative Data and Factors Affecting

### Normative Data

In situations where a child's growth is stunted or maturation is delayed, which is particularly true in children with chronic diseases, it may be more appropriate to determine whether BMC or aBMD results are appropriate for his or her body size by comparing the measurements with those of children of similar height or weight (see discussion above). However, these reference databases are not available on the DXA software and must be obtained from the pediatric literature.

Although numerous studies have included normative infant and toddler DXA data, the populations are typically small or highly selected based on specific population characteristics (Table 8.2). The largest studies providing age-specific reference data of the spine by fan-beam for infants and toddlers are those of Gallo et al. [58] (n=62, 0–360 days; Fig. 8.1) and Kalkwarf et al. [79] (n=308, 1–36 months; Fig. 8.2).

Pediatric reference values for DXA measurements obtained on 1554 U.S. children aged 5 years and older in five centers across the U.S. have been published [91] and are currently used as the normative data for Hologic devices. These data indicate that BMD measures are not necessarily normally-distributed and the use of the standard Z-scores may not be appropriate. The LMS modeling approach, used in the papers by Kalkwarf and others for both toddlers [91] and infants [79], does not require normally-distributed data and can provide greater accuracy in defining the upper and lower ends of the population distributions.

### Gestational Age and Birth Size

Intrauterine bone accretion is significant during the third trimester of pregnancy and preterm infant have decreased BMC later in life compared to term infants of similar postconceptional age [38, 92, 93]. Preterm infants are at risk for osteopenia due to postnatal nutritional deficits [94]. Appropriate feeding of these infants results in a catch-up in bone mineralization and their BMC is appropriate for their size [95–98], although preterm infants tend to be shorter and lighter than their peers [97, 99].

Small-for-gestational-age (SGA) infants also have decreased BMC even after controlling for body size. The exact mechanism is not clear, but reduced in utero bone turnover has been suggested as one possibility [100]. Alterations in IGF-1 are also thought to play a major role in the growth retardation and have been shown to persist into adulthood in approximately 10 % of the individuals born SGA [101]; growth hormone has been shown to increased final adult height in many of these children [102].

## Age, Sex, and Race

Whole body BMC and spine aBMD increase dramatically during the first year of life in healthy infants. Kalkwarf found that spine BMC increased fivefold between 1 and 36 months of age, while spine aBMD increased twofold [79]. BMC differs between the sexes, similar to weight and length, but the timing of this difference may vary by bone site. In general, males have higher BMC and aBMD than females prior to 1 year of age.

BMC and aBMD also differ by race, with higher bone measures in black than whites. However, the age at which these differences appear and at which bone sites is not evident. Garn reported a greater bone width in black children compared to white children 1–2 years of age [103] and Hammami et al. reported a greater whole body bone area in black neonates compared to white neonates [104]. Gilsanz and coworkers found no significant race differences in true volumetric density of the spine in older children until puberty [53]. Whole body BMC has been shown to be slightly higher in black infants compared to white infants aged 1–18 months [105], and forearm BMC measured by single photon absorptiometry was higher in black compared to white children 1–6 years of age [106]. A large study of infants and toddler 1–36 months of age found no race differences in either spine BMC or aBMD [79]. Studies of other race comparisons are not common. In one report Asian neonates had 29 % lower spine BMC compared to white neonates, whereas Native American neonates had intermediate values [107].

## Body Composition and Growth

At all ages BMC and aBMD are positively associated with weight and height, due in part to age-related increases in body and bone size combined with increased loads on the skeleton with increasing weight. Among infants and toddlers aged 1–36 months, weight-for-age (WAZ) and length-for-age Z-scores (LAZ) are associated with spine and whole body BMC and spine aBMD Z-scores [79]. Because of the strong influence on body size on bone DXA bone measures it is important to consider body size when interpreting scan results (see Chap. 5).

In older children and adolescents body composition, especially lean mass, has been found useful when interpreting whole body BMC measures [108, 109]. Gains in fat and lean mass may have different effects on bone accrual, with a positive relationship between gains in lean mass and bone accrual, but a negative relationship between gains in fat mass and bone accrual [110]. Although gains in fat mass are associated with decreased bone accrual in older children [110], a similar finding has not been observed in infants [111]. Sudhagoni and coworkers combined data from three separate longitudinal studies involving a total of 362 infants between the ages of 1 and 12 months and found that changes in both lean and fat mass were positively associated with whole body bone accrual, a finding that remained significant when body length was included as a covariate [111].

## Infant Feeding and Gross Motor Development/Bone Loading

Type of infant feeding and bone loading activities are both likely to influence bone accrual and aBMD early in life. Bone accretion rates have been shown to vary in the first year of life between human milk-fed and formula-fed infants with a greater bone accretion among formula-fed infants, especially formula with higher mineral content, compared to human milk [7, 79, 112, 113]. This effect does not persist and there is no evidence that human milk feeding is associated with decreased whole body BMC later in childhood [114–116].

Significant changes in gross motor skills and activities occur during infancy and the toddler years with the onset of crawling, standing, and walking. These developmental changes influence mechanical loading of the skeleton, which theoretically should increase bone accrual [33, 117–119]. A 1-year randomized trial of 72 infants enrolled at 6 months of age to either gross motor or fine motor activities found that calcium intake appeared to modify the effect of gross motor activity on bone accretion [118]. Infants in both gross motor and fine motor groups had similar bone accretion at moderately high calcium intakes, but at low calcium intakes infants in the gross motor group had lower BMC at 18 months of age than the infants in the fine motor group. These results suggest that calcium intake may modify the bone response to loading. Although differences in gross motor activity and age at walking have been proposed as an explanation for bone differences between term and preterm infants [92], other studies have not supported this explanation [38, 93].

## Who Should Be Scanned and Reporting Results

### Current Guidelines

The 2013 ISCD position paper includes guidelines related to densitometry in infants and young children (Table 8.3). The 2007 ISCD position paper did not include recommendations for clinical densitometry in infants and young children due to the

**Table 8.3**  Official ISCD 2013 positions: densitometry in infants and young children

- DXA is an appropriate method for clinical densitometry of infants and young children
- DXA whole body measurements are feasible and can provide reproducible measures of BMC and aBMD for   children ≥3 years
- DXA whole body BMC measurements for children <3 years of age are of limited clinical utility due to feasibility and lack of normative data. aBMD should not be used routinely due to difficulty in appropriate positioning
- DXA lumbar spine measurements are feasible and can provide reproducible measures of BMC and aBMD for infants and young children 0–5 years of age
- Forearm and femur measurements are technically feasible in infants and young children, but there is insufficient information regarding methodology, reproducibility, and reference data for these measurements sites to be clinically useful at this time

lack of normative data. The current guidelines include the appropriateness of DXA for infants and young children, with spine measurements being the most feasible and providing the most reproducible results for ages 0–5 years. Due to difficulties with positioning and movement artifacts resulting from the longer scan time and lack of normative data in infants and toddlers, whole body scans were considered feasible and reproducible in young children aged 3 years and older. Both forearm and femur measurements are technically feasible but are not currently thought to be clinically useful due to the lack of reference data and insufficient information regarding the methodology. As discussed previously, it also was recommended that the impact of growth delay should be considered when interpreting DXA results.

## Clinical Indications

Conditions that may place infants and toddlers at increased risk of low bone density include chronic inflammation, prolonged immobilization, and osteopenia on X-ray. Rare diseases also might place an infant or toddler at increased risk of low BMD and include extreme prematurity, congenital neutropenia, certain inborn errors of metabolism, Ehlers Danlos syndrome, Duchenne muscular dystrophy, cerebral palsy, osteogenesis imperfecta, and hypophosphatasia. Long-term use of corticosteroids also increases a child's risk of low bone density or fracture. High fracture rates (20–30%) reported in preterm infants in the 1970s and 1980s are less common today due to improvements in dietary management of preterm infants. The American Academy of Pediatrics recently published guidance related to assessment and management of bone status in preterm infants [120]. Due to variation among machines and the different pediatric reference databases and software programs that are available, it is important that clinicians consult with pediatric bone specialists before using DXA diagnostically.

Although bone densitometry is often ordered after fractures in infants or toddlers in whom nonaccidental trauma (NAT) is considered possible, scan results cannot be used to distinguish between underlying bone fragility and nonaccidental trauma. There is no established "fracture threshold" for aBMD in pediatrics and the risk for bone fragility likely increases along a continuum as bone density decreases. Furthermore, the presence of low bone density for age does not preclude the possibility of nonaccidental trauma resulting in fracture. This issue is discussed in more detail in Chap. 12.

## How Results Should Be Reported

The diagnosis of osteoporosis for adults is based on the WHO criterion that uses BMD T scores, which is defined as the standard deviation (SD) score of the observed aBMD compared with that of a normal young adult. A T-score of less than −1 SD in adults indicates osteopenia and a T-score of less than −2.5 SD indicates osteoporosis [121]. Because T-scores compare the observed aBMD with that of young adults they are *not appropriate* for growing children and should *never* be used.

A more appropriate method of comparison of aBMD in pediatrics is the use of the Z-score, defined as the SD score based on age- and sex-specific norms. The ISCD currently recommends that the pediatric bone density be evaluated based on Z-scores, with low-for-chronological-age being defined as a *Z-score less than −2.0* [12, 122].

In summary, the development of methods for assessing pediatric bone and the development of normative data bases have lead to the ability to quantify bone mass and to assess how various factors influence bone accretion in infants and toddlers.

## Summary Points

- DXA is currently the preferred method for assessing bone health in infants and toddlers.
- Normative data for infants and toddlers are available for whole body and spine scans.
- There are significant differences in results based on machine manufacturer and among different software versions. These differences need to be considered when using normative databases.
- Although low BMC or BMD is associated with fractures in older children, data on this relationship in infants and toddlers are limited.
- Anthropometric, demographic, and lifestyle (e.g., diet, activity levels) factors should be considered when evaluating scan results.
- DXA cannot be used to distinguish between underlying bone fragility and nonaccidental trauma.

# References

1. Lachman E. Osteoporosis: the potentialities and limitations of its roentgenologic diagnosis. Am J Roentgenol. 1955;74:712.
2. Greer FR, McCormick A. Bone growth with low bone mineral content in very low birth weight premature infants. Pediatr Res. 1986;20:925–8.
3. Moyer-Mileur L, Ledkemeier MJ, Chan GM. Physical activity enhances bone mass in very low birthweight infants. Pediatr Res. 1995;37:314A.
4. Koo W, Walters J, Carlson S. Delayed bone mineralization in preterm infants. J Bone Miner Res. 1995;10:S296.
5. Koo WWK, Gupta JM, Nayanar VV, Wilkinson M, Posen S. Skeletal changes in very low birth weight infants. Arch Dis Child. 1982;57:447–52.
6. Lapillonne AA, Glorieux FH, Salle BL, Braillon PM, Chambon M, Rigo J, et al. Mineral balance and whole body bone mineral content in very low-birth-weight infants. Acta Paediatr Suppl. 1994;405:117–22.
7. Specker BL, Beck A, Kalkwarf H, Ho M. Randomized trial of varying mineral intake on total body bone mineral accretion during the first year of life. Pediatrics. 1997;99:e12.
8. Rigo J, Nyamugabo K, Picaud JC, Gerard P, Peltain C, DeCurtis M. Reference values of body composition obtained by dual energy x-ray absorptiometry in preterm and term neonates. J Pediatr Gastro Nutr. 1998;27:184–90.
9. Mehta KC, Specker BL, Bartholmey S, Giddens J, Ho ML. Trial on timing of introduction to solids and food type on infant growth. Pediatrics. 1998;102:569–73.
10. Brunton JA, Saigal S, Atkinson SA. Growth and body composition in infants with broncho-pulmonary dysplasia up to 3 months corrected age: a randomized trial of a high-energy nutrient-enriched formula fed after hospital discharge. J Pediatr. 1998;133:340–5.
11. Butte N, Heinz C, Hopkinson J, Wong W, Shypailo R, Ellis K. Fat mass in infants and toddlers: comparability of total body water, total body potassium, total body electrical conductivity, and dual energy x-ray absorptiometry. J Pediatr Gastro Nutr. 1999;29:184–9.
12. Kalkwarf H, Abrams SA, DiMeglio LA, Koo WW, Specker BL, Weiler H. Bone densitometry in infants and young children: the 2013 ISCD pediatric official positions. J Clin Densit. 2014;17:243–57.
13. Baroncelli GI, Federico G, Vignolo M, Valerio G, del Puente A, Maghnie M, et al. Cross-sectional reference data for phalangeal quantitative ultrasound from early childhood to young-adulthood according to gender, age, skeletal growth, and pubertal development. Bone. 2006;39:159–73.
14. Zadik Z, Price D, Diamond G. Pediatric reference curves for multi-site quantitative ultrasound and its modulators. Osteoporos Int. 2003;14:857–62.
15. Dib L, Arabi A, Maalouf J, Nabulsi M, Fuleihan GEH. Impact of anthropometric, lifestyle, and body composition variables on ultrasound measurements in school children. Bone. 2005;36:736–42.
16. Zuccotti G, Vigano A, Cafarello L, Pivetti V, Pogliani L, Puzzovio M, et al. Longitudinal changes of bone ultrasound measurements in healthy infants during the first year of life: influence of gender and type of feeding. Calcif Tissue Int. 2011;89(4):312–7.
17. Teitelbaum JE, Rodriguez RJ, Ashmeade TL, Yaniv I, Osuntokun BO, Hudome S, et al. Quantitative ultrasound in the evaluation of bone status in premature and full-term infants. J Clin Densit. 2006;9:358–62.
18. Fielding KT, Nix DA, Bachrach LK. Comparison of calcaneus ultrasound and dual x-ray absorptiometry in children at risk of osteopenia. J Clin Densit. 2003;6:7–15.
19. van Rijn RR, van der Sluis IM, Lequin MH, Robben SG, de Muinck Keizer-Schrama SM, Hop WC, et al. Tibial quantitative ultrasound versus whole-body and lumbar spine DXA in a Dutch pediatric and adolescent population. Invest Radiol. 2000;35:548–52.

20. Pluskiewica W, Adamczyk P, Drozdzowska B, Szprynger K, Szczepanska M, Halaba Z, et al. Skeletal status in children, adolescents and young adults with end-stage renal failure treated with hemo-orperitoneal dialysis. Osteoporos Int. 2002;13:353–7.
21. Koo WWK, Bajaj M, Mosely M, Hammami M. Quantitative bone US measurements in neonates and their mothers. Pediatr Radiol. 2008;38:1323–9.
22. Bajaj M, Koo WWK, Hammami M, Hockman EM. Effect of subcutaneous fat on quantitative bone ultrasound in chicken and neonates. Pediatr Res. 2010;68:81–3.
23. Ferretti JL. Perspectives of pQCT technology associated with biomechanical studies in skeletal research employing rat models. Bone. 1995;17:353S–64.
24. Louis O, Willnecker J, Soykens S, Van den Winkel P, Osteaux M. Cortical thickness assessed by peripheral quantitative computed tomography: accuracy evaluated on radius specimens. Osteoporos Int. 1995;5:446–9.
25. Butz S, Wuster C, Scheidt-Nave C, Gotz M, Ziegler R. Forearm BMD as measured by peripheral quantitative computed tomography (pQCT) in a German reference population. Osteoporos Int. 1994;4:179–84.
26. Lettgen B. Peripheral quantitative computed tomography: reference data and clinical experiences in chronic diseases. In: Schoenau E, editor. Pediatric osteology: new developments in diagnostics and therapy. Amsterdam: Elsevier Science; 1996. p. 141–6.
27. Schiessl H, Ferretti JL, Tysarczyk-Niemeyer G, Willnecker J. Noninvasive bone strength index as analyzed by peripheral quantitative computed tomography (pQCT). In: Schoenau E, editor. Paediatric osteology: new developments in diagnostics and therapy. Amsterdam: Elsevier; 1996. p. 141–6.
28. Schoenau E. The development of the skeletal system in children and the influence of muscular strength. Horm Res. 1998;49:27–31.
29. Schoenau E, Werhahn E, Schiedermaier U, Mokow E, Schiessl H, Scheidhauer K, et al. Bone and muscle development during childhood in health and disease. In: Schoenau E, editor. Paediatric osteology: new developments in diagnostics and therapy. Amsterdam: Elsevier Science; 1996. p. 63–6.
30. Cowell CT, Lu PW, Lloyd-Jones SA, Briody JN, Allen JR, Humphries IR, et al. Volumetric bone mineral density—a potential role in paediatrics. Acta Paediatr Suppl. 1995;411:12–6.
31. De Schepper J, De Boeck H, Louis O. Measurement of radial bone mineral density and cortical thickness in children by peripheral quantitative computed tomography. In: Schoenau E, editor. Paediatric osteology: new developments in diagnostics and therapy. Amsterdam: Elsevier Science; 1996.
32. Binkley TL, Specker BL. pQCT measurement of bone parameters in young children: validation of technique. J Clin Densit. 2000;3:9–14.
33. Specker B, Binkley T. Randomized trial of physical activity and calcium supplementation on bone mineral content in 3-5 year old children. J Bone Miner Res. 2003;18:885–92.
34. Viljakainen HT, Saarnio E, Hytinantti T, Miettinen M, Surcel H, Makitie O, et al. Maternal vitamin D status determines bone variables in the newborn. J Clin Endocrinol Metabol. 2010;95:1749–57.
35. Viljakainen HT, Korhonen T, Hytinantti T, Laitinen EKA, Andersson S, Mäkitie O, et al. Maternal vitamin D status affects bone growth in early childhood—a prospective cohort study. Osteoporos Int. 2011;22(3):883–91.
36. Holmlund-Suila E, Viljakainen H, Hytinantti T, Lamberg-Allardt C, Andersson S, Maekitie O. High-dose vitamin D intervention in infants—effects on vitamin D status, calcium homeostasis, and bone strength. J Clin Endocrinol Metab. 2012;97:4139–47.
37. Binkley T, Johnson J, Vogel L, Kecskemethy HH, Henderson RC, Specker B. Bone measurements by peripheral quantitative computed tomography (pQCT) in children with cerebral palsy (CP). J Pediatr. 2005;147:791–6.
38. Abou-Samra H, Specker B. Walking age does not explain term versus preterm difference in bone geometry. J Pediatr. 2007;151:61–6.
39. Binkley T, Specker B, Wittig T. Centile curves for bone densitometry measurements in healthy males and females ages 5-22 years. J Clin Densit. 2002;5:343–53.

40. Neu CM, Manz F, Rauch F, Merkel A, Schoenau E. Bone densities and bone size at the distal radius in healthy children and adolescents: a study using peripheral quantitative computed tomography. Bone. 2001;28:227–32.
41. Binkley T, Specker B. Increased periosteal circumference remains present 12 months after an exercise intervention in preschool children. Bone. 2004;35:1383–8.
42. Johannsen N, Binkley T, Englert V, Niederauer G, Specker B. Bone response to jumping is site-specific in children: a randomized trial. Bone. 2003;33:533–9.
43. Macdonald H, Kontulainen S, Khan KM, McKay HA. Is a school-based physical activity intervention effective for increasing tibial bone strength in boys and girls? J Bone Miner Res. 2007;22:434–46.
44. Schoenau E, Neu CM, Mokov E, Wassmer G, Manz F. Influence of puberty on muscle area and cortical bone area of the forearm in boys and girls. J Clin Endocrinol Metab. 2000;85:1095–8.
45. Schoenau E, Neu CM, Rauch F, Manz F. Gender-specific pubertal changes in volumetric cortical bone mineral density at the proximal radius. Bone. 2002;31:110–3.
46. Binkley T, Parupsky E, Kleinsasser B, Weidauer L, Specker B. Feasibility, compliance, and efficacy of a randomized controlled trial using vibration in pre-pubertal children. J Musculoskelet Neuronal Interact. 2014;14(3):294–302.
47. Koo WW, Hammami M, Hockman EM. Use of fan beam dual energy x-ray absorptiometry to measure body composition of piglets. J Nutr. 2002;132:1380–3.
48. Chauhan S, Koo WW, Hammami M, Hockman EM. Fan beam dual energy X-ray absorptiometry body composition measurements in piglets. J Am Coll Nutr. 2003;22:408–14.
49. Damilakis J, Solomou G, Manios G, Karantanas A. Pediatric radiation dose and risk from bone density measurements using a GE Lunar Prodigy scanner. Osteoporos Int. 2013;24:2025–31.
50. Thomas S, Kalkwarf H, Buckley D, Heubi J. Effective dose of dual-energy x-ray absorptiometry scans in children as a function of age. J Clin Densit. 2005;8:415–22.
51. Recommendations on Limits for Exposure to Ionizing Radiation. National Council on Radiation Protection and Measurements., 1987 June 1, 1987. Report No.: 91.
52. Binkley TL, Berry R, Specker BL. Methods for measurement of pediatric bone. Rev Endocrin Metab Disord. 2008; DOI 10.1007/S11154-008-9073-5.
53. Gilsanz V, Roe TF, Mora S, Costin G, Goodman WG. Changes in vertebral bone density in black girls and white girls during childhood and puberty. N Engl J Med. 1991;325:1597–600.
54. Wang Q, Alén M, Nicholson P, Lyytikäinen A, Suuriniemi M, Helkala E, et al. Growth patterns at distal radius and tibial shaft in pubertal girls: a 2-year longitudinal study. J Bone Miner Res. 2005;20:954–61.
55. Prentice A, Parsons T, Cole T. Uncritical use of bone mineral density in absorptiometry may lead to size related artifacts in the identification of bone mineral determinants. Am J Clin Nutr. 1994;60:837–42.
56. Carter DR, Bouxsein ML, Marcus R. New approaches for interpreting projected bone densitometry data. J Bone Miner Res. 1992;7:137–45.
57. Short DF, Gilsanz V, Kalkwarf HJ, Lappe JM, Oberfield S, Shepherd JA, et al. Anthropometric models of bone mineral content and areal bone mineral density based on the bone mineral density in childhood study. Osteoporos Int. 2014; DOI 10.1007/s00198-014-2916-x.
58. Gallo S, Vanstone CA, Weiler HA. Normative data for bone mass in healthy term infants from birth to 1 year of age. J Osteopor. 2012;2012. ID672403.
59. Goksen D, Darcan S, Coker M, Kose T. Bone mineral density of helathy Turkish children and adolescents. J Clin Densit. 2006;9:84–90.
60. Zemel BS, Leonard MB, Kelly A, Lappe JM, Gilsanz V, Oberfield S, et al. Height adjustment in assessing dual energy x-ray absorptiometry measurements of bone mass and density in children. J Clin Endocrinol Metab. 2010;95:1265–73.
61. Chan GM, Hess M, Hollis J, Book LS. Bone mineral status in childhood accidental fractures. Am J Dis Child. 1984;138:569–70.

62. Goulding A, Cannan R, Williams SM, Gold EJ, Taylor RW, Lewis-Barned NJ. Bone mineral density in girls with forearm fractures. J Bone Miner Res. 1998;13:143–8.
63. Ma D, Jones G. The association between bone mineral density, metacarpal morphometry, and upper limb fractures in children: a population-based case-control study. J Clin Endocrinol Metab. 2003;88:1486–91.
64. Clark E, Ness AR, Bishop NJ, Tobias JN. Association between bone mass and fractures in children: a prospective cohort study. J Bone Miner Res. 2006;21:1489–95.
65. Ferrari SL, Chevalley T, Bonjour JP, Rizzoli R. Childhood fractures are associated with decreased bone mass gain during puberty: an early marker of persistent bone fragility? J Bone Miner Res. 2006;21:501–7.
66. Kalkwarf HJ, Laor T, Bean J. Fracture risk in children with a forearm injury is associated with volumetric bone density and cortical area (by peripheral QCT) and areal bone density (by DXA). Osteoporos Int. 2011;22:607–16.
67. Rizzoli R, Bianchi ML, Garabedian M, McKay HA, Moreno LA. Maximizing bone mineral mass gain during growth for the prevention of fractures in the adolescents and the elderly. Bone. 2010;46:294–305.
68. Amin S, Melton III JL, Achenback SJ, Atkinson EJ, Dekutoski MB, Kirmani S, et al. A distal forearm fracture in childhood is associated with an increased risk for future fragility fractures in adult men, but not women. J Bone Miner Res. 2013;28:1751–9.
69. Koo MWM, Yang K, Begeman P, Hammami M, Koo WWK. Prediction of bone strength in growing animals using noninvasive bone mass measurements. Calcif Tissue Int. 2001;68:230–4.
70. Mayranpaa MK, Makitie O, Kallio PE. Decreasing incidence and changing pattern of childhood fractures: a population-based study. J Bone Miner Res. 2010;25:2752–9.
71. Gordon CM, Bachrach LK, Carpenter TO, Crabtree N, Fuleihan GEH, Kutilek S, et al. Dual energy X-ray absorptiometry interpretation and reporting in children and adolescents: the 2007 ISCD pediatric official positions. J Clin Densit. 2008;11:43–58.
72. Heaney RP. Bone mienral content, not bone mineral density, is the correct bone measure for growth studies. Am J Clin Nutr. 2003;78:350–1.
73. Taylor A, Konrad PT, Norman ME, Harcke HT. Total body bone mineral density in young children: influence of head bone mineral density. J Bone Miner Res. 1997;12:652–5.
74. Courteix D, Lespessailles E, Obert P, Benhamou CL. Skull bone mass deficit in prepubertal highly-trained gymnast girls. Int J Sports Med. 1999;20:328–33.
75. Bikle DD, Halloran BP. The response of bone to unloading. J Bone Miner Rcs. 1999;17:233–44.
76. Arnaud S, Powell M, Vernikos-Danellis J, Buchanan P. Bone mineral and body composition after 30 day head down tilt bed rest. J Bone Miner Res. 1988;3:S119.
77. Zia-Ullah M, Koo WWK, Hammami M. Lumbar spine bone measurements in infants: whole-body vs lumbar spine dual x-ray absorptiometry scans. J Clin Densit. 2002;5:17–25.
78. Koo WWK, Hockman EM. Physiologic predictors of lumbar spine bone mass in neonates. Pediatr Res. 2000;48:485–9.
79. Kalkwarf HJ, Zemel BS, Yolton K, Heubi JE. Bone mineral content and density of the lumbar spine of infants and toddlers: influence of age, sex, race, growth, and human milk feeding. J Bone Miner Res. 2013;28:206–12.
80. Hazell TJ, Vanstone CA, Rodd CJ, Rauch F, Weiler HA. Bone mineral density measured by a portable x-ray device agrees with dual-energy x-ray absorptiometry at forearm in preschool aged children. J Clin Densit. 2013;16:302–7.
81. Zanchetta J, Plotkin H, Filgueira M. Bone mass in children: normative values for the 2-20 year old population. Bone. 1995;16:S393–9.
82. Willing MC, Torner JC, Burns TL, Janz KF, Marshall TA, Gilmore J, et al. Percentile distribution of bone measurements in Iowa children: the Iowa Bone Development Study. J Clin Densit. 2005;8:39–47.

83. Webber CE, Beaumont LF, Morrison J, Sala A, Barr RD. Age-predicted values for lumbar spine, proximal femur, and whole-body bone mineral density: results from a population of normal children aged 3 to 18 years. Can Assoc Radiol J. 2007;58:37.
84. Ausili E, Rigante D, Salvaggio E, Focarelli B, Rendeli C, Ansuini V, et al. Determinants of bone mineral density, bone mineral content, and body composition in a cohort of healthy children: influence of sex, age, puberty, and physical activity. Rheumatol Int. 2012;32:2737–43.
85. Gallo S, Comeau K, Vanstone CA, Agellon S, Sharma A, Jones G, et al. Effect of different dosages of oral vitamin D supplementation on vitamin D status in healthy, breastfed infants. JAMA. 2013;309(17):1785–92.
86. Specker BL, Namgung R, Tsang RC. Bone mineral acquisition in utero and during infancy and childhood. In: Marcus R, Feldman D, Kelsey J, editors. Osteoporosis. 2nd ed. San Diego: Academic; 2001. p. 599–620.
87. Hammami M, Koo WW, Hockman EM. Technical considerations for fan-beam dual-energy x-ray absorptiometry body composition measurements in pediatric studies. J Parenter Enteral Nutr. 2004;28:328–33.
88. Godang K, Qvigstad E, Voldner N, Isaksen GA, Froslie KF, Notthellen J, et al. Assessing body composition in healthy newborn infants: reliability of dual-energy x-ray absorptiometry. J Clin Densit. 2010;13:151–60.
89. Ay L, Jaddoe VWV, Hofman A, Moll HA, Raat H, Steegers EAP, et al. Foetal and postnatal growth and bone mass at 6 months: the generation R study. Clin Endocrinol. 2011;74:181–90.
90. Koo WWK, Massom LR, Walters J. Validation of accuracy and precision of dual energy x-ray absorptiometry for infants. J Bone Miner Res. 1995;10:1111–5.
91. Kalkwarf HJ, Zemel BS, Gilsanz V, Lappe JM, Horlick M, Oberfield S, et al. The bone mineral density in childhood study: bone mineral content and bone mineral density according to age, sex, and race. J Clin Endocrinol Metab. 2007;92:2087–99.
92. Specker BL, Johannsen N, Binkley T, Finn K. Total body bone mineral content and tibial cortical bone measures in preschool children. J Bone Miner Res. 2001;16:2298–305.
93. Abou-Samra H, Stevens D, Binkley T, Specker B. Determinants of bone mass and size in 7-year-old former term, late-preterm and preterm boys. Osteoporos Int. 2009;20:1903–10.
94. Lapillonne A, O'Connor DL, Wang D, Rigo J. Nutritional requirements for the late-preterm infant and the preterm infant after hospital discharge. J Pediatr. 2013;162:S90–100.
95. Schanler RJ, Burns PA, Abrams SA, Garza C. Bone mineralization outcomes in human milk-fed preterm infants. Pediatr Res. 1992;31:583–6.
96. Backstrom MC, Maki R, Kuusela AL, Sievanen H, Koivisto AM, Koskinen M, et al. The long-term effect of early mineral, vitamin D, and breast milk intake on bone mineral status in 9- to 11- year old children born prematurely. J Pediatr Gastroenterol Nutr. 1999;29:575–82.
97. Fewtrell MS, Prentice A, Jones SC, Bishop NJ, Stirling D, Buffenstein R, et al. Bone mineralization and turnover in preterm infants at 8-12 years of age: the effect of early diet. J Bone Miner Res. 1999;14:810–20.
98. van de Lagemaat M, Rotteveel J, van Weissenbruch MM, Lafeber HN. Increased gain in bone mineral content of preterm infants fed an isocaloric, protein-, and mineral-enriched postdischarge formula. Eur J Clin Nutr. 2013;52:1781–5.
99. Bowden LS, Jones CJ, Ryan SW. Bone mineralisation in ex-preterm infants aged 8 years. Eur J Pediatr. 1999;158:658–61.
100. Namgung R, Tsang RC, Specker BL, Sierra RI, Ho ML. Reduced serum osteocalcin and 1,25-dihydroxyvitamin D concentrations and low bone mineral content in small for gestational age infants: evidence of decreased bone formation rates. J Pediatr. 1993;122:269–75.
101. Verkauskiene R, Jaquet D, Deghmoun S, Chevenne D, Czernichow P, Lévy-Marchal C. Smallness for gestational age is associated with persistent change in insulin-like growth factor I (IGF-I) and the ratio of IGF-I/IGF-binding protein-3 in adulthood. J Clin Endocrinol Metab. 2005;90:5672–6.

102. Lem AJ, van der Kaay DCM, de Ridder MAJ, Bakker-van Waarde WM, van der Hulst FJPCM, Mulder JC, et al. Adult height in short children born SGA treated with growth hormone and gonadotropin releasing hormone analog: Results of a randomized, dose-response GH trial. J Clin Endocrinol Metab. 2012;97:4096–105.
103. Garn SM. Lifelong black-white differences in bone size and cortical area (letter). Am J Dis Child. 1990;144:750–1.
104. Hammami M, Koo WW, Hockman EM. Body composition of neonates from fan beam dual energy x-ray absorptiometry measurement. J Parenter Enteral Nutr. 2003;27:423–6.
105. Rupich RC, Specker BL, Lieuw-A-Fam N, Ho M. Gender and race differences in bone mass during infancy. Calcif Tissue Int. 1996;58:395–7.
106. Li JY, Specker BL, Ho ML, Tsang RC. Bone mineral content in black and white children 1 to 6 years of age. Am J Dis Child. 1989;143:1346–9.
107. Weiler HA, Fitzpatrick-Wong S, Schellenberg J. Bone mass in First Nations, Asian and white newborn infants. Growth Dev Aging. 2008;71(1):35–43.
108. Crabtree NJ, Kibirige MS, Fordham JN, Banks LM, Muntoni F, Chinn D, et al. The relationship between lean body mass and bone mienral content in paediatric health and disease. Bone. 2004;35:965–72.
109. Hogler W, Briody J, Woodhead H, Chan A, Cowell CT. Importance of lean mass in the interpretation of total body densitometry in children and adolescents. J Pediatr. 2003;143:81–8.
110. Wey HE, Binkley T, Beare T, Wey CL, Specker B. Cross-sectional versus longitudinal associations of lean and fat mass with pQCT bone outcomes in children. J Clin Endocrinol Metab. 2011;96:106–14.
111. Sudhagoni R, Wey HE, Djira GD, Specker B. Longitudinal effects of fat and lean mass on bone accrual in infants. Bone. 2012;50:638–42.
112. Steichen JJ, Tsang RC. Bone mineralization and growth in term infants fed soy-based or cow milk-based formula. J Pediatr. 1987;110:687–92.
113. Hillman LS. Bone mineral content in term infants fed human milk, cow milk-based formula, or soy-based formula. J Pediatr. 1988;113:208–12.
114. Jones G, Riley M, Dwyer T. Breastfeeding in early life and bone mass in prepubertal children: a longitudinal study. Osteoporos Int. 2000;11:146–52.
115. Harvey NC, Robinson SM, Crozier SR, Marriott LD, Gale CR, Cole ZA, et al. Breast-feeding and adherence to infant feeding guidelines do not influence bone mass at age 4 years. Br J Nutrit. 2009;102:915–20.
116. Fewtrell MS, Kennedy K, Murgatroyd PR, Williams JE, Chomtho S, Lucas A. Breast-feeding and formula feeding in healthy term infants and bone health at age 10 years. Br J Nutr. 2013;1106:1061–7.
117. Bailey DA, McKay HA, Mirwald RL, Crocker PRE, Faulkner RA. A six-year longitudinal study of the relationship of physical activity to bone mineral accrual in growing children: the University of Saskatchewan Bone Mineral Accrual Study. J Bone Miner Res. 1999;14:1672–9.
118. Specker BL, Mulligan L, Ho ML. Longitudinal study of calcium intake, physical activity, and bone mineral content in infants 6-18 months of age. J Bone Miner Res. 1999;14:569–76.
119. Janz KF, Letuchy EM, Eichenberger-Gimore JM, Burns TL, Torner JC, Willing MD, et al. Early physical activity provides sustained bone health benefits later in childhood. Med Sci Sports Exer. 2010;42:1072–8.
120. Abrams SA, Bhatia JJS, Corkins MR, de Ferranti SD, Golden NH, Silverstein J. Calcium and vitamin D requirement of enterally fed preterm infants. Pediatrics. 2013;131:e1676–83.
121. WHO. Assessment of fracture risk and its application to screening for postmenopausal osteoporosis: report of a WHO study group. Geneva: WHO Technical Report Series 843; 1994.
122. Leib ES, Lewiecki EM, Binkley N, Hamdy RC. Official positions of the International Society for Clinical Densitometry. J Clin Densit. 2004;7:1–5.
123. Brunton JA, Weiler HA, Atkinson SA. Improvement in the accuracy of dual energy x-ray absorptiometry for whole body and regional analysis of body composition: validation using piglets and methodologic considerations in infants. Pediatr Res. 1997;41:590–6.

124. Picaud JC, Lapillonne A, Pieltain C, Reygrobellet B, Claris O, Salle BL, et al. Software and scan acquisition technique-related discrepancies in bone mineral assessment using dual-energy X-ray absorptiometry in neonates. Acta Paediatr. 2002;91(11):1189–93.
125. Koo WW, Hockman EM, Hammami M. Dual energy X-ray absorptiometry measuements in small subjects: conditions affecting clinical measurements. J Am Coll Nutr. 2004;23(3):212–9.
126. Avila-Díaz M, Flores-Huerta S, Martínez-Muñiz I, Amato D. Increments in whole body bone mineral content associated with weight and length in pre-term and full-term infants during the first 6 months of life. Arch Med Res. 2001;32:288–92.
127. Koo WWK, Hammami M, Margeson DP, Nwaesei C, Montalto MB, Lasekan JB. Reduced bone mineralization in infants fed palm olein-containing formula: a randomized, double-blinded, prospective trial. Pediatrics. 2003;111:1017–23.
128. Koo WW, Hammami M, Hockman EM. Interchangeability of pencil-beam and fan-beam dual-energy X-ray absorptiometry measurements in piglets and infants. Am J Clin Nutr. 2003;78(2):236–40.
129. Fields DA, Demerath EW, Pietrobelli A, Chandler-Laney PC. Body composition at 6 months of life: comparison of air displacement plethysmography and dual-energy X-ray absorptiometry. Obesity. 2012;20(11):2302–6.
130. Venkataraman PS, Ahluwalia BW. Total bone mineral content and body composition by x-ray densitometry in newborns. Pediatrics. 1992;90:767–70.
131. Atkinson SA, Randall-Simpson J. Factors influencing body composition of premature infants at term-adjusted age. Ann NY Acad Sci. 2000;904:393–9.
132. Koo WWK, Bush AJ, Walters J, Carlson SE. Postnatal development of bone mineral status during infancy. J Am Coll Nutr. 1998;17(1):65–70.
133. Butte NF, Hopkinson JM, Wong WW, Smith EO, Ellis K. Body composition during the first 2 years of life: an updated reference. Pediatr Res. 2000;47(5):578–85.
134. Braillon PM, Salle BL, Brunet J, Gloricux FII, Delmas PD, Meunier PJ. Dual energy x-ray absorptiometry measurement of bone mineral content in newborns: validation of a technique. Pediatr Res. 1992;32:77–80.
135. Salle BL, Braillon P, Glorieux FH, Brunet J, Cavero E, Meunier PJ. Lumbar bone mineral content measured by dual energy x-ray absorptiometry in newborns and infants. Acta Paediatr. 1992;81:953–8.
136. Kurl S, Heinonen K, Jurvelin JS, Lansimies E. Lumbar bone mineral content and density measured using a Lunar DPX densitometer in healthy full-term infants during the first year of life. Clin Physiol Funct Imaging. 2002;22(3):222–5.

# Chapter 9
# DXA in Children with Special Needs

Heidi H. Kecskemethy, Elizabeth Szalay, and H. Theodore Harcke

## Introduction

Children with special needs include those with neuromuscular conditions, cognitive deficits, and/or some skeletal dysplasias. These conditions place the child at risk for suboptimal bone health due to any combination of limited or lack of weight-bearing, poor nutrition, lack of sun exposure, limited intake of and/or deficiencies of calcium or vitamin D, and use of medications that negatively affect bone metabolism. This combination of factors causes skeletal deficits in children with a variety of medical conditions ranging from cerebral palsy (CP), Rett Syndrome, Duchenne muscular dystrophy (DMD), spina bifida (SB), spinal muscular atrophy (SMA), and other genetic syndromes that cause neuromuscular problems [1–5].

Children who are unable to bear weight have increased risk for fracture and exhibit low bone mineral density (BMD) and content [6]. The mechanism for bone weakening due to immobility or weightlessness is well described in both adult and pediatric literature [7, 8]. The deleterious effect of reduced or absent weight bearing on bone is described in many circumstances, including after surgery [9], post spinal cord injury [10], weightlessness in space [11, 12], and immobilization from casting [13, 14]. The types of fractures that healthy children experience differ from those in

H.H. Kecskemethy, MS.Ed., R.D.N., C.S.P., C.B.D.T. (✉)
Departments of Biomedical Research and Medical Imaging, Nemours/A.I. duPont
Hospital for Children, 1600 Rockland Rd, Wilmington, DE 19803, USA
e-mail: hkecskem@nemours.org

E. Szalay, M.D. (Deceased)
Pediatric Orthopedic Surgery, Carrie Tingley Hospital, University of New Mexico,
2211 Lomas Blvd NE, Albuquerque, NM 87106, USA

H.T. Harcke, M.D., F.A.C.R., F.A.I.U.M.
Department of Medical Imaging, Nemours/A.I. duPont Hospital for Children,
1600 Rockland Road, Wilmington, DE 19086, USA
e-mail: tharcke@nemours.org

© Springer International Publishing Switzerland 2016                                   179
E.B. Fung et al. (eds.), *Bone Health Assessment in Pediatrics*,
DOI 10.1007/978-3-319-30412-0_9

non-ambulatory children with disabilities; healthy children sustain forearm fractures [15] while disabled children more commonly sustain lower extremity fractures [16, 17], with the majority occurring in the distal femur [17, 18]. The mechanism of fracture also differs: healthy children sustain fracture with trauma, while low energy fractures are common in non-ambulatory children with neuromuscular conditions [19]. In prospective studies of healthy children, DXA measures have been found to predict future fracture risk [20, 21]. Similarly in non-ambulatory children, lower extremity BMD has been associated with fracture in non-ambulatory children with CP and DMD [19].

In addition to immobilization disorders, other underlying medical conditions may also affect skeletal growth and development. Atypical skeletal development, morphology, and mineralization as seen the skeletal dysplasias including osteogenesis imperfecta (OI) and mucopolysacchridoses pose other unique issues with scan acquisition and interpretation of bone density results.

## Challenges of Measuring Children with Disabilities

The challenges in acquiring usable scans at the recommended body sites in pediatric dual-energy X-ray absorptiometry (DXA) in children with special needs stem from both positioning difficulties and from artifacts encountered that can be present on the scan. Acquiring and interpreting scans on these children requires more than an understanding of the medical condition and indication for the scan. With patience and creativity, a child deemed impossible to be assessed by DXA can be successfully studied. Disability refers to cognitive delays, physical (neuromuscular) disabilities, or both. Cognitive delays can affect the patient's ability to understand, follow instructions, and cooperate during the scan, whereas physical disabilities may affect positioning, cause involuntary movement, and compromise the validity of certain body sites for scan acquisition due to the presence of internal hardware. It is not unusual for a medical condition to have both cognitive and physical implications.

Some facilities use sedation to prevent movement or to allow the patient to relax enough for required positioning. Every center has its own rules on sedation and in some facilities, sedation may not be an option. The risk of sedation must be weighed against the potential benefit of the information obtained from the scan. Some DXA body sites, such as the total body, may require sedation while others do not; the importance of the information provided by the body site measured must considered by the clinician when ordering (sedation for) DXA. It may be prudent to limit the study to those sites that can be obtained without sedation. A conversation between the imaging center and the ordering clinician should occur to determine the center's familiarity measuring children with disabilities, scanning techniques they use, and results obtained when a DXA scan is ordered for a child with disabilities. Scanning centers that frequently scan children with disabilities will likely offer more options for scanning alternative body sites that typically do not require sedation.

Many centers use a questionnaire that gathers patient information necessary for the technologist to acquire optimal scans and to aid the clinician in proper interpretation of scan results (see Chap. 7 for details). Consideration of these factors allows for optimal decision making about scan site selection and will aid in correct interpretation of results.

Pre-scan patient information is used by the technologist to determine DXA scan site selection; specifics are discussed in the next sections. This information will also be helpful to the clinician interpreting the scan (Table 9.1).

## Positioning and Artifacts

It can be difficult if not impossible to scan the recommended body sites of whole body and PA lumbar spine in children who have joint contractures or limited mobility, dislocated hips, severe scoliosis, compression fractures, and limited range of motion, as can be seen in children with CP, muscular dystrophy (MD), certain genetic syndromes and conditions, and OI (Fig. 9.1). Movement disorders, lack of understanding due to limited cognitive abilities, and the inability to lie in a required position can pose additional challenges to obtaining usable scans. Lying flat on the back for the duration of the scan time, for instance, as is required for the total body scan may not be possible for some patients who have severe gastroesophageal reflux or respiratory compromise in that position. Severe scoliosis, kyphosis and/or lordosis can make appropriate positioning impossible for technically valid lumbar spine measurements.

The presence of internal metallic devices or hardware causes a fictitious increase in BMD results. Metallic artifacts commonly seen in children with disabilities can include any combination of rods, screws, plates, clips, and baclofen pumps (Fig. 9.2a, b). Other artifacts that can affect BMD include movement, positioning aids (wedges, pillows, sandbags), and tubes (IV's, button, ventriculoperitoneal shunt, feeding tube, portacath). When performing serial scans on patients with non-removable artifacts, careful attention should be paid to the appearance and position of the artifact which would affect the ability to compare serial studies and interpret change in BMD over time. If the artifacts are external (e.g. a lead running from the patient to a machine), the position of the artifact should be replicated to ensure better reproducibility.

**Table 9.1** Pre-scan patient information useful for technologist to determine DXA scan site selection and for clinician scan interpretation

| |
|---|
| • Diagnosis |
| • Fracture history |
| • Medication use (steroid, anticonvulsant, and bisphosphonate) |
| • Status of hips (dislocation, past surgery) |
| • Presence of nonremovable orthopedic or internal hardware and location (plates, screws, rods, baclofen pump, button, tracheostomy) |
| • Tubes (ventriculoperitoneal shunt, feeding tube, portacath) |
| • Scoliosis |
| • Use of contrast material for medical tests in the past 7 days may affect total body and lumbar spine values and require rescheduling |

**Fig. 9.1** Total body DXA in a 17-year-old male with CP. Head motion, contractures, severe scoliosis, and dislocated right hip are evident. Total body less head values unaffected by head movement

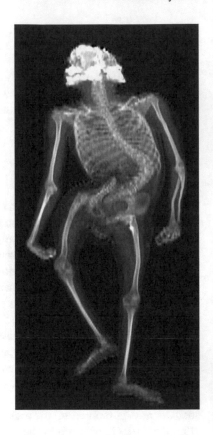

It is common to encounter a number of complicating factors in children with disabilities that can compromise scan quality or negate the value of the scan. Some DXA body sites are more prone to be problematic, such as the whole body. Other body sites, while obtainable, may give information of limited clinical value. Positioning concerns and the presence of artifact must be considered in scan site selection.

## Body Sites to Measure

Recommend body sites to measure by DXA in children are addressed in Chap. 5, and include the total body (less head) and PA lumbar spine. Other body sites such as the lateral distal femur and forearm may also be useful sites to measure by DXA in specific circumstances [22]. Alternative sites are sometimes the only sites that can be measured and for some populations may provide the most clinically relevant information about BMD in these children. This section describes the circumstances

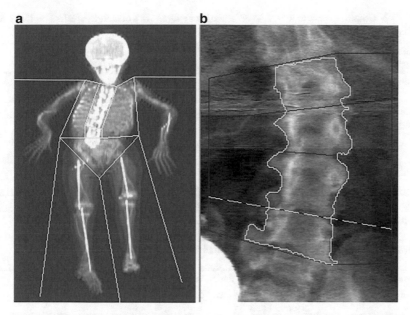

**Fig. 9.2** Metallic artifacts frequently encountered when measuring BMD in children with neuromuscular disabilities. (**a**) Total body DXA in 11-year-old female with OI: note spinal fusion and fixation of left forearm and lower extremities. Note increased density in distal femurs and proximal tibias due to bisphosphonate treatment. (**b**) Lumbar scoliosis and indwelling baclofen pump in lower right corner of scan on lumbar spine DXA in 18 year old male with CP. Scan successfully accomplished avoiding overlap of metallic pump with edge of vertebral bodies

commonly encountered while measuring children with special needs at the common and alternative pediatric DXA body sites (Table 9.2). Site-specific influences noted in Table 9.2 do not always mean that a measure from that site should be disregarded; rather, it should be accounted for in interpretation. It is important to obtain scans on as many body sites as feasible during the initial exam, because a body site may become of limited value over time as fractures occur or metal rods or hardware are inserted. Subregion analysis of a body site may allow the continued use of that site over time.

## Recommended DXA Sites for Children

### Lumbar Spine

Many patients with disabilities can cooperate for lumbar spine scan acquisition due to a short scan time (<30 s) and a stable position. The position required is comfortable for most because while patients are still on their back, their hips and knees are

**Table 9.2** Conditions encountered when scanning children with disabilities, effect on DXA scan, and body site affected

| Condition encountered | Problem created with scan | DXA site affected |
|---|---|---|
| Excessive movement | Movement artifact | All; least likely to affect LDF |
| Contractures | Inability to place correct regions of interest | TB; H |
| Scoliosis | Inability to place correct regions of interest | TB; LS |
| Metallic implant | Artifact—metal adds density | All; implants least likely in LDF |
| Feeding tube | Artifact—adds density or area | TB; likely LS |
| Baclofen pump | Artifact—metal adds density | TB; possibly LS |
| High muscle tone | Positioning problems; unable to lie flat | TB; H; rarely LDF |
| Startle reflex | Movement artifact when table and/or arm moves | All; most likely TB |
| Obesity | Patient exceeds width of table; excessive tissue thickness | TB; possibly LS |
| Cognitive delays | Patient unable to understand instructions | All; most likely TB |
| Dislocated hip | Atypical anatomy invalidates landmarks for valid analysis | H; possibly LDF |

*DXA* dual energy X-ray absorptiometry, *TB* total body, *LS* lumbar spine, *H* hip, *LDF* lateral distal femur
*Reprinted with permission.* Kecskemethy HH, Harcke HT. Assessment of bone health in children with Disabilities. J Pediatr Rehabil Med. 2014;7(2):111–24

in flexion and the knees are supported on a foam block which has the net effect of creating more trunk stability and less stress on contracted muscles with limited range of motion. Gastroesophgeal reflux and respiratory concerns may still be present, though they are typically not a concern due to the very short scan time. However, scoliosis, the presence of abdominal artifacts (tubes, shunts, pumps), and spinal compression fractures, and atypical skeletal morphology, as seen in the skeletal dysplasias, all have an effect on the scan analysis and must be considered for scan interpretation. Spinal fusion instrumentation to stabilize scoliosis may be present in the lumbar region and preclude measurement of some or all of the vertebral elements. Orthopedic hardware will artificially elevate BMD results.

## Total Body

Total body is usually the most problematic body site to measure by DXA in children with special needs for several reasons. The total body scan takes the longest to perform, running 1.5–55 min depending on the scanner used and size of the patient; holding still for the time required for scan acquisition can be challenging for young children, those with limited cognitive ability, and for patients with positioning limitations. Because of the longer scan time, this body site is most susceptible to movement artifact. A valid total body DXA scan requires the patient to lie flat on the scan table, which can be impossible for children with contractures. For many children with disabilities, lying supine creates discomfort and may be contraindicated due to gastroesopageal reflux or respiratory compromise that may be exacerbated by the position. Some children with special needs, particularly those with sensorimotor issues or high startle reflexes (as seen in spasticity) feel unstable on their back and fear that they may fall off the edge of the table. Indwelling artifacts from metallic hardware or tubes are frequently present somewhere in the body and because the entire body is being scanned, all nonremovable medical equipment in or on the patient will be evident on the scan and will affect results by elevating BMD values.

## Alternative DXA Sites

### Forearm

The forearm DXA scan is useful for children who exceed the weight limit of the table or who have metallic or other artifacts in body parts measured at other scan sites. In a group of 90 children with repeated forearm fractures, forearm DXA results (BMD and BMC) were found to be significantly reduced [23]. Usefulness of the forearm for monitoring site-specific changes has been demonstrated, and it correlates well to strength indices of peripheral quantitative computed tomography [24]. Compared to total body and spine, the forearm scan in children has the poorest precision [25]. The forearm is a resident scan modality for scan acquisition and analysis on bone densitometry machines. Normative data are available for children, but are limited to the Hologic scanner [26, 27].

The position requires the patient to place their forearm in the center of the scan table, typically leaning from a seated position alongside the table. For small children with special needs, the positioning may involve the child laying supine on the scan table with the arm extended. The hand must be flat on the scan table which can be problematic for children with hand contractures. If arm range of motion is limited due to contractures, extension of the arm in order to reach the proper position on the table may not be possible. For more adult-sized obese patients, like teenage boys with Duchenne Muscular Dystrophy, it may not be possible for the arm to reach the required position on the scan table due to excessive soft tissue around the torso, limited arm reach, and pain.

### Lateral Distal Femur

The lateral distal femur (LDF) was first described by Harcke et al. in 1998 and was developed specifically to measure BMD in children for whom the traditional sites were invalid or unobtainable due to the presence of hardware, contractures, scoliosis, or excessive movement [28]. The distal femur was chosen because it is the bone most likely to fracture in non-ambulatory children and therefore is the most clinically relevant site to assess [18, 29]. The lateral body placement allows for a comfortable, side-lying position for scan acquisition and it is well tolerated in children with a variety of disabilities including CP, SB, DMD, OI, spinal muscular atrophy, Rett syndrome, Pelizaeus-Merzacher Syndrome, and Mucopolysacchridosis IV (Morquio A & B) [9, 16, 19, 30–37]. Many times it is the only viable and valid site to measure in children with special needs [4].

The LDF scan modality is not available on any DXA scanner, so the scan is acquired in the forearm mode. Because the scan modality does not exist on any DXA system, specialized training on scan acquisition and scan analysis is required; acquisition and analysis techniques vary depending on manufacturer. Several pediatric centers in the United States and internationally have been trained and regularly utilize the LDF DXA scan. For scan analysis, the DXA technologist manually creates three subregions of interest for the LDF using a standardized approach that was designed to accommodate changes in bone due to growth. In addition, a correction factor is applied to adjust for technological system upgrades that can affect the aspect ratio of the scan image [38]. The three regions of interest represent three types of bone: Region 1, adjacent to the growth plate is the metaphyseal region, comprised primarily of trabecular bone; Region 2 is the metadiaphyseal region, and is a balanced aggregate of cortical and trabecular bone; and Region 3 is the diaphyseal region, comprised primarily of cortical bone (Fig. 9.3). Because Region 1 is primarily cancellous (trabecular) bone, it is the most sensitive area for noting bone turnover (gain or loss). The growth plate, where endochondral bone formation occurs, is highly affected by bisphosphonates [30].

The position requires the patient to lie on their side for the leg that is being measured. Positioning aids (foam blocks and a sand bag) are frequently used to elevate and support the leg that is not being measured. Bilateral measurements are recommended because there are side-to-side difference in non-ambulatory children and a high likelihood that one femur may fracture sometime during childhood [39, 40]. Lower extremity fracture is the most common site of fracture in non-ambulatory children with CP and within the lower extremities, the majority of are distal femur fractures [29, 41–43]. Most patients tolerate the position very well, as it is similar to a side-sleeping position, and when properly positioned, very stable and less susceptible to movement than other DXA sites (Fig. 9.4). However, some patients with dislocated hips may have difficulty lying on their side. Scan acquisition time is 20–40 s. Normative data are available for children, but are limited to the Hologic scanner [44].

More information about the LDF can be obtained at www.lateraldistalfemur.org.

**Fig. 9.3** LDF DXA
analysis protocol requires
placement of 3 subregions
of interest: Region 1 (distal
metaphysic) is primarily
trabecular bone; Region 2
(metadiaphyseal) is mixed
cortical and trabecular
bone; and Region 3
(diaphyseal) is mainly
cortical bone. Note
movement at the top of the
scan beyond regions of
interest: patient was able to
hold still long enough for
successful scan acquisition

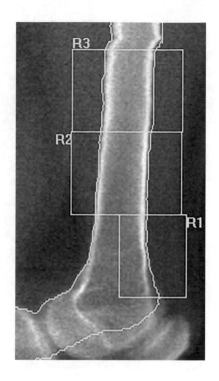

# Strategies for Scanning Children with Special Needs: Measurement and Analysis

When acquiring a DXA on a child with special needs, it is usually helpful to have the family or care providers stay in the room to help to reassure the child and assist with moving and positioning the child. They also usually know best how to help their child relax. If the child has a movement disorder, extra hands may be needed to help to hold the child during the scan. Prior to scanning, the DXA technologist should inform the child and care providers about what will happen during the exam, and how the machine moves and sounds during the scan.

Patients can present with chronic pain, dislocated hips, and the inability to move or control extremities. Large body habitus and knee contractures pose a challenge in positioning children with special needs—some are unable to fit within the parameters of the scanning table. If the patient exceeds the scanning width of the table, as can occur with large patients with Duchenne's Muscular Dystrophy (DMD) or in patients with knee flexion contractures, an approach called "offset scanning" should be used [45]. In offset scanning, the patient is positioned so the axis of the body is offset from the center axis of the scan table, thereby allowing one side of the patient to lie beyond the width of the scan table and ensuring that one side of the patient is completely scanned. If the patient has knee and hip contractures that will not allow them to straighten their legs for the total body measurement except in a wind-swept

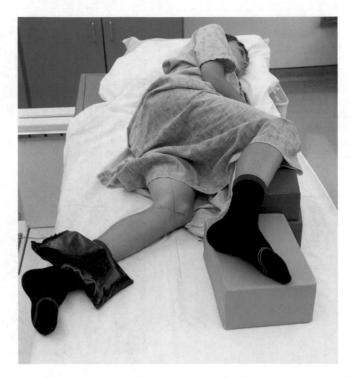

**Fig. 9.4** The side-lying position required for LDF DXA acquisition is comfortable for children with disabilities. The leg being measured (closest to the table) is positioned with femoral shaft following the long axis of the table. *LDF* lateral distal femur, *DXA* dual energy X-ray absorptiometry

or frog-legged position they can lie flat on the table; these leg positions can still yield valid total body scans. Similarly, if the child is not able to lie or keep their arms by their sides for the total body, care must be taken to ensure that the arms and hands remain flat on the table in whatever position is comfortable; care must be taken to keep the hands out the head region of interest for valid total body less head results.

Experienced bone densitometry technologists who are accustomed to acquiring images on children with special needs are familiar with ways to decrease anxiety for children and accompanying care providers. General tips for obtaining scans on children with disabilities are listed in Table 9.3. It is imperative that positioning is consistent at every body site measured to create valid, reproducible serial scans (described in Chap. 5).

During scan analysis, technologists should carefully review bone mapping and ROI placement, particularly if auto-analysis was used, making any necessary corrections. Errors are more apt to occur with auto-analysis when measuring atypical anatomy or with very low bone density. During analysis of whole body scans acquired using the "offset" technique, the values of the side that was completely

**Table 9.3** General tips for scanning children with disabilities

| Tip | Effect |
|---|---|
| Explain and show how the scanning table/arm moves | Helps the child know what to expect—see how machine moves; hear machine sounds |
| Low noise, dim lights | Lessen startle reflex from noises; calming atmosphere to promote relaxation |
| Parent/care provider stands beside child at head of table | Assures child that they will not roll or fall off of the machine table. Can provide help holding the child, if needed, for positioning and reassurance |
| Use sheet on table | Used as draw sheet to help with positioning |
| Have positioning aids handy | Pillows, foam blocks, wedges, sandbags can be useful for positioning, stabilization, and comfort |
| Take time; do not rush | Relaxed technologist=relaxed parent/care provider=better chance of relaxed child |
| Wait for patient to get used to new position | Tone is higher after repositioning; wait for tone to decrease |
| Avoid conversation during scan acquisition | Discourage response by child during scan to minimize movement and excitability. Parent/care provider should sing or calmly talk continuously to child to keep them relaxed and engaged |
| Wait until entire exam is complete to celebrate and shower child with praise | Share in great joy when study is complete! Calm, positive encouragement given after each scan during study. Excessive excitement between scans increases tone and child loses focus |
| Hands on | Strategically placed hands help stabilize, prevent movement artifact, and relax the child |
| Have scan ready to start before positioning | Quickly scanning once patient is positioned requires patient to hold position for less time |

*Reprinted with permission.* Kecskemethy HH, Harcke HT. Assessment of bone health in children with Disabilities. J Pediatr Rehabil Med. 2014;7(2):111–24

scanned are then mirrored for the extremities that were not included on the scan. This approach is deemed to be more accurate than ignoring the body parts that were excluded from the scan. The way that this "offsetting" is accomplished varies by machine brand: one manufacturer's machine allows for replacement of one limb exhibiting large differences in bone density with the BMD values from the contra-lateral limb and another manufacturer's software uses a mirroring technique of half of the body scan [45]. The general tips listed on Table 9.3 apply to any body site being measured.

## Specific Scanning Tips by Body Site

Following are specific tips, listed by body site, which can be helpful when measuring children with special needs.

## Lumbar Spine

The lumbar spine position is generally more comfortable and easily obtained than the total body. This provides an immediate success and lets the child understand the sounds and movement of the machine, which relaxes both child and care-provider and can help for the remainder of the exam. It is important to consider how well the child can control his legs. If muscle control is poor or nonexistent or if the child has uncontrolled movements, the technologist should keep his or her hands on the patient's legs during the scan and whenever the legs are on the positioning block to ensure patient safety. If the child has a g-tube, move or remove the extension tubing so that it is not overlapping the spine. If a baclofen pump is present and overlaps the edge of a vertebra on the scan, repositioning the child may decrease or eliminate overlap on the spine. Because the scan time is very quick, it can be useful to perform this scan first (Fig. 9.2b).

## Total Body

The whole body is generally the most difficult to acquire and the most challenging scan to analyze. Correct ROI placement may not be attainable depending on the positioning limitations of the patient (Fig. 9.1). Attempting to acquire this scan last will allow the child to get used to the sounds and movement of the machine, which can help them relax and decrease muscle tone for better positioning and reduce movement. It will also help the parent or care provider relax, which in turn helps the child to relax. It may not be possible to acquire a total body scan and successfully acquiring other scans first will make success in acquiring the total body less stressful. Assess for attached artifact-producing items and remove as many as possible. For example, some patients with SMA will continuously wear a pulse oximeter. Determine if it is possible to remove it for the scan duration. If it is not possible, minimize the amount of the lead on the table, and ensure that the device itself is not on the scan table.

The technologist should be familiar with the scan acquisition pattern of the machine and use this to determine how they make accommodations with explanation and/or strategic holding of body parts. For instance, some scanners acquire the total body scan in several full-length passes of the table, moving across the table from the patient's right to left. If the child is able to understand and can answer when asked if they will be able to hold their arm down by their side for a few seconds while the scan arm passes over that area, they may be able to temporarily hold that position, and then once that arm has been scanned, the technologist can carefully move the arm to a more comfortable position as long as it is in the scan field that has already been acquired. Tape can be useful to help the child temporarily hold a position, as long as the technologist has verified that it would be permissible to use tape and that the patient does not have a tape allergy. In order to position appendages flat on the table within the width of the table, and not overlying other body parts, it may be necessary to strategically move appendages *during the scan*. This requires explanation to the child that you will help them by doing this, their agreement, and the willingness of the technologist to be hands-on. It also requires the technologist to carefully keep an eye on both the scan arm as the scan is being acquired to see where the X-ray beam is relative to the body, and the computer screen to make sure the image is being acquired properly. Explaining to the child what is happening, when they might be touched or moved, and when the machine will move is important. For some children with high muscle tone or a strong startle reflex, the act of touching or moving one body part will cause involuntary movement in another. This possibility must be assessed prior to starting the scan.

## Forearm

Small children can lie prone of the table with their arm extended in order to properly position the forearm on the scanner table. For larger patients who must be seated alongside the table, using a chair without arms will allow them lean closer to the required location on the table. If the patient is in a wheel chair, inquire whether the arm can be removed on the side next to the table. Some wheel chairs have adjustable height seats and it may be necessary to adjust the seat height to assist with positioning. Once in the required position, holding the arm above the elbow can reduce the chance of movement. Tape can also be useful to hold the hand in position to minimize movement. If using tape, seek permission and verify that the patient has no tape allergy.

## Lateral Distal Femur

Because the LDF was developed for children with disabilities, it is generally very well tolerated. The position is side-lying, on the side being measured. It is imperative to have a pillow under the head and to support the knee and ankle of the leg not being measured by placing them on foam blocks which provides greater comfort, less stress on joints and facilitates relaxation. Watch to make sure that the pillow does not obstruct the child's face and that they are able to breathe. When positioning the child on the table for the LDF, the femur being measured should follow the long axis of the table. The body and other leg should be adjusted accordingly. It is not necessary to align the child's body to the axis of the table, only the leg being measured needs to be aligned to the axis of the table. It is frequently necessary for the child's back (head to rump) to run diagonally or nearly across the width of the table depending on hip flexion contractures. A draw sheet on the table is very useful for adjusting the patient's position on the table.

For children exhibiting muscular rigidity (high muscle tone in both flexor and extensor muscles), spasticity (hypertonia in one set of muscles), and severe contractures of the hip and leg joints, slow and small positioning adjustments should be made with the legs, allowing the child's muscles to relax and conform to the position before making the next adjustment. Rapid movements and extending a child to the limit of their range of motion can cause pain and frequently results in increased spasticity (activation of antagonist muscles) and reactionary jerking movements which cause movement and the inability to maintain a position. It can be extremely difficult for children with hypertonia and hip contractures to "scissor" their legs; a calm, nonhurried approach along with careful positioning by the technologist will yield positive results.

The LDF should be acquired with the distal femur in true anatomic lateral orientation; on the scan image, the condyles of the distal femur should be aligned posteriorly and the knee cap should not overlap the anterior margin of the femur. Slight positioning adjustments at the hips and shoulders as well as varying the height of the knee not being scanned can correct a femur that is not truly lateral. For children with athetosis resulting in excessive movement, with limited understanding, or who just cannot lie still, a hand firmly holding the hip with slight pressure toward the table will provide security and stability and minimize movement at the femur being measured. In children with very excessive movement and muscle spasms, the help of an extra person will be needed. One person can stabilize the hip and shoulder, and the second person hold can hold the proximal tibia just below the knee to isolate the area of interest being measured. This will allow for a valid scan even when the child is moving a body part outside the scan area. Contrary to expectation, attempting to hold the entire body still on patients with high muscle tone will yield even greater spasticity and movement.

For obese patients who may not have the ability to control their legs, such as teenage boys with DMD, SMA, or SB, positioning can be limited by the width of the scan table and their limited range of motion or muscle flaccidity. For safety, two people are needed to help move these patients from side to side for LDF positioning and they should remain during the scan to ensure that the child is stable and supported. Many very large patients who are unable to control their limbs could and will fear that they may fall off of the table if not properly supported.

## Scan Interpretation

### *Challenges*

Clinical condition and current and/or prior treatment must be considered when interpreting DXA scans for any age patient. In children with special needs, there are many clinical factors that can affect interpretation of results. Morphologic, developmental, and therapeutic parameters commonly encountered with these children include small stature and bone size, early or late onset of puberty affecting skeletal maturity, under or overweight, medication use that can affect BMD, history of fracture and surgery, atypical skeletal growth/mineralization, and altered functional activity. Because of the propensity of these children to fracture, bisphosphonate treatment is now often used in children with OI or idiopathic or disuse osteoporosis who have low BMD and history of fracture [30, 31, 46–48].

It is expected that BMD of non-ambulatory children will be lower than normal for age, as has been demonstrated in several populations including CP, DMD, SB, and Rett Sydrome [1, 3, 4, 19, 30–32, 34–37]. Impaired ambulation is one of the most significant risk factors for low BMD, but physical development is also relevant. Children with height and weight measures below the 5th percentile can be expected to have lower BMD than their normal sized peers of the same age. Examining bone mineral content in addition to BMD may provide additional insight into abnormal results. If results are unexpectedly normal or high when one would expect low values, contributory factors such as the presence of artifact or callus with healing fracture should be explored to rule out technical reasons for the unexpected findings.

It may or may not be appropriate to compare the patient's results with normative reference data depending on the child's medical condition and the quality of the scan. The appropriateness of comparing the bone density of children with disabilities (who may have smaller bones, bone loss, or abnormal bone metabolism) to children who are typically developing, normal sized, and ambulatory is currently under debate amongst pediatric bone experts.

## Size

Size of the child is an important factor, and adjustments to BMD based on size may be appropriate, however there is lack of consensus within the scientific community as to which adjustments to BMD are most appropriate and when they should be applied [22]. Size adjustments based on height should be considered with caution for conditions involving contractures, as obtaining accurate height measures on these children is extremely difficult. For patients with significantly reduced heights in comparison to their peers, like those with mucopolysacchridoses, adjusting BMD using a height correction can result in overcorrection [38]. Typically the height Z-score correction works well for children with height Z-scores between −2.5 and +2.5 (B. Zemel, personal communication).

## Skeletal Maturity

Assessment of stage in puberty or bone age, to gain a sense of skeletal maturation, provides insight into the interpretation of BMD results. Skeletal maturity is frequently assessed by radiologic assessment of the growth centers of the hand and wrist (bone age). Bone age is used as an indication of skeletal development with regard to chronologic age. This provides an indication of where the individual is on the pathway to skeletal maturity. Children with achondroplasia exhibit impaired bone growth without skeletal delay. Puberty is also used as an indicator of physical development and it is known that onset is normally associated with a period of rapid growth and increase in BMD. Pubertal development is assessed by evaluating and classifying the development of secondary sexual characteristics into five stages as defined by Tanner (Tanner stage). In children with cerebral palsy, early or delayed puberty is common [49]. BMD is influenced by gonadal sex steroids. For children with late or early onset of puberty, caution should be used when comparing BMD results to normal reference standards which are based on chronologic age and assume normal progression of puberty.

## Artifacts

The presence of metallic and nonmetallic artifacts overlying bone on scan images have the effect of increasing BMD values and depending on placement may alter bone edge detection and increase area. Movement artifact affects bone edge detection and negatively impacts reproducibility on serial scans. Infrequently, barium may be present in the intestine from earlier GI studies and this may appear on the total body or lumbar spine scan; barium superimposed on bone in DXA images increases BMD results and therefore invalidates the resulting values.

## Normative Values

In pediatrics, DXA scan results are compared to age, race, and gender-matched norms and are reported as Z-scores, as described in Chaps. 6 and 7. These normative data are based on large groups of typically developing healthy children. Normative values are available for all DXA body sites described in this chapter, however normative values for the LDF and forearm in children are limited to the Hologic scanner. Manufacturer-specific normative values are available for the total body and lumbar spine, though there are limited data for certain races and availability varies by body site. Attention should be paid to both the version of software being used for scan analysis (because with system upgrades, default scan acquisition settings can change) and changes in normative databases triggered by the software version. Changes in scan settings and reference norms can influence BMD values and Z-score values, respectively, on serial scans.

## Bisphosphonates

Bisphosponate therapy is generally restricted to patients who have sustained low trauma, fragility fractures in an attempt to improve BMD and reduce fracture occurrence [30, 31, 46, 50]. Bisphosponates are sometimes given to children to improve BMD and reduce fracture occurrence [30, 31, 46, 50]. When growing children

**Fig. 9.5** LDF DXA in a
14-year-old boy with
Pelizaeus Merzbacher
syndrome undergoing
pamidronate treatment.
Three subregions of
interest are placed
according to LDF analysis
protocol. In Region 1,
dense parallel bands reflect
treatment cycles. Migration
of bands reflects interval
growth

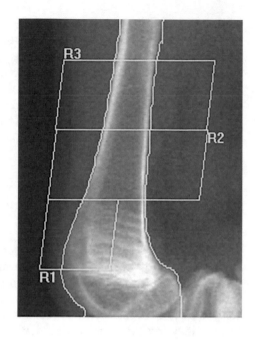

receive cyclical bisphosphonate treatments, dense metaphseal bands form at the growth plates of the long bones. With serial courses of treatment and growth they appear as dense parallel bands which can increase BMD. The bands are particularly evident on the LDF (Fig. 9.5). Bisphosphonates increase BMD at all 3 regions of the LDF but region 1, adjacent to the growth plate, exhibits that greatest increase, raising BMD as much as 89 % [30]. As the bone continues to grow, the bands migrate up the femoral shaft, eventually moving into region 2 and region 3, which then exhibit a larger increase in BMD than when the bands weren't in the region. If bisphosphonate treatment is stopped, the bands disappear over time as bone remodeling occurs. In some patients, the bands remain evident for several years after discontinuation of treatment.

## Atypical Skeletal Configuration or Morphology

Scoliosis is common in children with neuromuscular conditions. In severe scoliosis or lordosis it may be very challenging to obtain a valid scan image. The spine may barely fit within the ROI, vertebral bodies may overlap, or individual vertebral bodies may be so rotated that they appear nearly lateral on an anterior-posterior projection. Correct region of interest placement can be challenging and reproducibility on subsequent scans can be compromised as curvature increases.

Children with skeletal dysplasias have abnormal skeletal conformation due to atypical bone size, morphology, and mineralization. Most patients with mucopolysaccharide disorders exhibit abnormally shaped vertebrae, dislocated hips, and short stature. Correct positioning for the spine can be difficult due to overlapping vertebrae, making the validity of scan results. Lumbar spine DXA images are difficult to interpret for children with Mucoplysaccharidosis IV because vertebrae are bullet-shaped, beaked, and overlapping [51]. Children with OI exhibit atypical bone mineralization, morphometry, and short stature to varying degrees as determined by clinical severity and type of OI.

## Initial/Baseline Scan

The initial DXA scan allows for assessment of results in comparison to normal, healthy children of the same race, gender, and age; the goal is to establish a baseline against which subsequent scans will be compared. Artifacts present on scans will influence Z-scores. Review of results from multiple body sites will give an overall impression of the child's BMD. If there is discrepancy between ROIs, the clinical history may provide the reasons for this and should be discussed in the interpretation.

Subregion analyses may be necessary if valid body sites are limited and scan results are affected by poor positioning, movement, or the presence of artifact. In some children with multiple fractures, every body site measured by DXA will contain metal due to rod insertion to stabilize fractures. If the child is undergoing treatment with bisphosphonate, the treating clinician may elect to scan particular body sites despite the presence of metal, so results obtained, even though flawed, can be used to check for interval change. The patient in effect serves as his own control.

## Follow-Up Scans

It is important to determine whether changes that occur on serial scans are true changes in BMD or reflect variation in measurement due to the software machine or the operator. The positioning challenges described above can introduce a higher coefficient of variation. Positional differences and movement can introduce errors of 4–6% in bone mineral content which compromise interpretation of serial data [52, 53].

BMC and BMD are expected to increase with age in a growing child. Comparison of a child's BMD to normative reference data allows the clinician to assess whether or not gains in BMD have occurred at the expected rate for age. If increases in BMD are not as robust as those in healthy youth, the BMD Z-score may decrease. The decrease in Z-score need not indicate bone loss but rather suggests that accretion of bone did not occur at the expected rate (Fig. 9.6).

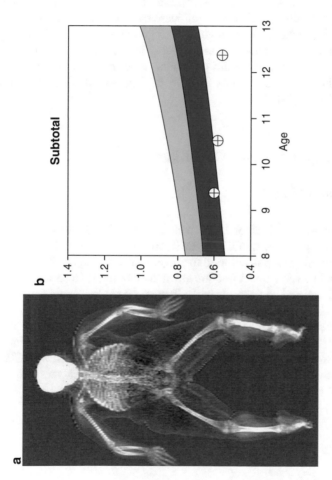

**Fig. 9.6** (a) Graphic display of serial scans of 12-year-old male with Duchenne Muscular Dystrophy shows progressive decrease in BMD over time. (b) Total body DXA of this patient shows positioning limitations and excessive adipose tissue with body fat measured at 59 %

When evaluating serial scans, prior scans should be reviewed for consistency in positioning and region of interest placement. Artifacts might have changed (added or removed) since the prior scan. Changes in clinical condition and treatment should be reviewed. A new fracture might have occurred and medications affecting BMD might have changed. Review of radiographs that have been taken in the interval between BMD studies may be helpful, as they can be correlated with scan images and used to explain why BMD in a particular area of the skeleton has changed.

Healing fractures will change over time, and can affect BMD results. As described earlier, bisphosphonates will increase BMD particularly at the LDF, impacting results in the different regions with growth (Fig. 9.5). If least significant change (LSC) has been calculated and is being used for interpretation (see details Chap. 5), the representative patient population used for that calculation should be considered. There may be greater variability in children with disabilities compared to unaffected individuals [34].

# Bone Fragility in Specific Conditions

## *Cerebral Palsy (CP)*

It is well documented that children with CP, particularly those who are non-ambulatory, have growth deficits, low BMD, and are at greater risk for fracture [54]. Fracture rate in this group is reported to range from 4 % [55] to 12 % [18] and children who sustain a low impact fracture are also more likely to sustain another fracture [34]. Children and adolescents with CP are prone to low energy (nontraumatic) fractures, with 74 % of fractures occurring in the distal femur [43].

Pamidronate was demonstrated to be effective in improving BMD at the lumbar spine and LDF in a small double blind, randomized control trial [30]. Pamidronate is effective at lowering rate of fracture in non-ambulatory children with CP: fracture rate was decreased from 30.6 %/year before treatment to 13 %/year after pamidronate treatment [42].

## *Spina Bifida (Myelomeningocele)*

Children with Spina Bifida often have limited to no ambulation and are susceptible to disuse osteoporosis characterized by low BMD and low energy fractures [56]. Reported annual fracture rate is 23–29 % among children and adolescents, respectively, and the lower extremities were the most common site of fracture [57]. Nearly 25 % of the patients experienced more than one fracture, and all who had multiple fractures were non-ambulatory.

BMD results in children with SB are directly related to degree of ambulation. Non- and partially ambulatory children had low LDF BMD and fully ambulatory children's BMD results were normal. The non-ambulators had worse BMD Z-scores than the partial ambulators [19, 36, 56]. Despite the low BMD and fracture rate well above normal, bisphosphonate treatment has not been well described in the literature and is limited to case studies and only a few patients.

## Duchenne Muscular Dystrophy

Children with DMD are typically treated with corticosteroids to attenuate loss of muscle function and preserve ambulation. With reduced ambulation, increasing muscle weakness, and glucocorticoid therapy, patients often become obese. These factors combined increase risk for fracture resulting in spinal compression fractures from chronic corticosteroid use [58, 59]. The muscle weakness can result in scoliosis. Annual fracture rate has not been described in the general DMD population, but in a group of 35 boys on corticosteroids, after 100 months of treatment, 75 % had sustained a vertebral fracture [60].

Lower extremity has been reported to be low in several studies examining LDF DXA. Non-ambulatory patients had the poorest BMD [16, 19, 36]. Few reports exist describing bisphosphonate use in boys with DMD, but preliminary results look promising: BMD of the LS was preserved despite disease progression, pain improved, and there was a demonstrated association between bisphosphonate use and improved life expectancy [61].

## Osteogenesis Imperfecta

OI is one of the most-studied conditions from a bone quality standpoint. Cyclic bisphosphonate use in children with OI was first reported in 1998. Since then numerous studies have been published utilizing a variety of bisphosphonates. Studies have focused on bisphosphonate effect on a variety of parameters including BMD, pain, vertebral body morphology, histomorphometric analyses, and fractures [62–69]. Current practice involves continuation of bisphosphonate therapy through adolescence once it has been initiated. Long term effects of continuous bisphosphonate therapy have shown positive effects on BMD but fractures continued [70]. Lower dose maintenance bisphosphonate therapy has been demonstrated to preserve the beneficial effects seen during the higher dose active treatment [71]. The effect of bisphosphonate holidays, currently being used in adults on long-term treatment, is unknown in pediatrics.

## Summary Points

- Children with neuromuscular and cognitive deficits present positioning difficulties and artifacts when DXA scans are performed.
- Traditionally acquired DXA sites, the total body and lumbar spine, may not be feasible in children with neuromuscular and cognitive deficits. The lateral distal femur is an informative and feasible alternative DXA site.
- Low bone mineral density is common in children with neuromuscular disabilities, particularly in those who are non-ambulatory.
- Fractures are found to occur in children with disabilities and low BMD, despite limited exposure to physical activities which might result in fracture.
- Bisphosphonate treatment is used in children with disabilities and frequent fracture; while fracture rates typically decrease with bisphosphonate therapy, BMD response varies by skeletal disorder and body site measured.
- Serial DXA scans are useful with a patient's first study serving as a reference.
- Reference data are obtained from normal, healthy children and DXA results in children with disabilities needs to be interpreted with this in mind.

## References

1. Apkon SD, Kecskemethy HH. Bone health in children with cerebral palsy. J Pediatr Rehabil Med. 2008;1(2):115–21.
2. Lee JJ, Lyne ED, Kleerekoper M, Logan MS, Belfi RA. Disorders of bone metabolism in severely handicapped children and young adults. Clin Orthop Relat Res. 1989;245:297–302.
3. Henderson RC, Kairalla J, Abbas A, Stevenson RD. Predicting low bone density in children and young adults with quadriplegic cerebral palsy. Dev Med Child Neurol. 2004;46(6):416–9.
4. Szalay EA, Cheema A. Children with spina bifida are at risk for low bone density. Clin Orthop Relat Res. 2011;469(5):1253–7.
5. Quan A, Adams R, Ekmark E, Baum M. Bone mineral density in children with myelomeningocele. Pediatrics. 1998;102(3):E34.
6. Henderson RC. Bone density and other possible predictors of fracture risk in children and adolescents with spastic quadriplegia. Dev Med Child Neurol. 1997;39(4):224–7.
7. Forwood MR. Mechanical effects on the skeleton: are there clinical implications? Osteoporos Int. 2001;12(1):77–83.
8. Behringer M, Gruetzner S, McCourt M, Mester J. Effects of weight-bearing activities on bone mineral content and density in children and adolescents: a meta-analysis. J Bone Miner Res. 2014;29(2):467–78.
9. Szalay EA, Harriman D, Eastlund B, Mercer D. Quantifying postoperative bone loss in children. J Pediatr Orthop. 2008;28(3):320–3.
10. Giangregorio L, McCartney N. Bone loss and muscle atrophy in spinal cord injury: epidemiology, fracture prediction, and rehabilitation strategies. J Spinal Cord Med. 2006;29(5):489–500.
11. Sibonga JD, Evans HJ, Sung HG, Spector ER, Lang TF, Oganov VS, Bakulin AV, Shackelford LC, LeBlanc AD. Recovery of spaceflight-induced bone loss: bone mineral density after long-duration missions as fitted with an exponential function. Bone. 2007;41(6):973–8.
12. Smith SM, Wastney ME, O'Brien KO, Morukov BV, Larina IM, Abrams SA, et al. Bone markers, calcium metabolism, and calcium kinetics during extended-duration space flight on the MIR space station. J Bone Miner Res. 2005;20(2):208–18.

13. Ceroni D, Martin X, Delhumeau C, Rizzoli R, Kaelin A, Farpour-Lambert N. Effects of cast-mediated immobilization on bone mineral mass at various sites in adolescents with lower-extremity fracture. J Bone Joint Surg Am. 2012;94(3):208–16.
14. Ceroni D, Martin X, Delhumeau-Cartier C, Rizzoli R, Kaelin A, Farpour-Lambert N. Is bone mineral mass truly decreased in teenagers with a first episode of forearm fracture? A prospective longitudinal study. J Pediatr Orthop. 2012;32(6):579–86.
15. Cooper C, Dennison EM, Leufkens H, Bishop N, van Staa TP. Epidemiology of childhood fractures in Britain: a study using the general practice research database. J Bone Miner Res. 2004;19:1976–81.
16. Larson CM, Henderson RC. Bone mineral density and fractures in boys with Duchenne muscular dystrophy. J Pediatr Orthop. 2000;20:71–4.
17. McIvor WC, Samilson RL. Fractures in patients with cerebral palsy. J Bone Joint Surg Am. 1966;48:858–66.
18. Leet AI, Mesfin A, Pichard C, Launay F, Brintzenhofeszoc K, Levey EB, Sponseller PD. Fractures in children with cerebral palsy. J Pediatr Orthop. 2006;26(5):624–7.
19. Henderson RC, Berglund LM, May R, Zemel BS, Grossberg RI, Johnson J, et al. The relationship between fractures and DXA measures of BMD in the distal femur of children and adolescents with cerebral palsy or muscular dystrophy. J Bone Min Res. 2010;25(3):520–6.
20. Clark EM, Ness AR, Bishop NJ, Tobias JH. Association between bone mass and fractures in children: a prospective cohort study. J Bone Miner Res. 2006;21:1489–95.
21. Goulding A, Jones IE, Taylor RW, Manning PJ, Williams SM. More broken bones: a 4-year double cohort study of young girls with and without distal forearm fractures. J Bone Miner Res. 2000;15:2011–8.
22. Crabtree NJ, Arabi A, Bachrach LK, Fewtrell M, El-Hajj Fuleihan G, Kecskemethy HH, Jaworski M, Gordon C. Dual-energy X-ray absorptiometry interpretation and reporting in children and adolescents: the revised 2013 ISCD Official Pediatric Positions. J Clin Densitom. 2014;17(2):225–42.
23. Goulding A, Grant AM, Williams SM. Bone and body composition of children and adolescents with repeated forearm fractures. J Bone Miner Res. 2005;20(12):2090–6.
24. Dowthwaite JN, Flowers PP, Scerpella TA. Agreement between pQCT- and DXA-derived indices of bone geometry, density, and theoretical strength in females of varying age, maturity, and physical activity. J Bone Miner Res. 2011;26(6):1349–57.
25. Shepherd JA, Wang L, Fan B, et al. Optimal monitoring time interval between DXA measures in children. J Bone Miner Res. 2011;26(11):2745–52.
26. Kalkwarf HJ, Zemel BS, Gilsanz V, Lappe JM, Horlick M, Oberfield S, Mahboubi S, Fan B, Frederick MM, Winer K, Shepherd JA. The Bone Mineral Density in Childhood Study (BMDCS): bone mineral content and density according to age, sex and race. J Clin Endocrinol Metab. 2007;92(6):2087–99.
27. Zemel BS, Kalkwarf HJ, Gilsanz V, Lappe JM, Oberfield S, Shepherd JA, Frederick MM, Huang X, Lu M, Mahboubi S, Hangartner T, Winer KK. Revised reference curves for bone mineral content and areal bone mineral density according to age and sex for black and non-black children: results of the bone mineral density in childhood study. J Clin Endocrinol Metab. 2011;96(10):3160–9.
28. Harcke HT, Taylor A, Bachrach S, Miller F, Henderson RC. Lateral femoral scan: an alternative method for assessing bone mineral density in children with cerebral palsy. Pediatr Radiol. 1998;28(4):241–6.
29. Presedo A, Dabney KW, Miller F. Fractures in patients with cerebral palsy. J Pediatr Orthop. 2007;27:147–53.
30. Henderson RC, Lark RK, Kecskemethy HH, Miller F, Harcke HT, Bachrach SJ. Bisphosphonates to treat osteopenia in children with quadriplegic cerebral palsy: a randomized, placebocontrolled clinical trial. J Pediatr. 2002;141(5):644–51.
31. Bachrach SJ, Kecskemethy HH, Harcke HT, Lark RK, Miller F, Henderson RC. Pamidronate treatment and posttreatment bone density in children with spastic quadriplegic cerebral palsy. J Clin Densitom. 2006;9(2):167–74.

32. Finbråten AK, Syversen U, Skranes J, Andersen GL, Stevenson RD, Vik T. Bone mineral density and vitamin D status in ambulatory and non-ambulatory children with cerebral palsy. Osteoporos Int. 2015;26(1):141–50.
33. Tryon E, Szalay EA. The lateral distal femoral DEXA scan in children: a chronology of growing bone? Orthopedics. 2008;31(11):1093.
34. Kecskemethy HH, Harcke HT. Assessment of bone health in children with Disabilities. J Pediatr Rehabil Med. 2014;7(2):111–24.
35. Haas RE, Kecskemethy HH, Lopiccolo MA, Hossain J, Dy RT, Bachrach SJ. Lower extremity bone mineral density in children with congenital spinal dysfunction. Dev Med Child Neurol. 2012;54(12):1133–7.
36. Harcke HT, Kecskemethy HH, Conklin D, Scavina M, Mackenzie WG, McKay CP. Assessment of bone mineral density in Duchenne's muscular dystrophy (DMD) using the lateral distal femur. J Clin Neuromusc Dis. 2006;8:1–6.
37. Roende G, Ravn K, Fuglsang K, Andersen H, Nielsen JB, Brøndum-Nielsen K, Jensen JE. DXA measurements in Rett syndrome reveal small bones with low bone mass. J Bone Miner Res. 2011;26(9):2280–6.
38. Polgreen LE, Thomas W, Fung E, et al. Low bone mineral content and challenges in interpretation of dual-energy x-ray absorptiometry in children with mucopolysaccharidosis types I, II and VI. J Clin Densiom Assess Manag Musculoskel Health. 2014;17(1):200–6.
39. Grissom LE, Kecskemethy HH, Bachrach SJ, McKay CP, Harcke HT. Bone densitometry in pediatric patients treated with pamidronate. Ped Radiol. 2005;35:511–7.
40. Henderson RC, Lark RK, Newman JE, Kecskemethy H, Fung EB, Renner JB, Harcke HT. Normal pediatric reference data for DXA measures of bone density in the distal femur. Am J Radiol. 2002;178:439–43.
41. Henderson RC, Lark RK, Gurka MJ, Worley G, Fung EB, Conaway M, et al. Bone density and metabolism in children and adolescents with moderate to severe cerebral palsy. Pediatrics. 2002;110(1 Pt 1):e5.
42. Bachrach SJ, Kecskemethy HH, Harcke HT, Hossain J. Decreased fracture incidence after 1 year of pamidronate treatment in children with spastic quadriplegic cerebral palsy. Dev Med Child Neurol. 2010;52(9):837–42.
43. Brunner R, Doderlein L. Pathological fractures in patients with CP. J Ped Orthop B. 1996;5:232–8.
44. Zemel B, Stallings V, Leonard M, Paulhamus D, Kecskemethy HH, Harcke HT, Henderson RC. Revised pediatric reference data for the lateral distal femur measured by dual energy X-ray absorptiometry. J Clin Densit. 2009;12:207–18.
45. Hangartner TN, Warner S, Braillon P, Jankowski L, Shepherd J. The official positions of the International Society for Clinical Densitometry: acquisition of dual-energy X-ray absorptiometry body composition and considerations regarding analysis and repeatability of measures. J Clin Densitom. 2013;16(4):520–36.
46. Castillo H, Samson-Fang L, American Academy for Cerebral Palsy and Developmental Medicine Treatment Outcomes Committee Review Panel. Effects of bisphosphonates in children with osteogenesis imperfecta: an AACPDM systematic review. Dev Med Child Neurol. 2009;51(1):17–29.
47. Forlino A, Cabral WA, Barnes AM, Marini JC. New perspectives on osteogenesis imperfecta. Nat Rev Endocronol. 2011;7(9):540–57.
48. El Maghraoui A, Do Santos Zounon AA, Jroundi I, Nouijai A, Ghazi M, Achemlal L, Bezza A, Tazi MA, Abouqual R. Reproducibility of bone mineral density measurements using dual X-ray absorptiometry in daily clinical practice. Osteoporos Int. 2005;16(12):1742–8.
49. Worley G, Houlihan CM, Herman-Giddens ME, O'Donnell ME, Conaway M, Stallings VA, Chumlea WC, Henderson RC, Fung EB, Rosenbaum PL, Samson-Fang L, Liptak GS, Calvert RE, Stevenson RD. Secondary sexual characteristics in children with cerebral palsy and moderate to severe motor impairment: a cross-sectional survey. Pediatrics. 2002;110(5):897–902.
50. Sbrocchi AM, Rauch F, Jacob P, McCormick A, McMillan HJ, Matzinger MA, et al. The use of intravenous bisphosphonate therapy to treat vertebral fractures due to osteoporosis among boys with Duchenne muscular dystrophy. Osteoporos Int. 2012;23(11):2703–11.

51. Kecskemethy HH, Kubaski F, Harcke HT, Tomatsu S. Bone mineral density in MPS IV A (Morquio Syndrome Type A). Mol Genet Metab. 2016;117(2):144–9.
52. Henderson RC, Lark RK, Renner JB, Fung EB, Stallings VA, Conaway M, et al. Dual X-ray absorptiometry assessment of body composition in children with altered body posture. J Clin Densitom. 2001;4(4):325–35.
53. Koo WW, Walters J, Bush AJ. Technical considerations of dual-energy X-ray absorptiometry-based bone mineral measurements for pediatric studies. J Bone Miner Res. 1995;10(12):1998–2004.
54. Mughal MZ. Fractures in children with CP. Current Osteoporosis Rep. 2014;12:313–8.
55. Stevenson RD, Conaway M, Barrington JW, Cuthill SL, Worley G, Henderson RC. Fracture rate in children with cerebral palsy. Pediatr Rehabil. 2006;9:396–403.
56. Rosenstein BD, Greene WB, Herrington RT, Blum AS. Bone density in myelomeningocele: the effects of ambulatory status and other factors. DevMed Child Neurol. 1987;29(4):486–94.
57. Dosa NP, Eckrich M, Katz DA, Turk M, Liptak GS. Incidence, prevalence, and characteristics of fractures in children, adolescents, and adults with spina bifida. J Spinal Cord Med. 2007;30 suppl 1:S5–9.
58. Mayo AL, Craven BC, McAdam LC, Biggar WD. Bone health in boys with Duchenne muscular dystrophy on long-term daily deflazacort therapy. Neuromuscu Disord. 2012;22:1040–5.
59. King WM, Ruttencutter R, Nagaraja HN, et al. Orthopedic outcomes of long-term daily corticosteroid treatment in Duchenne muscular dystrophy. Neurology. 2007;68:1607–13.
60. Bothwell JE, Gordon KE, Dooley JM, MacSween J, Cummings EA, Salisbury S. Vertebral fractures in boys with Duchenne muscular dystrophy. Clin Pediatr (Phila). 2003;42(4):353–6.
61. Boyce AM, Tosi LL, Paul SM. Bisphosphonate treatment for children with disabling conditions. PM R. 2014;6(5):427–36.
62. Astrom E, Soderhall S. Beneficial effect of long term intravenous bisphosphonate treatment of osteogenesis imperfecta. Arch Dis Child. 2002;86:356–64.
63. Plotkin H, Rauch F, Bishop NJ, et al. Pamidronate treatment of severe osteogenesis imperfecta in children under 3 years of age. J Clin Endocrinol Metabol. 2000;85:1846–50. 37.
64. Zacharin M, Bateman J. Pamidronate treatment of osteogenesis imperfecta—lack of correlation between clinical severity, age at onset of treatment, predicted collagen mutation and treatment response. J Pediatr Endocrinol Metab. 2002;15:163–74.
65. Rauch F, Plotkin H, Zeitlin L, Glorieux FH. Bone mass, size, and density in children and adolescents with osteogenesis imperfecta: effect of intravenous pamidronate therapy. J Bone Miner Res. 2003;18:610–4.
66. Arikoski P, Silverwood B, Tillmann V, Bishop NJ. Intravenous pamidronate treatment in children with moderate to severe osteogenesis imperfecta: assessment of indices of dual-energy x-ray absorptiometry and bone metabolic markers during the first year of therapy. Bone. 2004;34:539–46.
67. Sumnik Z, Land C, Rieger-Wettengl G, Korber F, Stabrey A, Schoenau E. Effect of pamidronate treatment on vertebral deformity in children with primary osteoporosis. A pilot study using radiographic morphometry. Hormone Res. 2004;61:137–42.
68. Glorieux FH, Bishop NJ, Plotkin H, Chabot G, Lanoue G, Travers R. Cyclic administration of pamidronate in children with severe osteogenesis imperfecta. N Engl J Med. 1998;339:947–52.
69. Rauch F, Travers R, Plotkin H, Glorieux FH. The effects of intravenous pamidronate on the bone tissue of children and adolescents with osteogenesis imperfecta. J Clin Invest. 2002;110:1293–9.
70. Palomo T, Fassier F, Ouellet J, Sato A, Montpetit K, Glorieux FH, Rauch F. Intravenous bisphosphonate therapy of young children with osteogenesis imperfecta: skeletal findings during follow up throughout the growing years. J Bone Miner Res. 2015. doi:10.1002/jbmr.2567 [Epub ahead of print].
71. Biggin A, Zheng L, Briody JN, Coorey CP, Munns CF. The long-term effects of switching from active intravenous bisphosphonate treatment to low-dose maintenance therapy in children with osteogenesis imperfecta. Horm Res Paediatr. 2015;83(3):183–9. doi:10.1159/000369582. Epub 2015 Feb 10.

# Chapter 10
# Bone Mineral Density as a Predictor of Vertebral Fractures in Children and Adolescents

**Leanne M. Ward and Jinhui Ma**

## Abbreviations

| | |
|---|---|
| ABQ | Algorithm-based qualitative method |
| ALL | Acute lymphoblastic leukemia |
| BMD | Bone mineral density |
| CT | Computed tomography |
| DMD | Duchenne muscular dystrophy |
| DXA | Dual energy X-ray absorptiometry |
| GC | Glucocorticoid(s) |
| LS | Lumbar spine |
| MRI | Magnetic resonance imaging |
| OI | Osteogenesis imperfecta |
| SDI | Spinal deformity index |
| VF | Vertebral fracture(s) |
| VFA | Vertebral fracture assessment |

L.M. Ward, M.D., F.A.A.P., F.R.C.P.C. (✉)
Division of Endocrinology and Metabolism, Department of Pediatrics, Children's Hospital of Eastern Ontario, University of Ottawa, 401 Smyth Road, Ottawa, ON, Canada K1H 8L1
e-mail: lward@cheo.on.ca

J. Ma, Ph.D.
School of Epidemiology, Public Health and Preventive Medicine, University of Ottawa, Children's Hospital of Eastern Ontario Research Institute, Room 250E, 401 Smyth Road, Ottawa, ON, Canada K1H 8L1
e-mail: jma@cheo.on.ca

© Springer International Publishing Switzerland 2016
E.B. Fung et al. (eds.), *Bone Health Assessment in Pediatrics*,
DOI 10.1007/978-3-319-30412-0_10

# Introduction

While typically considered a disease of the aging, it is now well-established that children can present with fractures due to osteoporosis for a variety of different reasons throughout the pediatric years. Osteogenesis imperfecta (OI), a heritable form of bone fragility, is considered the prototypic osteoporotic condition of childhood given its potential for severe consequences. OI has readily identifiable features including limb deformity, loss of ambulation, chronic pain, scoliosis, craniofacial and dental abnormalities as well as debilitating bone fragility. Osteoporosis can also occur in childhood as a result of serious systemic disorders and their treatment, particularly diseases requiring glucocorticoid (GC) therapy such as leukemia, rheumatic disorders, and Duchenne Muscular Dystrophy (DMD), and those which adversely impact mobility (for example, neuromuscular disorders including cerebral palsy) as discussed in Chaps. 1 and 4.

Although the term "fragility fractures" usually conjures an image of an arm or leg fracture along with casts and crutches, vertebral fractures (VF) are a key manifestation of osteoporosis in childhood, underscored by the fact that VF can be the first manifestation of a serious diagnosis such as childhood leukemia [1] or inflammatory bowel disease [2]. In fact, VF are often the earliest sign of osteoporosis in at-risk children, with the potential to occur well before or even in the absence of long bone fractures. This observation, combined with the current standard of care for pediatric osteoporosis management (predicated upon secondary prevention—i.e. intervention at the earliest signs of bone fragility in those with persistent risk factors), highlights the importance of VF detection as part of the bone health assessment in childhood.

Bone mineral density (BMD) testing by dual energy X-ray absorptiometry (DXA) has been in widespread, practical use as part of the pediatric bone health evaluation for over two decades. As an osteoporosis monitoring and diagnostic tool, BMD is highly attractive given its broad availability, rapid execution, high reproducibility, and low radiation. Countless studies have been carried out in children over the past 2 decades to assess the impact of underlying diseases or their treatment on BMD, with BMD serving as the sole or main bone health outcome. However, the knowledge arising from this approach has been insufficient to fully guide clinicians in the practical use of BMD during routine pediatric bone health care. As a result, the diagnosis and monitoring of osteoporosis in children increasingly focuses on a functional approach with emphasis on evaluation of fragility fractures. The knowledge gained from this approach has been helpful in guiding practitioners on the use of BMD as a clinical tool during routine care. The current chapter focuses on the following aspects of the pediatric bone health assessment: (a) VF as a manifestation of osteoporosis in children (diagnostic methods, prevalence, and incidence in various disease states), (b) clinical and laboratory predictors of VF, including BMD, (c) BMD restitution and vertebral body reshaping of previously fractured vertebral bodies as indices of recovery, and (d) the impact of the relationship between BMD and VF on clinical practice. These discussion points will assist clinicians in the diagnosis and monitoring of bone health in at-risk children, and in making decisions around optimal candidates for bone-targeted treatment.

# The Diagnosis of Vertebral Fractures in Children

## *The Definition of Pediatric Vertebral Fractures*

The first published, standardized assessment method for VF in adults was quantitative vertebral morphometry which involves direct measurement of vertebral body shape through six-point vertebral morphometry [3, 4]. With this method, points are placed in the superior and inferior endplates at the anterior, middle, and posterior aspects of the vertebral bodies. The ratios that are generated are then compared to cut-off values based on standard deviation reductions from the healthy population mean. The VF type is then determined by which vertebral height is most diminished (i.e. wedge, biconcave, or crush). Using ratios is preferable to absolute height values, since vertebral bodies farther away from the film can be falsely magnified depending on the distance of the X-ray tube from the patient. This method has not been adapted to children since normative data for vertebral height ratios at all vertebral levels do not exist; furthermore, the technique is highly laborious, time-consuming, and does not take into account the expertise of an experience reader/radiologist in ruling out non-VF pathology or normal variants.

The most widely used tool for the assessment of VF in both children and adults is the Genant semiquantitative method [5] (Fig. 10.1). According to the Genant method, the definition of a VF is loss of more than 20 % in vertebral height ratio regardless the different VF morphology. With this method, VF are subjectively graded by trained readers according to the magnitude of the reduction in vertebral body height ratios, without direct measurement. Vertebral height ratios are used when the anterior vertebral height is compared with the posterior height (for an anterior wedge fracture), middle height to the posterior height (biconcave fracture), and posterior height to the posterior height of adjacent vertebral bodies (crush fracture). The Genant scores correspond to the following reductions in height ratios: grade 0 (normal), ≤20 %; grade 1 fracture (mild), >20–25 %; grade 2 fracture (moderate), >25–40 %; grade 3 fracture (severe), >40 %. Using the Genant scores at each vertebral level for an individual patient, the Spinal Deformity Index (SDI) can be calculated by summing the individual vertebral body grades [6], providing a useful index of the overall VF status for a given child with multiple fractures. The Genant semiquantitative method is preferred over quantitative (6-point) vertebral morphometry since it is faster, and takes into consideration the expertise of an experienced reader by ensuring that normal variants are not mistaken for deformities resulting from fractures.

A number of recent studies have provided validity for the Genant approach in children given the following key observations. First, Genant-defined VF in children give rise to a bimodal distribution of fractures from T4 to L4 similar to the known distribution in adults [7–10], with a predilection for the mid-thoracic region (T5 to T8, the site of the natural kyphosis) and the thoracolumbar junction (the site of the natural lordosis) [1, 10] (Fig. 10.2). Secondly, a number of biologically relevant clinical predictors of Genant-defined VF have been identified, including back pain, low lumbar spine (LS) BMD Z-scores, longitudinal decreases in LS BMD Z-scores, and GC exposure [1, 11, 12].

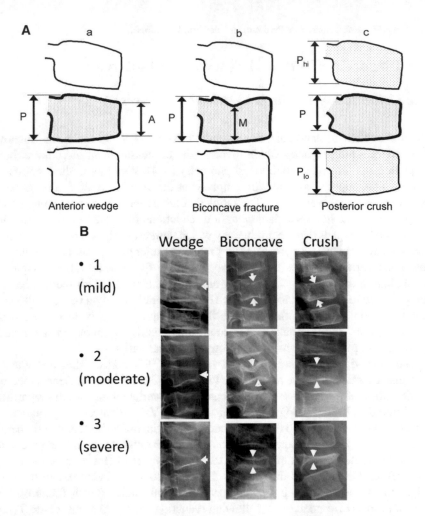

**Fig. 10.1** (a) A pictorial review of the Genant semiquantitative method for vertebral fracture assessment: (a) Anterior wedge fracture: measure the anterior height loss relative to posterior height (i.e. ratio $= (P-A)/P \times 100\%$). (b) Biconcave fracture: measure the minimum central vertebral body height relative to posterior height (i.e. ratio $=(P-M)/P \times 100\%$). Note that this fracture description is a misnomer because in many cases only one endplate is involved; the term is retained for fidelity with the original Genant grading system. (c) Posterior crush fracture: this height should be measured relative to the posterior height of the adjacent vertebrae because the posterior body wall is altered in this type of fracture and cannot serve as its own reference. The lower of the two ratios $(P_{hi}-P)/P_{hi}$ and $(P_{lo}-P)/P_{lo}$ is recorded as a percentage. Because L4 is the lowest level scored in Genant, at L4 only the L3 posterior height is used for comparison. Genant grades are: 0, height loss 20% or less; 1 (mild), >20–25%; 2 (moderate), >25–40%; 3 (severe), >40%. (**b**) Examples of actual fractures of each subtype in the Genant semiquantitative grading system. All images are sagittal radiographs of thoracolumbar vertebrae oriented with anterior to the right. Top row: 5-year-old girl with acute lymphoblastic leukemia; 9-year-old girl with acute lymphoblastic leukemia; 6-year-old boy with acute lymphoblastic leukemia. Middle row: 10-year-old girl with acute lymphoblastic leukemia; 10-year-old girl with osteogenesis imperfecta; 5-year-old girl with acute lymphoblastic leukemia. Bottom row: 9-year-old girl with acute lymphoblastic leukemia; 8-year-old girl with acute lymphoblastic leukemia; 10-year-old boy with histiocytosis. Arrows indicate the fracture in each image. In the image of the grade 2 crush fracture, note also the grade 1 wedge fracture at the vertebra below (with permission from Jaremko et al. and the Canadian STOPP Consortium, Pediatr Radiol, 2015)

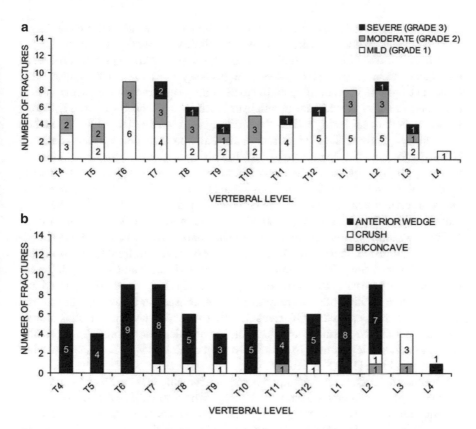

**Fig. 10.2** (**a**) The frequency and location of vertebral fractures in children with acute lymphoblastic leukemia at diagnosis in relation to the number of fractures identified as mild (grade 1), moderate (grade 2), and severe (grade 3) at each vertebral level. Most vertebral fractures occur in the mid-thoracic region and at the thoraco-lumbar junction. (**b**) The morphology of vertebral fractures in relation to location and frequency among children with ALL at diagnosis (an anterior wedge fracture is the most common morphology in children) (with permission from Halton et al. and the Canadian STOPP Consortium, J Bone Min Res, 2009)

A key observation to assert the validity of this approach in children is that Genant-defined VF at leukemia diagnosis are a robust clinical predictor of incident (new) VF in the 3 years following chemotherapy initiation [12, 13]. Even grade I (mild) VF at GC initiation independently predict incident VF over the ensuing 3 years in children [12, 13]. This observation lends credence to the cut-off of at least 20 % loss of vertebral height ratio to define a pediatric VF by the Genant method. Gaca et al. [14] have shown that 95 % of healthy children had anterior wedging at the thoraco-lumbar junction that did not exceed an 11 % reduction in anterior:posterior height ratio. This observation is consistent with the traditional radiology teaching that normal physiological rounding of vertebral bodies, which is frequently observed in children prior to the appearance of the ring apophysis around the time of puberty, does not exceed about 10 % [15]. Taken together, the critical threshold of a 20 % loss in vertebral height ratio to define a VF in children appears valid, and is increasingly used in clinical practice, research studies, and clinical consensus statements [16].

A third VF assessment method has been developed, which addresses the issue that quantitative or semiquantitative morphometry does not fully capture other important signs of VF, including endplate deformity (interruption), anterior cortical buckling, and loss of endplate parallelism (with loss of vertical continuity along vertebral bodies anteriorly). The "algorithm-based qualitative (ABQ)" method developed by Jiang et al. [17] is based on the assumption that the vertebral endplate is always deformed in the presence of a VF. This method asserts that the endplate is always centrally depressed (whether concave, wedge, or crushed), and that vertebral height ratios can be diminished in non-VF states such as oblique image projections and with certain anatomical variants (such as Cupid's bow deformity). The ABQ method uses a flowchart to systematically rule out non-VF deformities that mimic VF by examining various distinct radiological characteristics of the vertebral bodies. A radiologist skilled in the ABQ method is needed to differentiate accurately between VF and non-VF deformities or normal variants. The Canadian STeroid-induced Osteoporosis in the Pediatric Population (STOPP) Consortium, a national pediatric bone health working group that was established to understand the natural history of VF in the pediatric GC-treated setting, recently published an atlas of non-VF deformities and normal variants in children which can mimic VF. This atlas serves as a valuable resource to radiologists and clinicians who assess spine radiographs in children [18] (Fig. 10.3).

Overall, the Genant semiquantitative method remains in widest use, including in children. The Genant method has the advantages that it quantifies the severity of VF (an important predictor of the potential for spontaneous vertebral body reshaping following VF in children) and it permits calculation of the SDI (a measure of the child's global spine morbidity as discussed). The kappa statistics for intra- and inter-observer agreement are similar for children compared to adults using the Genant semiquantitative method [5, 19, 20]. In general, the ABQ method shows low to moderate agreement with other methods [17].

## *Imaging Methods for Vertebral Fracture Detection*

To date, the most common imaging tool for VF detection in childhood (also the technique upon which the Genant semiquantitative method was pioneered) has been lateral thoracolumbar spine radiographs from T4 to L4. These vertebral levels are typically targeted since T1 to T3 can be difficult to visualize due to overlying lung, and L5 has normal posterior wedging that can be confused with a fracture. However, if T1 to T3 are well-visualized and more than 20% loss of vertebral height ratio is observed, then this finding should also be reported by the radiologist.

In view of the high radiation exposure from spine radiographs, nonradiographic imaging techniques have been developed which use the scoring methods described above. One such technique is "vertebral fracture assessment" (VFA), using images

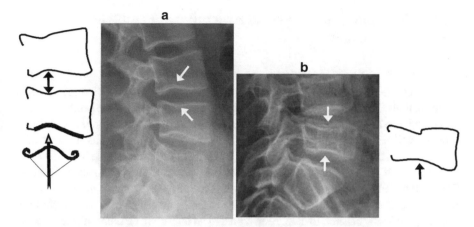

**Fig. 10.3** Normal variants mimicking fractures in children with glucocorticoid-treated diseases. (**a**) Cupid's bow vs. biconcave fracture: Diagram and lateral radiograph depict Cupid's bow or balloon disk at multiple levels in a 17-year-old boy treated with glucocorticoids for vasculitis. This normal variant is a curved indentation centered at the posterior third of the endplate (*arrows*). The shape resembles Cupid's bow (diagram, *bottom*), and when present at adjacent endplates it gives the impression of disk expansion, hence it is also known as "balloon disk." (**b**) Biconcave endplate fracture at L5, in a 10-year-old boy treated with glucocorticoids for acute lymphoblastic leukemia. There is interruption of the superior endplate of L5, the endplate concavities are centered at the mid-disk rather than the posterior third, there is overall height loss, and adjacent levels are not affected (with permission from Jaremko et al. and the Canadian STOPP Consortium, Pediatr Radiol, 2015)

captured on a lateral spine DXA. VFA is extremely attractive as a VF assessment tool, given its low radiation and the fact that fan-beam technology facilitates capture of the entire spine on a single image without divergent beam issues due to parallax. Newer DXA machines have a rotating "c-arm" which obviates the need to re-position the patient from the supine to the lateral position. Recently, it has been shown that image quality varies significantly depending on the densitometer [21]. Using a Hologic Discovery A machine, Mayranpaa et al. [22] showed low diagnostic accuracy for VFA compared to lateral spine radiographs and suboptimal image quality for children. Specifically, only 36% of VF identified on lateral spine radiographs were evident by VFA. Pediatric studies on newer DXA machines to determine the validity of this approach are presently underway [23]. Since the prevalence and incidence of VF in children with various osteoporotic conditions is clinically significant, validation of DXA-based VFA in the pediatric population is a meritorious endeavor.

Magnetic resonance imaging (MRI) is a three-dimensional evaluative tool without ionizing radiation that can demonstrate bone marrow edema, and is therefore useful in distinguishing acute versus old fractures. The disadvantage of MRI detection of VF is the long imaging time and high costs. Images produced by computed tomography (CT) have much higher spatial resolution than MRI and DXA; however, it has been shown that sagittal reformations are needed to demonstrate VF [24] and the dose of radiation is substantial with CT.

## The Epidemiology of Vertebral Fractures in Pediatric Osteoporotic Conditions

A number of studies have underscored that VF are an important, yet frequently over-looked manifestation of osteoporosis in children. This is particularly true in children with OI and in children with GC-treated disorders given the predilection of GC therapy to adversely impact the trabecular-rich spine. At the same time, children who are GC naïve are not exempt from VF, as the VF prevalence has been shown; for example, 25 % of children with motor disabilities have detectable VF [25].

Pediatric VF frequently go undetected in this population for two main reasons. First, VF are often asymptomatic in children [1, 12, 26–29], even in the presence of moderate and severe collapse [1]. Secondly, routine surveillance in at-risk children with a spine X-ray has not, to date, been signaled an important element of osteoporosis monitoring guidelines. However, the 2014 guidelines developed by the International Society for Clinical Densitometry have stated that the diagnosis of osteoporosis can be made in children with at least one vertebral fracture without BMD criteria [16], thereby advocating that spine health monitoring beyond BMD is needed in at-risk children.

In adults, only about one third of all VF come to clinical attention and 2/3 go undetected [30]; this observation is consistent with reports in children [1, 12, 27, 29]. The importance of identifying even asymptomatic VF is evident in the adult literature since both symptomatic and nonsymptomatic VF are associated with decreased quality of life [31, 32] and increased mortality [33]. While similar studies have not been carried out in children to determine the relationship between VF and quality of life measures or mortality risk, it is conceivable that this might be true in younger patients. Large, prospective studies are needed to investigate these relationships in more detail.

### Osteogenesis Imperfecta

The severity of bone fragility in OI spans a broad spectrum, ranging from asymptomatic individuals to perinatal lethality. In most cases, OI is caused by autosomal dominant mutations in either the *COL1A1* or *COL1A2* genes, interfering with either the synthesis or the structure (or both) of type I procollagen alpha1 or alpha2 chains [34]. Less often OI is due to recessive mutations, most of which interfere with post-translational processing and trafficking of type I procollagen [34].

VF are one of the hallmarks of OI, present in most patients with severe forms and a large proportion of those with the milder type I OI. Despite the common occurrence of VF in OI, there are few data on the prevalence of VF and none reporting the incidence of VF during the pediatric years. Ben Amor et al. [35] recently studied a large cohort of children with OI due to *COL1A1* haploinsufficiency. Haploinsufficiency results in about one-half of the normal amount of collagen type I protein. Mutations giving rise to haploinsufficiency are associated with a milder form of OI characterized by normal or near-normal stature and milder degrees of long bone and craniofacial deformity. However, 41 of 58 children (71 %) had VF on lateral spine radiographs [35]. The authors noted that this proportion does not represent a true prevalence, since some patients only underwent spine radiographs in the setting of back pain. Nevertheless, these estimates suggest the true prevalence is likely to be high. Girls had a median of 4 VF (range 0–14) while boys had a median of 1 VF (range 0–8), despite the fact that LS BMD Z-scores were slightly higher in girls compared to boys. The higher BMD in girls with VF and OI may be related to the fact that, according to trans-iliac histomorphometry studies, bone turnover is lower in girls compared to boys [36].

## Childhood Leukemia

Skeletal morbidity has long been associated with acute lymphoblastic leukemia (ALL), occurring at diagnosis, during treatment, and in the years after therapy [1, 12, 37]. Since current leukemia therapy results in a cure rate that approaches 80 % [38], ALL represents a transient threat to bone health for most children and adolescents. Although many children with skeletal morbidity with ALL show evidence of recovery [39], some are left with permanent skeletal abnormalities [40]. This underscores the importance of identifying those at risk for long-term sequelae and implementing appropriate treatment and prevention strategies.

At diagnosis, skeletal abnormalities are evident on plain radiographs in up to 75 % of children [41]. They include metaphyseal lucencies from aggressive osteolysis [42–44], periosteal separation, metaphyseal growth arrest lines and pathological extremity fractures [41–44]. Based on data from retrospective [41, 45, 46] and prospective [47] studies, the prevalence of low trauma non-VF ranges from 3 to 10 %. VF can cause a limp or inability to walk as a presenting feature of the disease. Incident VF also occur frequently around the time of diagnosis in childhood ALL; a prospective VF surveillance study confirmed that the spine fracture prevalence is 16 % at this time point [1]. Bone fragility at the time of ALL diagnosis has been linked to increased bone resorption resulting from cytokines released by the leukemic cells causing osteoclast hyperactivity [48].

The incidence of VF (both asymptomatic and symptomatic) is highest in the first year of chemotherapy for ALL; 16 % of patients developed VF within the first 12 months of chemotherapy [13]. The 4-year cumulative VF incidence in ALL was 35 % in one study. Over half of the patients reported an absence of back pain in the 12 months preceding the annual spine surveillance radiographs for fracture detection [13].

## Glucocorticoid-Treated Inflammatory Disorders

Children with rheumatic disorders are also fracture-prone, both at diagnosis and following GC initiation. In rheumatic disorders, the prevalence of VF at the time of GC initiation is 7 %, with a prevalence ranging from 10 to 23 % after long-term GC therapy [49–51]. The rate of incident VF ascertained by annual spine radiograph surveillance was 6% after 12 months of GC treatment in a large cohort of children with a variety of rheumatic disorders; 40% of the children with incident VF had juvenile dermatomyositis [29]. The 3-year cumulative VF incidence following GC initiation increases to 13% [11], and those with juvenile idiopathic arthritis have a 50% to threefold increased risk of a fracture (all types) during the pediatric years [52]. In a prospective study of children with a variety of GC-treated rheumatic disorders, one child with a normal lateral spine radiograph at GC initiation presented with painful, grade 1 and 2 VF after only 4 months of GC therapy, highlighting that overt bone morbidity can be evident soon after GC initiation [29] (Fig. 10.4). In keeping with other recent observations that VF are an under-recognized but nevertheless discrete manifestation of osteoporosis in children with inflammatory disorders [27, 29, 50, 53], VF occurred more frequently in an 80 patient cohort of children and adolescents with inflammatory bowel disease (11% prevalence after an average of 3 years from diagnosis, compared to 3% in healthy controls, $p=0.02$).

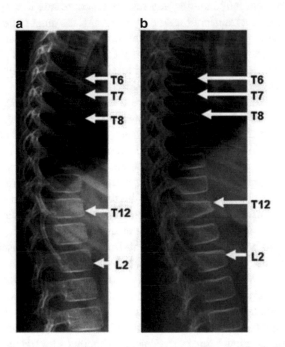

**Fig. 10.4** Spine radiographs from a 7-year-old girl with mixed connective tissue disease. At study entry, (**a**) her spine radiograph showed no signs of vertebral fractures; however, she manifested multiple painful vertebral fractures after only 4 months of glucocorticoid therapy. (**b**) This patient's clinical course was distinguished by Cushingoid features and a dramatic increase in body mass index (by 3.1 SD) in the first 3 months of glucocorticoid therapy. This was despite similar glucocorticoid exposure compared to the other children with rheumatic diseases and incidence VF in the first year following glucocorticoid initiation. An increase in body mass index Z-score in the first 6 months of glucocorticoid therapy is a known predictor of incident vertebral fractures over the following 3 years (see Table 10.1) (with permission from Rodd et al. and the Canadian STOPP Consortium, Arth Care Res, 2012)

## Neuromuscular Disorders

GC-treated Duchenne Muscular Dystrophy (DMD) is a "perfect storm" for severe osteoporosis with the combined threats of progressive myopathy and GC therapy. VF in pediatric DMD can be associated with severe chronic back pain; in addition, both spine and leg fractures can lead to premature, permanent loss of ambulation. While the annual incidence of fractures remains unknown, a few reports describing estimates of VF prevalence in pediatric DMD have been carried out [54–56]. These cross-sectional studies have shown that up to 30 % of boys with DMD develop symptomatic VF, and 20–60 % sustain extremity fractures. The fact that only symptomatic VF have been reported represents a knowledge gap in pediatric DMD, since we know that VF are frequently asymptomatic [12, 29]. Whether asymptomatic or not, VF are strongly associated with an increased risk of future fractures [12].

Children with cerebral palsy represent another group with an increased risk of VF. The overall prevalence of fractures (all types) in this condition is reported between 4 and 12 % [57]. A cross-sectional study of children with cerebral palsy and Gross Motor Function Classification System scores II or higher who underwent lateral spine radiographs showed that 7/37 (19 %) had VF; the back pain status in these patients was not reported. Since children with cerebral palsy are often nonverbal, even symptomatic VF may go undetected in this population.

## Nephrotic Syndrome

In contrast to pediatric ALL, DMD and rheumatic disorders, GC-treated nephrotic syndrome is considered an in vivo model of the impact of GC therapy on bone, since the underlying disease itself is not known to have a deleterious effect on the developing skeleton. Two studies have evaluated the prevalence and incidence of VF in GC-treated nephrotic syndrome [26, 28]. The first prospective study found the prevalence of VF within 37 days of GC initiation was 8 %, all of which were mild and asymptomatic [26]. There was an inverse relationship between GC exposure and LS BMD Z-scores even after just 37 days of GC therapy, testament to the expected rapidity with which GC exert their effect [58]. The second prospective study reported a 6 % incidence of VF after 12 months of GC therapy; LS BMD Z-scores improved in the majority by 12 months as many children entered remission and discontinued GC therapy. A disproportionate number of children had LS BMD Z-scores ≤1.0 at 12 months; further study of these children revealed that their lower LS BMD Z-scores at 12 months were inversely associated with GC exposure in the first 3 months of therapy, despite similar GC dosing compared to the rest of the cohort. This observation suggests that some children are more sensitive to the osteotoxic effects of GC therapy compared to others, possibly reflecting that polymorphisms in the GC receptor gene are associated with GC dependence in pediatric nephrotic syndrome [59].

## Organ Transplantation

In children with hepatic diseases requiring transplantation, the overall fracture prevalence in retrospective studies ranges between 10 and 40 % of children prior to transplant [60–66] and from 12 to 50 % following transplant [60, 62, 63, 67]. A recent retrospective study of 40 children and adolescents post-liver transplant assessed patients' VF statuses through VFA on a Hologic machine (model not specified) [60]. A lateral spine radiograph was performed in those with spine BMD Z-scores ≤−2 SD, those with VFA images suggesting a VF, or when vertebral bodies were not sufficiently visible by VFA. With this approach, 73 % of patients required lateral thoracolumbar spine radiographs in addition to VFA and 7/40 patients (18 %) had prevalent VF. A study of pediatric liver, kidney, and bone marrow transplant recipients [62] reported a sixfold higher fracture rate for all fracture types and a 160-fold higher rate of VF compared to controls. Fifty percent of the pediatric patients with VF in this series were asymptomatic, consistent with the high frequency of asymptomatic VF in other pediatric chronic illnesses [1, 12, 29].

## Bone Mineral Density and Other Clinical Predictors of Vertebral Fractures

As shown in Table 10.1, a number of studies have been sufficiently powered to assess clinical predictors of VF in bi- or multivariable models or through nonparametric analyses. Most of these studies have been retrospective or cross-sectional; very few studies have assessed the frequency of incident VF in relation to the evolving clinical course of the child. A detailed description of the clinical predictors in the various disease states according to the published literature is provided in Table 10.1, along with the criteria for carrying out a VF assessment in a given population of children, the method and imaging modality for VF detection, and the overall incidence and prevalence rates. Note that if specific clinical criteria triggered VF assessment (such as a low BMD or back pain), then the estimate of VF prevalence or incidence in that cohort was only relevant to children with the same clinical profile. These heterogeneous methodologies need to be taken into account when comparing prevalence and incidence rates across studies with similar disease groups.

A number of clinically useful themes have emerged from these studies. First of all, GC exposure is a consistent predictor of both prevalent and incident VF. Both cumulative and average daily GC dose predict VF in a number of different diseases; short courses of high dose GC ("pulse" GC therapy) in children with leukemia also predict VF. Secondly, in leukemia it was also observed that prevalent VF around the time of diagnosis and GC initiation are highly predictive of future fractures, a phenomenon known as "the vertebral fracture cascade" [12, 13]. Even mild (grade 1) VF were independent predictors of future VF, highlighting the importance of identifying early signs of vertebral collapse [12, 13]. While back pain predicted

**Table 10.1** Relationship between clinical predictors and prevalent/incident vertebral fractures

| Disease | Publication and study design | Inclusion criteria | Number, age (yrs), and male (%) of patients | Clinical criteria for carrying out the VF assessment[a] | VF assessment method and imaging modality | VF prevalence/ incidence and time point | Clinical predictors of prevalent or incident VF from univariate or multivariable models (with effect size and 95 % CI) or statistical tests for comparing children with and without VF[b] |
|---|---|---|---|---|---|---|---|
| *Steroid-treated diseases* | | | | | | | |
| Leukemia | • Halton (STOPP) (2009) <br> • Prospective, observational | • Age from 1 month to 17 yrs with ALL <br> • Bone health assessment initiated within 30 days of chemotherapy initiation | • N=186 <br> • Age: median (IQR)=5.3 (3.4, 9.7) at chemotherapy initiation <br> • Male: 58 % | • Assessed at baseline and then annually for every patient | • Lateral spine X-ray <br> • Genant method | • Prevalence: 16 % <br> • Time: within 30 days of chemotherapy initiation | Multivariable model: <br> • Back pain: OR=4.7 (1.5, 14.5) <br> • ↓Second metacarpal percent cortical area Z-score: OR=2.0 (1.0, 3.2) <br> • ↓LSBMD Z-score: OR=1.8 (1.1, 2.9) |
| Leukemia | • Alos (STOPP) (2012) <br> • Prospective, observational | • Age from 1 month to 17 yrs with ALL <br> • Bone health assessment initiated within 30 days of chemotherapy initiation | • N=155 <br> • Age: median (min, max)=6.4 (2.2, 18.0) at 12 months after chemotherapy initiation <br> • Male: 59 % | • Assessed at baseline and then annually for every patient | • Lateral spine X-ray <br> • Genant method | • Incidence: 16 % <br> • Time: 12 months after chemotherapy initiation | Multivariable models: <br> • Prevalent VF (yes vs. no): OR=7.30 (2.30, 23.14) <br> • ↓LSBMD Z-score: OR=1.8 (1.2, 2.7) <br> • Prevalent VF (mild vs. none): OR=7.6 (1.8, 31.8) <br> • Prevalent VF (moderate/severe vs. none): OR=7.0 (1.6, 30.2) |

(continued)

**Table 10.1** (continued)

| Disease | Publication and study design | Inclusion criteria | Number, age (yrs), and male (%) of patients | Clinical criteria for carrying out the VF assessment[a] | VF assessment method and imaging modality | VF prevalence/incidence and time point | Clinical predictors of prevalent or incident VF from univariate or multivariable models (with effect size and 95% CI) or statistical tests for comparing children with and without VF[b] |
|---|---|---|---|---|---|---|---|
| Leukemia | • Cummings (STOPP) (2015)<br>• Prospective, observational | • Age from 1 month to 17 yrs with ALL<br>• Bone health assessment initiated within 30 days of chemotherapy initiation | • $N = 186$<br>• Age: median (IQR) = 5.3 (3.4, 9.7) at chemotherapy initiation<br>• Male: 58 % | • Assessed at baseline and then annually for every patient | • Lateral spine X-ray<br>• Genant method | • Incidence: 8.7 per 100 person-years<br>• Cumulative incidence: 26.4 %<br>• Time: over 4 years after chemotherapy initiation | Multivariable models:<br>• Prevalent VF (mild vs. none): HR = 4.2 (1.9, 9.6)<br>• Prevalent VF (moderate/severe vs. none): HR = 6.2 (3.4, 11.4)<br>• ↑Average daily GC (10 mg/m²): HR = 5.9 (3.0, 11.8)<br>• ↓LSBMD Z-score at the time of VF assessment: HR = 1.6 (1.2, 2.2)<br>• ↓age: HR = 1.1 (1.0, 2.2)<br>• ↑recent (12 months preceding VF assessment) average daily GC (10 mg/m²): HR = 5.1 (2.8, 9.5)<br>• ↑Recent GC dose intensity (10 mg/m²): HR = 1.2 (1.1, 1.4) |

| | | | | | | | |
|---|---|---|---|---|---|---|---|
| Rheumatic diseases | • Huber (STOPP) (2010)<br>• Prospective, observational | • Age from 1 month to 17 yrs<br>• Within 30 days of first-time GC therapy for the treatment of underlying rheumatic diseases including JDM, JIA (excluding systemic arthritis), SLE, JIA (systemic arthritis), SV, and others | • $N=134$<br>• Age: median (min, max) = 10.0 (1.4, 16.9)<br>• Male: 35 % | • Assessed at baseline and then annually for every patient | • Lateral spine X-ray<br>• Genant method | • Prevalence: 7 %<br>• Time: within 30 days of first-time GC therapy | Univariate model:<br>• Back pain: OR = 10.6 (2.1, 53.8) |
| Juvenile arthritis | • Markula-Patjas (2012)<br>• Cross-sectional | • Age <19 yrs<br>• Polyarticular JIA for ≥5 years, or systemic arthritis for ≥3 yrs | • $N=50$<br>• Age: median (range) = 14.8 (7.0, 18.7)<br>• Male: 18 % | • Assessed following enrollment into the study | • Lateral spine X-ray<br>• Method proposed by Makitie[c] | • Prevalence: 22 %<br>• Time: after enrollment into the study | Univariate model:<br>• Cumulative GC dose >75 mg/kg: OR = 7.2 (1.37, 38.0)<br>• Disease activity (CHAQ>0.5): OR = 7.2 (1.58, 32.9)<br>• BMI Z-score>2: OR = 4.7 (1.13, 19.21) |

(continued)

**Table 10.1** (continued)

| Disease | Publication and study design | Inclusion criteria | Number, age (yrs), and male (%) of patients | Clinical criteria for carrying out the VF assessment[a] | VF assessment method and imaging modality | VF prevalence/ incidence and time point | Clinical predictors of prevalent or incident VF from univariate or multivariable models (with effect size and 95% CI) or statistical tests for comparing children with and without VF[b] |
|---|---|---|---|---|---|---|---|
| Juvenile arthritis | • Varonos (1987)<br>• Retrospective, case-control | Group with VF:<br>• Age <16 yrs<br>• With juvenile chronic arthritis treated with GC<br>• Developed at least one vertebral collapse<br>Group without VF:<br>• With juvenile chronic arthritis<br>• Without fractures<br>• Received GC for at least 1 year<br>• At some time point in time had mean daily dose at least 5 mg of prednisolone | Group with VF:<br>• N=23<br>• Age: mean (min, max) =4.8 (1.3, 9.9)<br>• Male: % not reported<br>Group without VF:<br>• N=23<br>• Age: mean (min, max) =3.8 (0.9, 11.9)<br>• Male: % not reported | • Routinely performed annually from beginning of GC for every patient<br>• More frequently if chest pain or loss of height occurred | • Lateral spine X-ray<br>• Method proposed by Jensen and Tougaard[d] | N/A | Statistical test for comparing children with and without VF:<br>• ↑Average daily dose of GC<br>• ↑ Weight-adjusted average daily dose of GC |

| | | | | | | | |
|---|---|---|---|---|---|---|---|
| Rheumatic diseases | • Nakhla (2009)<br>• Cross-sectional | • ≤18 yrs<br>• Had earlier or current exposure to methotrexate, corticosteroids, or both<br>• Had the following diagnosis: JIA, CTD (including SLE, JDM, and SV) | • N=90<br>• Age: median (min, max)=13.1 (4.3, 18.0)<br>• Male: 24 % | • Assessed after enrollment into the study for every patient | • Lateral spine X-ray<br>• Genant method | • Prevalence: 19 %<br>• Time: after enrollment into the study | Multivariable models (predictors of the number of VF events):<br>• Sex (Male vs. Female): OR=6.04 (2.85, 12.81)<br>• ↑Cumulative GC (g/kg): OR=4.50 (1.42, 14.28)<br>• ↑BMI Z-score: OR=1.49 (1.05, 2.09) |
| Rheumatic diseases | • Rodd (STOPP) (2012)<br>• Prospective, observational | • Age from 1 month to 17 yrs<br>• Within 30 days of first-time GC therapy for the treatment of underlying rheumatic diseases including JDM, JIA (excluding systemic arthritis), SLE, JIA (systemic arthritis), SV, and others | • N=117<br>• Age: median (min, max)=11.0 (2.3, 17.9) at 12 months after GC initiation<br>• Male: 37 % | • Assessed at baseline and then annually for every patient | • Lateral spine X-ray<br>• Genant method | • Incidence: 5 %<br>• Time: 12 months after GC initiation | Statistical test for comparing children with and without VF:<br>• ↑BMI Z-score, study entry to 6 months<br>• ↑Weight Z-score, study entry to 6 months<br>• ↓LSBMD Z-score, study entry to 6 months<br>• LSBMD Z-score <−2.0 at 12 months<br>• ↑Cumulative GC<br>• ↑Average daily GC |

(continued)

**Table 10.1** (continued)

| Disease | Publication and study design | Inclusion criteria | Number, age (yrs), and male (%) of patients | Clinical criteria for carrying out the VF assessment[a] | VF assessment method and imaging modality | VF prevalence/ incidence and time point | Clinical predictors of prevalent or incident VF from univariate or multivariable models (with effect size and 95% CI) or statistical tests for comparing children with and without VF[b] |
|---|---|---|---|---|---|---|---|
| Rheumatic diseases | LeBlanc (2015)<br>• Prospective, observational | • Age from 1 month to 17 yrs<br>• Within 30 days of first-time GC therapy for the treatment of underlying rheumatic diseases including JDM, JIA (excluding systemic arthritis), SLE, JIA (systemic arthritis), SV, and others | • $N = 134$<br>• Age: mean (SD) = 9.9 (4.4) at the time of GC initiation<br>• Male: 35% | • Assessed at baseline and then annually for every patient | • Lateral spine X-ray<br>• Genant method | • Incidence: 4.4 per 100 person-years<br>• Cumulative incidence: 12.4%<br>• Time: over 3 year after GC initiation | Multivariable models:<br>• ↑Average daily GC dose (0.5 mg/kg): HR = 2.0 (1.1, 3.5)<br>• ↑VAS score, baseline to 12 months: HR = 1.4 (1.1, 1.7)<br>• ↑BMI Z-score in the first 6 months preceding each annual VF assessment: HR = 3.2 (1.6, 6.5)<br>• ↓LSBMD Z-score, baseline to 6 months: HR = 3.0 (1.1, 8.1)<br>• ↑Duration (month) of GC therapy in the preceding 12 months of each VF assessment: HR = 1.2 (1.1, 1.4) |

| | | | | | | |
|---|---|---|---|---|---|---|
| Solid organ transplant | • Helenius (2006)<br>• Retrospective chart review followed by a prospective observation | • <18 yrs old<br>• Received kidney, liver, or heart transplants | • $N=196$<br>• Age at transplant: mean (min, max) = 6.5 (0.4, 18.1)<br>• Male: 62 % | • Assessed at the final follow-up visit (5-yrs after enrollment into the study) for every patient | • DXA-based VFA or Lateral spine X-ray<br>• Method proposed by Makitie[c] | • Incidence: 18 %<br>• Time: at 10-yrs follow-up after transplant | Multivariable model:<br>• BMI ≥19 kg/m² at transplant: RR=4.30 (1.26, 9.97)<br>• Age (5–12 vs. 0–4 yrs): RR = 2.32 (1.07, 5.05)<br>• Age (13–20 vs. 0–4 yrs): RR=4.16 (1.60, 10.81) |
| Solid organ transplant | • Helenius (2006)<br>• Cross-sectional | • Young adult who received kidney, liver, or heart transplant as children | • $N=40$<br>• Age at transplant: mean (min, max) = 10.6 (1.1, 17.1)<br>• Male: 65 % | • Assessed following enrollment into the study | • MRI<br>• Method proposed by Makitie[c] | • Prevalence: 35 %<br>• Time: at a mean follow-up of 11.2 years after transplant | Statistical test for comparing children with and without VF:<br>• Male<br>• Treated for acute rejection |
| Renal transplant | • Vautour (2004)<br>• Retrospective medical records review & prospective follow-up | • Received a first renal transplant between Jan. 1, 1965 and Dec. 31, 1995 according to the Rochester Epidemiology Project database | • $N=86$<br>• Age at transplant: median (min, max)=36 (5, 77)<br>• Male: 69 % | • Diagnosis of VF was accepted on the basis of a radiologist's report | • Radiologist's report<br>• No specific criteria stated | • Cumulative Incidence: 20 %<br>• Among 15-year survivors | Multivariable model:<br>• ↑Age: HR=1.8 (1.2, 2.7)<br>• Prior diagnosis of osteoporosis: HR=9.5 (2.6, 35) |

(continued)

**Table 10.1** (continued)

| Disease | Publication and study design | Inclusion criteria | Number, age (yrs), and male (%) of patients | Clinical criteria for carrying out the VF assessment[a] | VF assessment method and imaging modality | VF prevalence/ incidence and time point | Clinical predictors of prevalent or incident VF from univariate or multivariable models (with effect size and 95 % CI) or statistical tests for comparing children with and without VF[b] |
|---|---|---|---|---|---|---|---|
| Renal transplant | • Valta (2009)<br>• Retrospective data collection and cross-sectional assessment of skeletal health | • Undergo renal transplant before 18 yrs old and 6 months before enrollment<br>• 4–20 years of age at the time of study | • N = 106<br>• Age at transplant: median (min, max) = 3.4 (0.7, 16.4)<br>• Male: 61 % | • DXA-based VFA for each patient<br>• Lateral spine radiograph for those with LSBMD Z-score ≤−2, or VF was suspected on a DXA image, or DXA image could not be reliably visualized | • DXA-based VFA and Lateral spine X-ray<br>• Method proposed by Makitie[c] | • Prevalence: 8 %<br>• Time: at a median follow-up of 5.1 years after transplant | Statistical test for comparing children with and without VF:<br>• Older age at the time of study<br>• Longer time since transplant |

| | | | | | | |
|---|---|---|---|---|---|---|
| Liver transplant | • Valta (2008)<br>• Cross-sectional & longitudinal | • Undergo liver transplant before 16 yrs old and 6 months before enrollment<br>• 4–20 years of age at the time of study | • $N=40$<br>• Age at transplant: median (min, max) =2.1 (0.4, 15.3)<br>• Male: 53 % | • DXA-based VFA for each patient<br>• Lateral spine X-ray if LSBMD Z-score ≤ −2 or VF was suspected in DXA image or DXA image could not be reliably visualized | • DXA-based VFA and Lateral spine X-ray<br>• Method proposed by Makitie[c] | • Prevalence: 18 %<br>• Time: at a median follow-up of 7 yrs after transplant | Statistical test for comparing children with and without VF:<br>• Older age at transplant<br>• More recently transplanted<br>• Higher BMI<br>• Higher whole body fat percentage<br>• Lower cumulative weight-adjusted GC dose<br>• Lower LSBMD Z-score<br>• Lower femoral head BMD Z-score<br>• Lower whole body BMD Z-score |
| DMD | • King (2007)<br>• Retrospective chart review | • With genetically confirmed DMD<br>• Followed at Ohio State University from 2000 to 2003 | Patients with GC treatment ≥1 year<br>• $N=75$<br>• Age: mean (SD) =16.9 (5.6)<br>• Male: 100 %<br>Patients with GC treatment <1 year<br>• $N=68$<br>• Age: mean (SD) =14.4 (8.1)<br>• Male: 100 % | • Data were obtained through chart review | • Presence and type of VF were determined by radiologist using accepted criteria<br>• Criteria not stated | • Prevalence: 32 % among patients with GC treatment ≥1 year; 0 % among patients with GC treatment <1 year<br>• Time: by the time of the study | Statistical test for comparing children with and without VF:<br>• GC treatment ≥1 year |

(continued)

Table 10.1 (continued)

| Disease | Publication and study design | Inclusion criteria | Number, age (yrs), and male (%) of patients | Clinical criteria for carrying out the VF assessment[a] | VF assessment method and imaging modality | VF prevalence/incidence and time point | Clinical predictors of prevalent or incident VF from univariate or multivariable models (with effect size and 95% CI) or statistical tests for comparing children with and without VF[b] |
|---|---|---|---|---|---|---|---|
| NS | • Feber (2012) <br> • Prospective, observational | • Age from 1 month to 17 yrs <br> • Within 30 days of first-time GC therapy for the treatment of NS | • N=80 <br> • Age: median (min, max)=4.4 (1.3, 16.9) <br> • Male: 58% | • Assessment at baseline and then annually for every patient | • Lateral spine X-ray <br> • Genant method | • Prevalence: 8% <br> • Time: within 30 days of GC initiation | Statistical test for comparing children with and without VF: <br> • Vitamin D daily intake <50% DRI |
| *Non-steroid-treated diseases* | | | | | | | |
| OI | • Ben Amor (2013) <br> • Retrospective chart review & cross-sectional assessment of skeletal health | • With known nonsense or frameshift mutations in *COL1A1* <br> • Evaluated at the Shriners Hospital for Children in Montreal between March 1992 and August 2010 | Entire cohort <br> • N=86 <br> • Age: mean (SD)=13.3 (13.9) <br> • Male: 42% <br> Patients in the absence of prior bisphosphonate treatment and age ≤21 yrs <br> • N=58 <br> • Age: mean (min, max)=7.4 (0.6, 18) <br> • Male: 47% | • VF assessment was limited to patients ≤21 yrs old | • Lateral spine X-ray <br> • Genant method | • Prevalence: 71% among patients in the absence of prior bisphosphonate treatment and age ≤21 yrs <br> • Time: after enrollment into the study | Multivariable model: <br> • ↓LSBMD Z-score: OR=2.5 (1.1, 5.0) <br> • Female: 6.6 (1.5, 28.3) |

| Thalassemia syndromes | • Engkakul (2013)<br>• Retrospective chart review and cross-sectional assessment | • With thalassemia syndromes, aged 10–60<br>• Attending the Hematology Clinic at the Faculty of Medicine, Ramathibodi Hospital, Mahidol University during the years 2010 and 2011 | • N=150<br>• Age at diagnosis: median (min, max)=3.0 (0.1, 36.0)<br>• Age by the time of this study: median (min, max)=15.7 (10.0, 59.8)<br>• Male: 47% | • Assessed following enrollment into the study | • Lateral spine X-ray<br>• Genant method | • Prevalence: 13%<br>• Time: after enrollment into the study | Multivariable model:<br>• Severe thalassemia: OR=5.7 (2.0, 16.8)<br>• Age (20 yrs or older): OR=5.0 (1.7, 14.0) |
|---|---|---|---|---|---|---|---|
| Recurrent fractures in otherwise healthy children | • Mayranpaa (2012)<br>• Prospective, observational | Healthy children over 4 years of age, who had sustained:<br>• At least two long-bone fractures before age 10 years<br>• At least three long-bone fractures before age 16 years<br>• At least one vertebral fracture | • N=66<br>• Age: mean (min, max)=10.7 (4.4, 16.8) at the time of evaluation<br>• Male: 67% | • Assessed during a 12-month period after enrolment into the study for every patient | • Lateral spine X-ray<br>• Method proposed by Makitie[c] | • Prevalence: 29%<br>• Time: within 12 months after enrollment into the study | Statistical test for comparing children with and without VF:<br>• Lower S-250HD<br>• Less long-bone fractures per child<br>• Lower LSBMD<br>• Z-score |

GC glucocorticoid(s), IQR interquartile range, LSBMD lumbar spine bone mineral density, CI confidence interval, OR odds ratio, HR hazard ratio, RR relative risk, VF vertebral fracture, DXA dual-energy X-ray absorptiometry, VFA vertebral fracture assessment, VAS Visual analog scale for disease activity, RC rheumatic conditions, OI osteogenesis imperfect, NS nephrotic syndrome, DRI dietary reference intake, ALL acute lymphoblastic leukemia, CHAQ Childhood Health Assessment Questionnaire, DMD Duchenne musclular dystrophy, JDM juvenile dermatomyositis, JIA juvenile idiopathic arthritis, SLE systemic lupus erythematosus, SV systemic vasculitis, MRI magnetic resonance imaging, CTD connective tissue disease, yrs years, min minimum, max maximum, N/A not relevant

[a]Note that if the patients were selected for a VF assessment from a larger pool of patients with the same condition according to certain clinical criteria, then the results are not true estimates of the overall prevalence or incidence for that condition, but rather they are estimates of the frequency of VF for a subgroup with the condition

[b]Note that if the association between predictors and VF was assessed using statistical tests for comparing those with and without VF, the effect size will not be available and presented

[c]Makitie O, Doria AS, Henriques F, Cole WG, Compeyrot S, Silverman E, Laxer R, Daneman A, Sochett EB 2005 Radiographic vertebral morphology: A diagnostic tool in pediatric osteoporosis. J Pediatr 146:395–401

[d]Jensen KK, Tougaard L (1981) A simple X-ray method for monitoring progress of osteoporosis, Lancet ii: 19–20

prevalent VF in two studies of children with GC-treated leukemia and rheumatic disorders [1, 27], back pain was not associated with incident VF in others [11, 13]. A lack of back pain does not rule out the presence of VF in at-risk children.

The fact that prevalent VF around the time of GC initiation predict future VF draws attention to the importance of the skeletal phenotype early in the child's disease course. In children with rheumatic disorders, clinical features early in the GC-treatment course were independent predictors of VF in the 3 years following GC initiation. These include increases in disease activity scores in the first 12 months of GC therapy as well as increases in body mass index Z-scores, and decreases in LS BMD Z-scores in the first 6 months of GC therapy [11]. These observations highlight the importance of understanding the child's bone health trajectory beginning *early* in the disease and GC-treatment course.

In summary, in children with GC-treated leukemia and rheumatic conditions, robust predictors of incident VF include a history of prior VF, low or declining BMD Z-scores in the first 6 months of GC therapy, increases in BMI Z-scores over the same time period, GC exposure (average daily dose, cumulative dose, and intensity of dosing), and back pain. In children with solid organ transplantation, older age was also a consistent predictor of an increased VF risk [60, 62, 68, 69].

With clear evidence now that BMD is a consistent predictor of VF in children, a key question is whether the relationship between BMD and VF risk varies depending on the normative database that is used to generate the Z-scores. The Canadian STOPP Consortium addressed this issue by describing the magnitude of the disparity in LS BMD Z-scores generated by both Hologic and Lunar machines [70] in children with ALL at diagnosis. The disparity in results between manufacturers was as much as 2.0 SD depending upon which database was used to generate the Z-scores. This study also showed that children with VF and leukemia at diagnosis frequently had BMD Z-scores better than −2.0 regardless of the reference database that was used, and that the proportion of children assigned a BMD Z-score above or below −2.0 SD varied considerably.

These disparate results in BMD Z-scores depending on the reference database that is used suggest that the use of a LS BMD Z-score cut-off as part of the definition of osteoporosis in children with VF is unnecessary [16]. In the International Society for Clinical Densitometry 2013 position statement on the definition of osteoporosis in children, attaining a BMD Z-score threshold of −2 or worse is no longer required to diagnose osteoporosis in a child with a VF; in fact, there are no longer BMD Z-score requirements at all in the setting of a low-trauma VF. Interestingly, Henderson et al. made a similar observation in children with neuromuscular disorders, showing that up to about 15 % of those with extremity fractures had lateral distal femur BMD Z-scores better than −2.0 [71]. In our opinion, Henderson's report also calls into question the retention of a BMD Z-score threshold as part of the definition of osteoporosis in at-risk children with extremity fractures [16].

In addition to highlighting the disparity in LS BMD Z-score generated by Lunar and Hologic machines, Ma et al. [70] showed in children with ALL at diagnosis using three different statistical approaches that the relationships between LS BMD Z-scores and VF are consistent regardless of the reference databases that are used to generate the Z-scores. This is not surprising, given that the available reference databases are all highly correlated with one another (with $r$ values ranges from 0.85 to 0.99) [70]. These findings suggest that while the use of a LS BMD Z-score threshold is invalid in the diagnosis of osteoporosis in children with VF, and that this is likely also true for other BMD sites in children with extremity fractures [71], the use of LS BMD Z-scores as a risk factor for VF in clinical research studies nevertheless remains a valid approach.

## Reshaping of Previously Fractured Vertebral Bodies and Bone Mineral Density Restitution as Indices of Recovery from Transient Bone Health Threats

The pediatric skeleton is a dynamic structure with the capability to not only undergo reclamation of BMD lost during transient bone health threats, but also to reshape vertebral bodies. Both indices are important measures of recovery in children, either spontaneously or following bone-targeted therapy (such as bisphosphonate treatment). Since vertebral body reshaping is exclusively growth-mediated, it is important to understand that bisphosphonate therapy does not directly bring about reshaping per se (since reshaping is growth-mediated, and bisphosphonates do not cause bone growth); rather bisphosphonate therapy has a permissive effect on growth-mediated reshaping by preventing further vertebral body collapse and thereby allowing the growth process to induce reshaping.

The disease that has been best-studied for signs of recovery from skeletal insult is pediatric ALL. This is not surprising, since ALL represents a transient threat to bone health in the majority of patients undergoing contemporary treatment strategies. Mostoufi-Moab [39] assessed children by tibia peripheral quantitative CT within 2 years following chemotherapy cessation and then again a year later. The study found that trabecular and cortical BMD Z-scores were significantly reduced compared to healthy controls within 2 years post-chemotherapy cessation, but that significant improvements (on average 0.5 SD) were evident a year later. Cortical dimensions also subsequently increased, followed by increases in cortical BMD. Other studies have also shown recovery in bone mass and density in the years following chemotherapy [72, 73]. Lack of BMD restitution is predicted by cranial and spinal radiation, particularly doses $\geq 24$ Gy [73], although the differences in spine BMD among those with radiation exposure compared to those without appear to arise in part from hormone deficiency-related short stature. Other risk factors for incomplete BMD restitution include untreated hypogonadism, vitamin D deficiency, hypophosphatemia, low IGF-binding protein-3, and reduced physical activity [74].

Recovery has been even more dramatically evident in leukemia survivors by evidence for reshaping of previously fractured vertebral bodies, both during and following leukemia chemotherapy [75] (Fig. 10.5). The fact that reshaping can occur during chemotherapy (i.e. during high dose GC therapy) is hypothesized to result from the saltatory pattern of GC exposure with current treatment protocols. On the

**Fig. 10.5** Spontaneous vertebral body reshaping in a child with leukemia. (**a**) X-ray of a 6-year-old boy at day 79 following initiation of chemotherapy. Collapse of the thoracic and lumbar vertebrae is shown. (**b**) X-ray after completion of chemotherapy showing vertebral body reshaping (with permission from Kakihara, Pediatr Int, 2002)

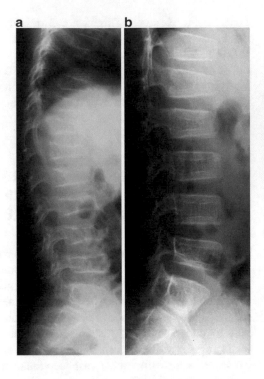

other hand, children with ALL who have insufficient residual growth potential can be left with permanent vertebral deformity after vertebral collapse. The long-term consequences of permanent vertebral deformity following chemotherapy remain unstudied; however, reports in adults indicate compromised quality of life due to pain and functional limitation [31, 32]. In order to understand which children with ALL and VF require bone-targeted intervention to prevent permanent vertebral deformity, the Canadian STOPP Consortium has assessed predictors of complete vertebral body reshaping (quantified by a decrease in a positive SDI by 100 % in the 4 years following chemotherapy initiation). Preliminary results suggest that moderate or severe vertebral collapse as well as older age are negative predictors of complete vertebral body reshaping; children with incomplete vertebral body reshaping were on average $8.7 \pm 3.8$ years compared to $5.6 \pm 4.2$ years for those with 100 % reshaping [76]. These data suggest the importance of identifying VF in a timely fashion, particularly in older children and in children with moderate and severe collapse. The next question is whether pharmacologic skeletal therapy with a bisphosphonate or other agent can prevent permanent vertebral deformity in older children with VF or in a child of any age with moderate and severe collapse. Trials to address this question are currently underway. In our experience, children with VF and ongoing GC exposure or other potent risk factors for VF such as immobilization/progressive myopathy typically do not demonstrate spontaneous vertebral body reshaping. Such patients are prime candidates for inclusion in much-needed osteoporosis primary prevention trials.

## Influence on Clinical Practice: The Impact of VF as a Manifestation of Osteoporosis in Childhood and of the Relationship Between Clinical Predictors and Vertebral Fractures

It is now well-established that VF are a frequent manifestation of osteoporosis in at-risk children. Clinical predictors of both VF and spontaneous recovery have been identified. With this knowledge, we can make logical decisions regarding the approach to bone health monitoring in at-risk children and identify optimal candidates for bone-targeted therapy.

Bone health monitoring should be considered an integral component of the care plan in children with serious chronic illnesses. Recently, the approach to the monitoring of osteoporosis in children has moved towards a functional approach, including an evaluation of the child's growth, pubertal status, pain, mobility, muscle strength, VF and non-VF statuses, as well as the potential for spontaneous recovery. Patients initiating treatment with GC for 3 or more months should undergo a baseline spine radiograph (or high quality DXA-based VFA, if available) at the time of GC initiation. Studies should be repeated at 12 months when the annual incidence of VF is highest in GC-treated children. Annual to biannual imaging for VF is advised thereafter among children with ongoing GC exposure, depending upon the magnitude of the risk factors for compromised bone health and changes in BMD Z-score. As previously discussed, a number of clinical predictors have been elucidated which assist the clinician in deciding the frequency of follow-up VF assessments beyond 12 months, including: ongoing GC exposure, low or declining LS BMD Z-scores in the first 6–12 months of GC therapy, increases in disease activity scores in the first year of GC therapy, back pain, and increases in BMI Z-scores in the first 6 months of GC therapy.

Among children with risk factors for bone fragility in the absence of GC exposure such as those with immobilization disorders, the same principles apply. The patient needs to be assessed for both non-VF *and* VF. For example, in children with chronic immobilization (such as cerebral palsy), a spine radiograph is recommended no later than 8 years of age and then annually to biannually thereafter until the end of growth, or sooner in the presence of back pain. Eight years of age is proposed as the latest age at which to begin monitoring for VF since older age negatively predicts vertebral body reshaping [76]. The purpose of an initial evaluation at this time point is to consider treatment while there sufficient residual growth potential for vertebral body reshaping.

While the child's functional and bone fragility statuses are focal points of the bone health assessment, BMD remains a valuable adjuvant tool in the overall evaluation. Serial DXA measurements assist the clinician in understanding the child's overall bone health trajectory and thereby making logical decisions about the need for ongoing monitoring, discharge from care or intervention. It is recommended that a BMD is carried out at least as frequently as spine radiographs according to the above guidelines.

Given the potential for spontaneous recovery from osteoporosis (including reshaping of vertebral bodies), primary prevention with bone-targeted medications such as bisphosphonate is not recommended at the present time. Instead, careful monitoring according to the guidelines above is recommended, as well as institution of bone-targeted therapy in those with VF who are also at risk for permanent vertebral deformity in the absence of therapy. Secondary prevention seeks to mitigate disease progression and foster recovery in those with vertebral collapse in its early stages. The most appropriate disease groups for eventual primary prevention are the progressive neuromuscular diseases such as GC-treated DMD. Here, there is an urgent cry for well-designed, bone-targeted prevention trials on sufficient numbers of patients to effectively assess functional outcomes, including VF in the context of primary prevention trials.

Ultimately, the goal of monitoring and intervention strategies is to prevent VF from occurring in the first place. However, in the absence of data from well-designed trials to support primary prevention at the present time, careful monitoring to identify earlier rather than late signs of bone fragility followed by bone-active treatment targeting children with more limited potential for spontaneous recovery (including vertebral body reshaping) remain the current cornerstones of bone health care.

## Future Directions

There has been significant progress in our understanding of the natural history of VF and associated risk and protective factors in children with osteoporotic conditions in recent years. This knowledge has allowed us to develop logical approaches to the diagnosis, monitoring, and timing of intervention in this setting. Given that VF are clearly an important manifestation of osteoporosis in childhood, low-radiation-conferring methods to diagnose VF are needed. Validation studies of techniques such as VFA are currently underway. Studies which assess the impact of VF on quality of life and mortality in pediatric chronic illnesses are also needed. Current management strategies include monitoring at-risk children to identify and then treat early signs of vertebral collapse in those with less potential for spontaneous vertebral body reshaping (i.e. a secondary prevention approach). Trials addressing primary prevention are also needed for children with both a high likelihood of developing VF and with persistent risk factors. While BMD is no longer the focus of the diagnosis of osteoporosis in children, it nevertheless provides important, adjuvant information about the child's overall bone health trajectory, signaling a child who is at increased risk for VF or who is showing signs of spontaneous recovery from a transient bone health threat.

## Summary Points

- VF are an important manifestation of osteoporosis in children with genetic disorders predisposing to bone fragility (such as OI) and in children with serious chronic illnesses such as GC-treated diseases and neuromuscular disorders.
- VF in children are frequently asymptomatic and may go undetected without routine surveillance among those at risk.

- Clinical characteristics that predict incident VF early in the course of illness or treatment include prevalent VF at diagnosis or GC initiation, GC exposure, back pain, increases in disease activity, declines in LS BMD Z-scores and increases in BMI Z-scores. These factors should be considered in determining the need for follow-up radiographs to detect VF.
- Children with transient bone health threats (such as those with short-term GC therapy) have the potential to undergo complete, growth-mediated vertebral body reshaping following VF (as well as BMD restitution), obviating the need for bone-targeted intervention.
- One of the goals of monitoring is to identify VF in a timely fashion, so that children with VF and less potential for spontaneous reshaping can be considered for bone-targeted intervention in order to prevent permanent vertebral deformity.
- LS BMD Z-scores are most useful when assessed over time to determine a child's overall bone health trajectory (that is, to determine whether the child is at risk for incident VF associated with declines in LS BMD Z-scores or whether the child is showing evidence of increments in BMD and thereby recovery).
- A LS BMD Z-score threshold (cut-off) value as part of the definition of osteoporosis in children is not valid for reasons discussed in this chapter. This has been recognized by the International Society for Clinical Densitometry recently in a position statement that recommends BMD criteria are no longer required to diagnose osteoporosis in the presence of a low-trauma vertebral fracture [16]. On the other hand, the relationship (i.e. odds for VF) between LS BMD Z-scores and VF is consistent regardless of the normative database that is used, providing validity for the use of BMD Z-scores as a VF predictor in clinical studies.
- Future research is needed validate the accuracy of DXA-based "VFA" to detect VF.
- Primary prevention trials are needed in children with a high incidence of VF and limited potential for spontaneous vertebral body reshaping.

**Acknowledgements**  Dr. Ward has been supported by a CIHR New Investigator Award (2004–2009), by a Canadian Child Health Clinician Scientist Career Enhancement Award (2007–2010), by a University of Ottawa Research Chair Award (2011 to current) and by the Children's Hospital of Eastern Ontario Department of Surgery, Division of Orthopedics (2009 to current). Dr. Ma is supported by the Children's Hospital of Eastern Ontario Research Institute. Drs. Ward and Ma would like to thank Victor Konji for his support in carrying out literature searches and preparing figures for this chapter and Poppy DesClouds and Liz Sykes for editorial work.

# References

1. Halton J, Gaboury I, Grant R, Alos N, Cummings EA, Matzinger M, Shenouda N, Lentle B, Abish S, Atkinson S, Cairney E, Dix D, Israels S, Stephure D, Wilson B, Hay J, Moher D, Rauch F, Siminoski K, Ward LM, The Canadian STOPP Consortium. Advanced vertebral fracture among newly diagnosed children with acute lymphoblastic leukemia: results of the Canadian Steroid-Associated Osteoporosis in the Pediatric Population (STOPP) research program. J Bone Miner Res. 2009;24:1326–34.

2. Thearle M, Horlick M, Bilezikian JP, Levy J, Gertner JM, Levine LS, Harbison M, Berdon W, Oberfield SE. Osteoporosis: an unusual presentation of childhood Crohn's disease. J Clin Endocrinol Metab. 2000;85:2122–6.
3. Eastell R, Cedel SL, Wahner HW, Riggs BL, Melton 3rd LJ. Classification of vertebral fractures. J Bone Miner Res. 1991;6:207–15.
4. McCloskey EV, Spector TD, Eyres KS, Fern ED, O'Rourke N, Vasikaran S, Kanis JA. The assessment of vertebral deformity: a method for use in population studies and clinical trials. Osteoporos Int. 1993;3:138–47.
5. Genant HK, Wu CY, van Kuijk C, Nevitt MC. Vertebral fracture assessment using a semiquantitative technique. J Bone Miner Res. 1993;8:1137–48.
6. Kerkeni S, Kolta S, Fechtenbaum J, Roux C. Spinal deformity index (SDI) is a good predictor of incident vertebral fractures. Osteoporos Int. 2009;20:1547–52.
7. Rea JA, Chen MB, Li J, Blake GM, Steiger P, Genant HK, Fogelman I. Morphometric X-ray absorptiometry and morphometric radiography of the spine: a comparison of prevalent vertebral deformity identification. J Bone Miner Res. 2000;15:564–74.
8. Vallarta-Ast N, Krueger D, Wrase C, Agrawal S, Binkley N. An evaluation of densitometric vertebral fracture assessment in men. Osteoporos Int. 2007;18:1405–10.
9. Wu C, van Kuijk C, Li J, Jiang Y, Chan M, Countryman P, Genant HK. Comparison of digitized images with original radiography for semiquantitative assessment of osteoporotic fractures. Osteoporos Int. 2000;11:25–30.
10. Siminoski K, Lee KC, Jen H, Warshawski R, Matzinger MA, Shenouda N, Charron M, Coblentz C, Dubois J, Kloiber R, Nadel H, O'Brien K, Reed M, Sparrow K, Webber C, Lentle B, Ward LM. Anatomical distribution of vertebral fractures: comparison of pediatric and adult spines. Osteoporos Int. 2012;23:1999–2008.
11. LeBlanc C, Ma J, Taljaard M, Roth J, Scuccimarri R, Miettunen P, Lang B, Huber AM, Houghton K, Jaremko J, Ho J, Shenouda N, Matzinger M, Lentle B, Stein R, Sbrocchi A, Oen K, Rodd C, Jurencak R, Cummings E, Couch R, Cabral D, Atkinson S, Alos N, Rauch F, Siminoski K, Ward LM, Canadian STOPP Consortium. Incident vertebral fractures and risk factors in the first three years following glucocorticoid initiation among pediatric patients with rheumatic disorders. J Bone Miner Res. 2015;30:1667–75.
12. Alos N, Grant RM, Ramsay T, Halton J, Cummings EA, Miettunen PM, Abish S, Atkinson S, Barr R, Cabral DA, Cairney E, Couch R, Dix DB, Fernandez CV, Hay J, Israels S, Laverdiere C, Lentle B, Lewis V, Matzinger M, Rodd C, Shenouda N, Stein R, Stephure D, Taback S, Wilson B, Williams K, Rauch F, Siminoski K, Ward LM. High incidence of vertebral fractures in children with acute lymphoblastic leukemia 12 months after the initiation of therapy. J Clin Oncol. 2012;30:2760–7.
13. Cummings E A, Ma J, Fernandez CV, Halton J, Alos N, Miettunen PM, Jaremko JL, Ho J, Shenouda N, Matzinger M, Lentle B, Stephure D, Stein R, Sbrocchi AM, Rodd C, Lang B, Israels S, Grant RM, Couch R, Barr R, Hay J, Rauch F, Siminoski K, Ward LM, The Canadian STOPP Consortium. Incident vertebral fractures in children with leukemia during the four years following diagnosis. J Clin Endocrinol Metab. 2015. J Clin Endocrinol Metab. 2015; 100:3408–17.
14. Gaca AM, Barnhart HX, Bisset 3rd GS. Evaluation of wedging of lower thoracic and upper lumbar vertebral bodies in the pediatric population. Am J Roentgenol. 2010;194:516–20.
15. Ebel KD, Blickman H, Willich E, Richter E. Abnormalities in vertebral body shape and size. In: Differential diagnosis in pediatric radiology. New York: Thieme Publishers; 1999.
16. Bishop N, Arundel P, Clark E, Dimitri P, Farr J, Jones G, Makitie O, Munns CF, Shaw N. Fracture prediction and the definition of osteoporosis in children and adolescents: the ISCD 2013 Pediatric Official Positions. J Clin Densitom. 2014;17:275–80.
17. Jiang G, Eastell R, Barrington NA, Ferrar L. Comparison of methods for the visual identification of prevalent vertebral fracture in osteoporosis. Osteoporos Int. 2004;15:887–96.
18. Jaremko JL, Siminoski K, Firth GB, Matzinger MA, Shenouda N, Konji VN, Roth J, Sbrocchi AM, Reed MH, O'Brien MK, Nadel H, McKillop S, Kloiber R, Dubois J, Coblentz C, Charron M, Ward LM. Common normal variants of pediatric vertebral development that

mimic fractures: a pictorial review from a national longitudinal bone health study. Pediatr Radiol. 2015;45:593–605.

19. Genant HK, Jergas M, Palermo L, Nevitt M, Valentin RS, Black D, Cummings SR. Comparison of semiquantitative visual and quantitative morphometric assessment of prevalent and incident vertebral fractures in osteoporosis. The Study of Osteoporotic Fractures Research Group. J Bone Miner Res. 1996;11:984–96.

20. Siminoski K, Lentle B, Matzinger MA, Shenouda N, Ward LM. Observer agreement in pediatric semiquantitative vertebral fracture diagnosis. Pediatr Radiol. 2014;44:457–66.

21. Buehring B, Krueger D, Checovich M, Gemar D, Vallarta-Ast N, Genant HK, Binkley N. Vertebral fracture assessment: impact of instrument and reader. Osteoporos Int. 2010;21: 487–94.

22. Mayranpaa MK, Helenius I, Valta H, Mayranpaa MI, Toiviainen-Salo S, Makitie O. Bone densitometry in the diagnosis of vertebral fractures in children: accuracy of vertebral fracture assessment. Bone. 2007;41:353–9.

23. Divasta AD, Feldman HA, Gordon CM. Vertebral fracture assessment in adolescents and young women with anorexia nervosa: a case series. J Clin Densitom. 2014;17:207–11.

24. Williams AL, Al-Busaidi A, Sparrow PJ, Adams JE, Whitehouse RW. Under-reporting of osteoporotic vertebral fractures on computed tomography. Eur J Radiol. 2009;69:179–83.

25. Kilpinen-Loisa P, Paasio T, Soiva M, Ritanen UM, Lautala P, Palmu P, Pihko H, Makitie O. Low bone mass in patients with motor disability: prevalence and risk factors in 59 Finnish children. Dev Med Child Neurol. 2010;52:276–82.

26. Feber J, Gaboury I, Ni A, Alos N, Arora S, Bell L, Blydt-Hansen T, Clarson C, Filler G, Hay J, Hebert D, Lentle B, Matzinger M, Midgley J, Moher D, Pinsk M, Rauch F, Rodd C, Shenouda N, Siminoski K, Ward LM. Skeletal findings in children recently initiating glucocorticoids for the treatment of nephrotic syndrome. Osteoporos Int. 2012;23:751–60.

27. Huber AM, Gaboury I, Cabral DA, Lang B, Ni A, Stephure D, Taback S, Dent P, Ellsworth J, LeBlanc C, Saint-Cyr C, Scuccimarri R, Hay J, Lentle B, Matzinger M, Shenouda N, Moher D, Rauch F, Siminoski K, Ward LM. Prevalent vertebral fractures among children initiating glucocorticoid therapy for the treatment of rheumatic disorders. Arthritis Care Res (Hoboken). 2010;62:516–26.

28. Phan V, Blydt-Hansen T, Feber J, Alos N, Arora S, Atkinson S, Bell L, Clarson C, Couch R, Cummings EA, Filler G, Grant RM, Grimmer J, Hebert D, Lentle B, Ma J, Matzinger M, Midgley J, Pinsk M, Rodd C, Shenouda N, Stein R, Stephure D, Taback S, Williams K, Rauch F, Siminoski K, Ward LM. Skeletal findings in the first 12 months following initiation of glucocorticoid therapy for pediatric nephrotic syndrome. Osteoporos Int. 2014;25:627–37.

29. Rodd C, Lang B, Ramsay T, Alos N, Huber AM, Cabral DA, Scuccimarri R, Miettunen PM, Roth J, Atkinson SA, Couch R, Cummings EA, Dent PB, Ellsworth J, Hay J, Houghton K, Jurencak R, Larche M, LeBlanc C, Oen K, Saint-Cyr C, Stein R, Stephure D, Taback S, Lentle B, Matzinger M, Shenouda N, Moher D, Rauch F, Siminoski K, Ward LM. Incident vertebral fractures among children with rheumatic disorders 12 months after glucocorticoid initiation: a national observational study. Arthritis Care Res (Hoboken). 2012;64:122–31.

30. Cooper C, Shah S, Hand DJ, Adams J, Compston J, Davie M, Woolf A. Screening for vertebral osteoporosis using individual risk factors. The Multicentre Vertebral Fracture Study Group. Osteoporos Int. 1991;2:48–53.

31. Burger H, Van Daele PL, Grashuis K, Hofman A, Grobbee DE, Schutte HE, Birkenhager JC, Pols HA. Vertebral deformities and functional impairment in men and women. J Bone Miner Res. 1997;12:152–7.

32. Nevitt MC, Ettinger B, Black DM, Stone K, Jamal SA, Ensrud K, Segal M, Genant HK, Cummings SR. The association of radiographically detected vertebral fractures with back pain and function: a prospective study. Ann Intern Med. 1998;128:793–800.

33. Bliuc D, Nguyen ND, Milch VE, Nguyen TV, Eisman JA, Center JR. Mortality risk associated with low-trauma osteoporotic fracture and subsequent fracture in men and women. JAMA. 2009;301:513–21.

34. Marini JC, Reich A, Smith SM. Osteogenesis imperfecta due to mutations in non-collagenous genes: lessons in the biology of bone formation. Curr Opin Pediatr. 2014;26:500–7.
35. Ben Amor IM, Roughley P, Glorieux FH, Rauch F. Skeletal clinical characteristics of osteo-genesis imperfecta caused by haploinsufficiency mutations in COL1A1. J Bone Miner Res. 2013;28:2001–7.
36. Rauch F, Lalic L, Roughley P, Glorieux FH. Relationship between genotype and skeletal phe-notype in children and adolescents with osteogenesis imperfecta. J Bone Miner Res. 2010; 25:1367–74.
37. van der Sluis IM, van den Heuvel-Eibrink MM, Hahlen K, Krenning EP, de Muinck Keizer-Schrama SM. Altered bone mineral density and body composition, and increased fracture risk in childhood acute lymphoblastic leukemia. J Pediatr. 2002;141:204–10.
38. Pui CH, Robison LL, Look AT. Acute lymphoblastic leukaemia. Lancet. 2008;371:1030–43.
39. Mostoufi-Moab S, Brodsky J, Isaacoff EJ, Tsampalieros A, Ginsberg JP, Zemel B, Shults J, Leonard MB. Longitudinal assessment of bone density and structure in childhood survivors of acute lymphoblastic leukemia without cranial radiation. J Clin Endocrinol Metab. 2012;97: 3584–92.
40. Mandel K, Atkinson S, Barr RD, Pencharz P. Skeletal morbidity in childhood acute lympho-blastic leukemia. J Clin Oncol. 2004;22:1215–21.
41. Riccio I, Marcarelli M, Del Regno N, Fusco C, Di Martino M, Savarese R, Gualdiero G, Oreste M, Indolfi C, Porpora G, Esposito M, Casale F, Riccardi G. Musculoskeletal problems in pedi-atric acute leukemia. J Pediatr Orthop B. 2013;22:264–9.
42. Baty JM, Vogt EC. Bone changes of leukemia in children. Am J Roentgenol. 1935;34:310–3.
43. Willson JK. The bone lesions of childhood leukemia; a survey of 140 cases. Radiology. 1959;72:672–81.
44. Simmons CR, Harle TS, Singleton EB. The osseous manifestations of leukemia in children. Radiol Clin North Am. 1968;6:115–30.
45. Rogalsky RJ, Black GB, Reed MH. Orthopaedic manifestations of leukemia in children. J Bone Joint Surg. 1986;68-A:494–501.
46. Silverman FN. The skeletal lesions in leukemia; clinical and roentgenographic observations in 103 infants and children, with a review of the literature. Am J Roentgenol Radium Ther. 1948;59:819–44.
47. Halton JM, Atkinson SA, Fraher L, Webber CE, Cockshott WP, Tam C, Barr RD. Mineral homeostasis and bone mass at diagnosis in children with acute lymphoblastic leukemia. J Pediatr. 1995;126:557–64.
48. Jayanthan A, Miettunen PM, Incoronato A, Ortiz-Neira CL, Lewis VA, Anderson R, Frohlich DE, Narendran A. Childhood acute lymphoblastic leukemia (ALL) presenting with severe osteolysis: a model to study leukemia-bone interactions and potential targeted therapeutics. Pediatr Hematol Oncol. 2010;27:212–27.
49. Regio P, Bonfa E, Takayama L, Pereira R. The influence of lean mass in trabecular and cortical bone in juvenile onset systemic lupus erythematosus. Lupus. 2008;17:787–92.
50. Nakhla M, Scuccimarri R, Duffy KN, Chedeville G, Campillo S, Duffy CM, Azouz EM, Shenouda N, Sharma AK, Rodd C. Prevalence of vertebral fractures in children with chronic rheumatic diseases at risk for osteopenia. J Pediatr. 2009;154:438–43.
51. Valta H, Lahdenne P, Jalanko H, Aalto K, Makitie O. Bone health and growth in glucocorticoid-treated patients with juvenile idiopathic arthritis. J Rheumatol. 2007;34:831–6.
52. Burnham JM, Shults J, Weinstein R, Lewis JD, Leonard MB. Childhood onset arthritis is asso-ciated with an increased risk of fracture: a population based study using the General Practice Research Database. Ann Rheum Dis. 2006;65:1074–9.
53. Varonos S, Ansell BM, Reeve J. Vertebral collapse in juvenile chronic arthritis: its relationship with glucocorticoid therapy. Calcif Tissue Int. 1987;41:75–8.
54. Larson CM, Henderson RC. Bone mineral density and fractures in boys with Duchenne mus-cular dystrophy. J Pediatr Orthop. 2000;20:71–4.

55. McDonald DG, Kinali M, Gallagher AC, Mercuri E, Muntoni F, Roper H, Jardine P, Jones DH, Pike MG. Fracture prevalence in Duchenne muscular dystrophy. Dev Med Child Neurol. 2002;44:695–8.
56. King WM, Ruttencutter R, Nagaraja HN, Matkovic V, Landoll J, Hoyle C, Mendell JR, Kissel JT. Orthopedic outcomes of long-term daily corticosteroid treatment in Duchenne muscular dystrophy. Neurology. 2007;68:1607–13.
57. Mughal MZ. Fractures in children with cerebral palsy. Curr Osteoporos Rep. 2014;12:313–8.
58. Canalis E, Mazziotti G, Giustina A, Bilezikian JP. Glucocorticoid-induced osteoporosis: pathophysiology and therapy. Osteoporos Int. 2007;18:1319–28.
59. Teeninga N, Kist-van Holthe JE, van den Akker EL, Kersten MC, Boersma E, Krabbe HG, Knoers NV, van der Heijden AJ, Koper JW, Nauta J. Genetic and in vivo determinants of glucocorticoid sensitivity in relation to clinical outcome of childhood nephrotic syndrome. Kidney Int. 2014;85:1444–53.
60. Valta H, Jalanko H, Holmberg C, Helenius I, Makitie O. Impaired bone health in adolescents after liver transplantation. Am J Transplant. 2008;8:150–7.
61. Okajima H, Shigeno C, Inomata Y, Egawa H, Uemoto S, Asonuma K, Kiuchi T, Konishi J, Tanaka K. Long-term effects of liver transplantation on bone mineral density in children with end-stage liver disease: a 2-year prospective study. Liver Transpl. 2003;9:360–4.
62. Helenius I, Remes V, Salminen S, Valta H, Makitie O, Holmberg C, Palmu P, Tervahartiala P, Sarna S, Helenius M, Peltonen J, Jalanko H. Incidence and predictors of fractures in children after solid organ transplantation: a 5-year prospective, population-based study. J Bone Miner Res. 2006;21:380–7.
63. Hill SA, Kelly DA, John PR. Bone fractures in children undergoing orthotopic liver transplantation. Pediatr Radiol. 1995;25 Suppl 1:S112–7.
64. Shneider BL, Neimark E, Frankenberg T, Arnott L, Suchy FJ, Emre S. Critical analysis of the pediatric end-stage liver disease scoring system: a single center experience. Liver Transpl. 2005;11:788 95.
65. Bales CB, Kamath BM, Munoz PS, Nguyen A, Piccoli DA, Spinner NB, Horn D, Shults J, Leonard MB, Grimberg A, Loomes KM. Pathologic lower extremity fractures in children with Alagille syndrome. J Pediatr Gastroenterol Nutr. 2010;51:66–70.
66. Klein GL, Soriano H, Shulman RJ, Levy M, Jones G, Langman CB. Hepatic osteodystrophy in chronic cholestasis: evidence for a multifactorial etiology. Pediatr Transplant. 2002;6:136–40.
67. D'Antiga L, Moniz C, Buxton-Thomas M, Cheeseman P, Gray B, Abraha H, Baker AJ, Heaton ND, Rela M, Mieli-Vergani G, Dhawan A. Bone mineral density and height gain in children with chronic cholestatic liver disease undergoing transplantation. Transplantation. 2002;73: 1788–93.
68. Valta H, Makitie O, Ronnholm K, Jalanko H. Bone health in children and adolescents after renal transplantation. J Bone Miner Res. 2009;24:1699–708.
69. Vautour LM, Melton 3rd LJ, Clarke BL, Achenbach SJ, Oberg AL, McCarthy JT. Long-term fracture risk following renal transplantation: a population-based study. Osteoporos Int. 2004;15:160–7.
70. Ma J, Siminoski K, Alos N, Halton J, Ho J, Lentle B, Matzinger M, Shenouda N, Atkinson S, Barr R, Cabral DA, Couch R, Cummings EA, Fernandez CV, Grant RM, Rodd C, Sbrocchi AM, Scharke M, Rauch F, Ward LM. The choice of normative pediatric reference database changes spine bone mineral density Z-scores but not the relationship between bone mineral density and prevalent vertebral fractures. J Clin Endocrinol Metab. 2015;100:1018–27.
71. Henderson RC, Berglund LM, May R, Zemel BS, Grossberg RI, Johnson J, Plotkin H, Stevenson RD, Szalay E, Wong B, Kecskemethy HH, Harcke HT. The relationship between fractures and DXA measures of BMD in the distal femur of children and adolescents with cerebral palsy or muscular dystrophy. J Bone Miner Res. 2010;25:520–6.

72. Marinovic D, Dorgeret S, Lescoeur B, Alberti C, Noel M, Czernichow P, Sebag G, Vilmer E, Leger J. Improvement in bone mineral density and body composition in survivors of childhood acute lymphoblastic leukemia: a 1-year prospective study. Pediatrics. 2005;116:e102–8.
73. Gurney JG, Kaste SC, Liu W, Srivastava DK, Chemaitilly W, Ness KK, Lanctot JQ, Ojha RP, Nottage KA, Wilson CL, Li Z, Robison LL, Hudson MM. Bone mineral density among long-term survivors of childhood acute lymphoblastic leukemia: results from the St. Jude Lifetime Cohort Study. Pediatr Blood Cancer. 2014;61:1270–6.
74. Makitie O, Heikkinen R, Toiviainen-Salo S, Henriksson M, Puukko-Viertomies LR, Jahnukainen K. Long-term skeletal consequences of childhood acute lymphoblastic leukemia in adult males: a cohort study. Eur J Endocrinol. 2013;168:281–8.
75. Pandya NA, Meller ST, MacVicar D, Atra AA, Pinkerton CR. Vertebral compression fractures in acute lymphoblastic leukaemia and remodelling after treatment. Arch Dis Child. 2001; 85:492–3.
76. Ward LM. Bone mass effects and fracture risk in children receiving glucocorticoid therapy—steroid-induced osteoporosis in the pediatric population—Canadian incidence study. E-PAS 2015:268OA: invited symposium, Pediatric Academic Sciences Annual Meeting, Vancouver, BC; 2014.

# Chapter 11
# Lessons Learned from Clinical Research Using QCT, pQCT, and HR-pQCT

Heather M. Macdonald, Heather A. McKay, and Mary B. Leonard

## Abbreviations

| | |
|---|---|
| aBMD | Areal bone mineral density (g/cm² by DXA) |
| BMC | Bone mineral content (g) |
| BMD | Bone mineral density (mg/cm³ by QCT methods) |
| BSI | Bone strength index (mg²/mm⁴ by QCT methods) |
| BV/TV | Bone volume fraction |
| CD | Crohn's disease |
| CSA | Cross-sectional area (cm² by QCT methods) |
| DXA | Dual energy X-ray absorptiometry |
| GC | Glucocorticoid |
| HR-pQCT | High-resolution pQCT |
| PHV | Peak height velocity |
| pQCT | Peripheral quantitative computed tomography |
| QCT | Quantitative computed tomography |
| SSI_p | Polar strength-strain index (mm³ by QCT methods) |
| SSNS | Steroid-sensitive nephrotic syndrome |

H.M. Macdonald, Ph.D. (✉)
Department of Family Practice and Centre for Hip Health and Mobility, University of British Columbia, 2635 Laurel Street, Vancouver, BC, Canada V5Z 1M9
e-mail: heather.macdonald@ubc.ca

H.A. McKay, Ph.D.
Departments of Orthopaedics and Family Practice, Centre for Hip Health and Mobility, 7th Floor, 2635 Laurel Street, Vancouver, BC, Canada V5Z 1M9
e-mail: heather.mckay@ubc.ca

M.B. Leonard, M.D., M.S.C.E.
Department of Pediatrics, Stanford University School of Medicine, 300 Pasteur Drive, H310, Stanford, CA 94305, USA
e-mail: leonard5@stanford.edu

© Springer International Publishing Switzerland 2016
E.B. Fung et al. (eds.), *Bone Health Assessment in Pediatrics*,
DOI 10.1007/978-3-319-30412-0_11

TNF-α      Tumor necrosis factor-α
2D         Two-dimensional
3D         Three-dimensional

# Introduction

As is evident from the first ten chapters of this book, dual energy X-ray absorptiometry (DXA) is a valid and reliable clinical and research tool that is widely used to monitor bone mass and density in the growing skeleton. Studies that utilized DXA to describe bone mineral accrual in healthy children and clinical populations or to evaluate bone's response to various interventions, have served to advance our understanding of pediatric bone physiology. However, given the key role that bone health during growth plays in determining adult bone status and ultimately fracture risk, we must consider more specific properties that confer bone its strength. Thus, with the advent of sophisticated three-dimensional (3D) imaging techniques, research focus has shifted toward bone strength, the "bottom line" of fracture prevention [1, 2].

Bone strength, or the ultimate load that a bone can withstand before breaking, is a function of its material properties (e.g., tissue density), the arrangement of this material at the macro (e.g., bone cross-sectional area or shape) and micro level (e.g., trabecular number and thickness) as well as overall bone size or mass [3, 4]. Although DXA-derived areal bone mineral density (aBMD) predicts fracture risk [5], this "catch-all" measure does not permit us to investigate the hierarchical nature of bone or describe the specific configurations of bone structure that underpin gains in bone strength during growth. Furthermore, childhood chronic diseases and their therapies may impact discrete components of bone density and structure that cannot be defined using DXA.

Advances in imaging modalities, specifically quantitative computed tomography (QCT)-based devices, permits us to noninvasively examine aspects of bone (micro) structure and volumetric BMD (BMD) in the growing skeleton. In Chap. 2, Ward and colleagues provided an excellent summary of the technical aspects of QCT, peripheral QCT (pQCT), and high-resolution pQCT (HR-pQCT), the common 3D imaging tools used in pediatric bone research. Thus, we aim to complement (rather than replicate) Chap. 2 by providing an overview of lessons learned from studies that assessed pediatric bone strength (including micro- and macro-structure and BMD), using QCT-based instruments. First, we summarize what is currently known about the acquisition of bone strength, structure, and density in healthy children, highlighting key QCT studies that have informed our understanding of these processes. Second, we review key determinants of bone strength acquisition during growth. Third, we describe the influence of chronic disease and medications on bone strength acquisition. Finally, we highlight challenges that confront researchers who use medical imaging techniques to assess children, and offer specific research questions that might guide further study.

## What Do We Know About Bone Strength Acquisition During Growth?

As reviewed in Chap. 1, our current understanding of bone acquisition during growth is based largely on results from several key longitudinal DXA studies that examined the timing and magnitude of bone mass accrual in boys and girls [6–9]. In addition to documenting significant sex differences in bone accrual, these studies highlighted adolescence as a critical period for development of a healthy skeleton.

As of yet we are unable to similarly map the growth trajectory for bone strength, (micro)structure, and density (acquired using 3D imaging techniques), as data from long-term prospective studies that utilized QCT-based imaging across all periods of growth and development in boys and girls do not exist. However, the field continues to advance with reports from large cross-sectional [10–14], short-term longitudinal studies [15] and one recent mixed-longitudinal study [16] that highlight sex- and maturity-related differences in bone strength acquisition. Current estimates suggest that the magnitude of the increase in bone strength during growth may be as high as 100–400 %, depending on skeletal site measured [10, 12, 14]. It is also clear that during puberty boys attain a bone strength advantage, compared with girls [10–12, 14, 15]. This benefit is sustained into older age and contributes to men's lower fracture risk [17]. These observational studies also illustrate how changes in BMD and bone structure during growth influence substantial gains in bone strength. We discuss these studies, below.

As in Chap. 2, we refer to common QCT-derived indices of bone strength. These include the bone strength index (BSI), which is a function of both BMD and bone area and provides an estimate of bone strength in compression at distal ends of long bones, and the polar strength-strain index ($SSI_p$), a density weighted section modulus which provides an estimate of bone strength in torsion at shaft sites of long bones. In HR-pQCT studies, finite element analysis is commonly applied to 3D images to estimate bone strength under uniaxial compression [18] (see Chap. 13 for a detailed description of finite element analysis). Bone strength of the vertebral bodies can also be estimated using finite element analysis applied to vertebral QCT scans [19]; however, this technique has not been used in pediatric studies.

At the *distal ends of long bones (metaphyseal sites)* compressive loads predominate. Bone strength at these sites is a function of the amount of bone material and bone size [20]. The distal radius and tibia are rich in trabecular bone. However, trabecular BMD (by pQCT) or trabecular bone volume (BV/TV by HR-pQCT) appears to change very little as girls advance through maturity [11, 21]. These same parameters may not change at all [11] or may increase only slightly during later stages of puberty in boys [10, 22]. Maturity-related gains in BV/TV in boys are likely due to increased trabecular thickness rather than trabecular number [10, 22]. Similarly, boys have greater BV/TV compared with girls, beginning in early puberty and persisting through postpuberty. This advantage appears to be a function of boys' thicker trabeculae, rather than a larger number of trabecular struts [10, 11, 22]. Together, these structural differences contribute to boys' greater bone strength at distal sites compared with girls. The bone strength advantage conferred boys, may approach 10–38 %, depending on maturity stage [10, 11].

These reports also speak to site specificity of bone development, as results differed from those reported for vertebral bodies, assessed by Gilsanz and colleagues using QCT. To illustrate, in both girls and boys vertebral trabecular (or cancellous) BMD remained relatively constant prior to puberty, increased with advancing maturity and remained constant once sexual maturity was reached [23, 24]. Further, trabecular BMD in the lumbar spine did not differ between boys and girls [24]. Variability between studies may reflect site-specific differences in trabecular BMD or may be due to the different imaging modalities used to measure bone in the growing skeleton.

The cortical shell in growing bone is very thin at metaphyseal regions such as the distal radius. Despite this, it is a key determinant of bone strength [25]. However, partial volume effects (discussed in Chap. 2) hamper our ability to accurately assess cortical bone properties at metaphyseal sites using pQCT (0.2–0.5 mm voxel size). HR-pQCT partially overcomes this limitation, as its resolution (62–82 μm) is sufficient to evaluate not only cortical BMD and thickness, but also estimate cortical porosity. Cortical BMD, a product of mean material density and porosity, appears to increase in the later stages of puberty in girls and boys, as does cortical area (Fig. 11.1) [10, 11, 22]. Conversely, cortical bone porosity appears to decline [10, 11, 22]. Further, with advancing maturity a clear sex difference emerges with girls developing denser and less porous cortices compared with boys during early and peripuberty [10, 11, 22]. This likely reflects higher rates of intracortical remodeling in boys associated with their greater rates of linear growth that elicits an increased demand for calcium [26].

Rapid changes observed in cortical bone at the distal radius during adolescent growth may lead to a transient period of bone fragility and an elevated risk of fracture [27]. Cross-sectional data from studies that used HR-pQCT suggest that the peak in cortical porosity aligns with the timing of peak forearm fracture incidence in girls and boys [10]. It is thought that despite very high rates of endocortical apposition at the distal radius metaphysis during adolescent growth, bone apposition may be insufficient to increase cortical thickness to a level needed to ensure bone's strength can withstand mechanical challenges [27]. Thus, it is not surprising that cortical thickness was identified as a risk factor for forearm fractures in children and adolescents [28, 29]. Timing of maturity may also play a role as later menarche was associated with thinner cortices in young adult women [30]. These cross-sectional reports have not been corroborated using prospective data. Thus, longitudinal studies are needed to better characterize changes in cortical bone structure at clinically relevant sites such as the distal radius, and to determine how these changes relate to timing of key maturational events.

At *diaphyseal or shaft sites of long bones*, resistance to the dominant bending and torsional forces is primarily a function of the distribution and material stiffness of cortical bone [2]. Thus, growth-related gains in bone strength at shaft sites are due, in large part, to increases in bone size resulting from periosteal apposition. This was evident in the early radiographic studies of the second metacarpal by Stanley

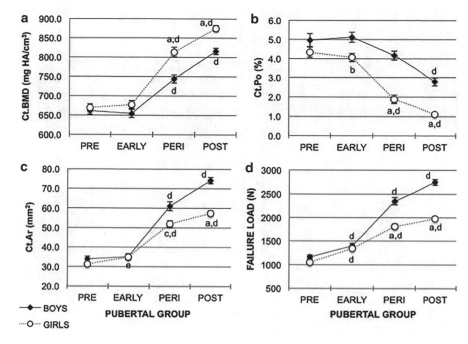

**Fig. 11.1** Plots of cortical bone mineral density (Ct.BMD; (**a**), cortical porosity (Ct.Po; **b**), cortical area (Ct.Ar; **c**), and failure load (**d**) measured at the distal radius with high-resolution peripheral quantitative computed tomography (HR-pQCT) in pre, early, peri, and postpubertal girls and boys. Error bars represent the standard error. (a) $p < 0.001$; (b) $p < 0.01$; (c) $p < 0.05$: significant difference between girls and boys within the same pubertal group. (d) $p < 0.001$; (e) $p < 0.01$; significant difference between pubertal group and the prepubertal group within sex. All $p$ values are after Bonferroni correction. Reproduced from Nishiyama et al. [11] with permission from John Wiley and Sons

Garn and colleagues [31, 32]. Periosteal apposition rates (predicted from cross-sectional data) mirrored the trajectory of linear growth, and were greater in boys compared with girls. In a recent 12-year mixed longitudinal study, periosteal apposition (represented by an increase in total bone cross-sectional area by pQCT) at the tibial shaft was greater in boys compared with girls both pre- and post-age at PHV (Fig. 11.2) [16]. Similar findings were also observed over a shorter timeframe across all maturity groups (early, peri, and postpubertal) [15]. Importantly, these data show that boys' bone size advantage may be apparent as early as prepuberty [12–14, 33]. However, the precise timing of bone strength accrual likely varies by skeletal site [34] and may be influenced by mechanical loads in combination with key hormones such as estrogen, testosterone, and growth hormone [35–37].

Notably, the positive exponential relationship between growth in bone width and bone bending strength serves to offset the inverse relationship between bone length and bone strength (Fig. 11.3). Growth in bone length occurs via endochondral ossification at the growth plate and without periosteal expansion slender bones are at an

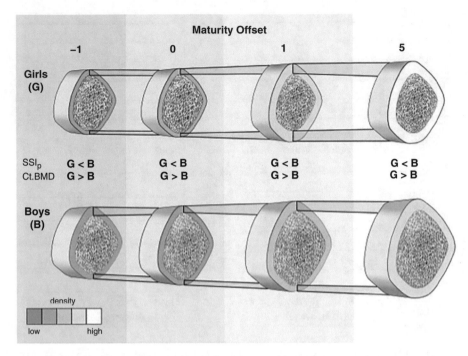

**Fig. 11.2** A schematic representation of differences in total area (Tt.Ar), medullary area (Me.Ar), cortical area (Ct.Ar), and cortical bone mineral density (Ct.BMD) in boys and girls in relation to maturity offset at −1, 0, 1, and 5 years (from age at peak height velocity). Significant differences between girls and boys are shown for strength-strain index (SSI$_p$), where boys' values exceeded girls' at all time points, and Ct.BMD, where girls' values exceeded boys' at all time points. (Diagram not exact scale). Reproduced from Gabel et al. [16] with permission from John Wiley and Sons

increased risk of fracture [38]. The apparent synchrony between increased bone width (total cross-sectional area) and bone length was illustrated in a 7-year longitudinal study of adolescent girls that used pQCT to assess the tibial shaft [39]. The growth trajectories of bone area and length were similar and both peaked approximately 20 months prior to menarche. This concerted growth may be necessary to avoid potential biomechanical challenges during periods of peak linear growth. Further study is needed to understand the mechanisms underlying this phenomenon and to determine if this relationship is also apparent in boys.

Whereas sex differences in magnitude and duration of periosteal apposition are the driving force behind boys' bone strength advantage at diaphyseal sites, adaptations on the endosteal surface must also be considered. The early work of Garn and colleagues indicated that girls might experience a greater degree of endosteal bone formation as a result of the pubertal surge in estrogen. A narrower marrow cavity and thicker cortex would in turn provide a calcium reservoir for later reproductive needs. However, some more recent studies that used QCT to revisit these surface-specific changes found something different. Whereas some studies supported Garn's

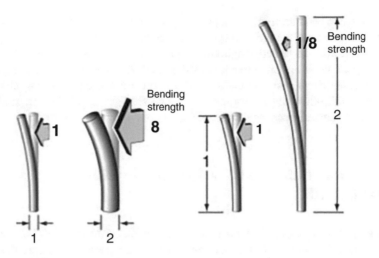

**Fig. 11.3** Illustration of the opposite effects of increases in bone width and bone length on bone bending strength. The two rods on the left have the same length, but the larger rod has twice the diameter of the thinner rod; therefore, bone bending strength is eight times greater in the larger rod. The two rods on the right have the same diameter, but a doubling of the rod length decreases bone strength to one eighth of the original value. Reproduced from Rauch [38] with permission

theory [14, 39, 40], others observed increased area of the marrow cavity, a surrogate for endosteal resorption, in *both* boys and girls [33, 34, 41]. For example, across 12-years of adolescent growth, medullary area at the tibial shaft (by pQCT) increased in boys and girls both pre- and post-PHV suggesting net endosteal bone resorption in both sexes [16] (Fig. 11.2). It is likely that discrepancies across studies represent a combination of differences in skeletal sites assessed, imaging modalities used, and study design.

Compared with the magnitude of the surface-specific changes that occur during growth, changes in cortical BMD are considerably smaller. In fact, earlier studies that used QCT to assess the mid-femur [42] and the radial shaft [43] reported that cortical BMD remained constant in girls aged 6–15 years. In contrast, results from cross-sectional studies that used pQCT suggest that at the tibial midshaft, cortical BMD is greater in girls compared with boys as early as prepuberty [13] and this sex difference may be more pronounced in the later stages of puberty [14]. Further, more recent evidence from longitudinal studies suggests that gains in cortical BMD (by pQCT at the tibial shaft) occur in both girls [39, 44] and boys [44] during puberty, although to a greater extent in girls (2–4 % over 20-months in girls versus 1 % in peri-pubertal boys). This provides further support for the hypothesis that in the female skeleton, consolidation of cortical bone during puberty provides calcium stores for later reproductive needs. Increased cortical density in girls may also serve to offset the bone strength disadvantage conferred to boys through their larger bone size, on average.

We have learned a great deal from studies that utilized QCT, pQCT, or HR-pQCT to evaluate the growing skeleton. However, the field is relatively young and numerous questions related to the trajectory of bone strength accrual in boys and girls have yet to be answered. An important gap in knowledge relates to the implications of these sex and maturation specific differences for short-term and long-term fracture risk. Well-designed longitudinal studies would serve to clarify the tempo and timing of gains in bone strength at different skeletal sites in boys and girls. In addition, researchers and clinicians must account for the confounding effects of maturation and other key determinants of bone strength acquisition in studies of childhood chronic disease, as discussed below.

# What Factors Influence Bone Strength Acquisition During Growth?

Although genetics largely determines our skeletal blueprint [45–49], bone accrual during growth is controlled by functional requirements needed to ensure that bone maintains its mechanical integrity. Conceptually, Rauch and Schoenau's functional model of bone development [50] is based on Harold Frost's mechanostat theory [51]. This model purports that increased bone length and muscle force are two major "challenges" that contribute to bone's integrity during growth. The model suggests that factors such as hormones, nutrition, and physical activity influence bone development through *direct* effects on the mechanostat strain setpoint or through *indirect* effects on longitudinal bone growth and muscle force [50]. A comprehensive review of determinants of bone strength accrual is beyond the scope of this chapter and we direct the reader to other excellent reviews of this area [52, 53]. Below, we focus on those factors that have been most frequently assessed in QCT-based studies in recent years.

## *Muscle*

During growth, muscle forces generated during muscular contractions impose the largest loads on the skeleton. This results from muscle continuously working against unfavorable lever arms [51, 54]. In turn, bone must adapt its mass, structure, and ultimately, its strength, to maintain its mechanical competence. The first study that used pQCT to assess bone, noted a strong association between grip strength and distal radius bone area and strength (BSI) in healthy children [55]. Since then numerous cross-sectional [13, 14, 56–60] and prospective studies [15, 39, 61, 62] have investigated the muscle-bone relationship at various skeletal sites using QCT-based imaging. Across these studies, muscle CSA (by pQCT) and lean body mass (excluding BMC, by DXA) were commonly used surrogates of muscle force and were more closely related to bone macrostructure (e.g., total and cortical bone area) and estimates of bone strength, than was BMD.

Should muscle be the primary driver of bone development, gains in muscle force (or a surrogate) during growth would peak prior to the peak for gains in bone strength. This timing differential between muscle and bone was nicely illustrated using cross sectional DXA and hip structure analysis data from the Saskatchewan Pediatric Bone Mineral Accrual Study cohort [63]. However, the only longitudinal study to examine the timing of the muscle-bone relationship (using pQCT) observed something quite different. Growth velocity of muscle CSA (a surrogate of muscle force) peaked 1–8 months earlier than did total BMC and cortical BMD at the tibial shaft. Importantly, this peak was 1 year after the peak in tibial length and total bone CSA in adolescent girls [39]. This suggests a potential differential influence of muscle on specific parameters of bone development. That is, growth in bone size may be less dependent on muscle force whereas bone mineral accrual may be highly dependent on muscle.

There are muscle properties beyond what imaging can assess that likely also play a role. Muscle CSA (by pQCT), as a surrogate of muscle force, may not adequately represent factors such as fiber type and pennation angle that contribute to muscle's force producing capacity during growth and thus, may not accurately define the loads to which bone is subjected to [58, 64]. In addition, chronic diseases may impact muscle quality, as we describe below. Functional measures of muscle force and power such as those obtained with jumping mechanography or dynamometry should be considered in future studies that aim to assess the muscle-bone relationship.

## *Nutrition*

Intake of total energy as well as specific nutrients such as protein and calcium is essential for optimal musculoskeletal development. These nutritional factors act indirectly on the theoretical mechanostat through their influence on key hormones such as growth hormone (GH) and IGF-1 [53]. However, due to its permissive nature, nutrition likely has the most profound influence on the mechanostat when there is a nutrient deficit. To date, no supplementation trial has investigated the effect of calcium alone on BMD, bone structure, or bone strength. However, there is some evidence to suggest that calcium combined with vitamin D may enhance trabecular BMD at metaphyseal sites in adolescent girls [65, 66].

Similar to calcium, there is insufficient evidence to support beneficial effects of vitamin D supplementation alone on bone structure and strength in the growing skeleton [67]. However, the widespread prevalence of vitamin D deficiency among US children and adolescents [68, 69] may be of particular concern for musculoskeletal health. Vitamin D deficiency may negatively affect bone mass accrual [70] and may also lead to myopathy and subsequent reduced skeletal loading [71]. In the only randomized controlled trial to examine the influence of vitamin D alone, 12-months of supplementation (four doses of 150,000 IU) in postmenarcheal girls did not lead to better bone geometry or strength at distal and shaft sites of the tibia compared with the placebo group, despite improved serum vitamin D levels [71]. We do not yet know whether vitamin D supplementation may benefit bone strength accrual in the less mature skeleton or in children who are vitamin D deficient or insufficient.

## Adiposity

We live in an era that has experienced a dramatic rise in childhood overweight and obesity; from 5 % in the 1960s to 32 % in the 1990s [72]. A 33 % higher risk of forearm fracture in overweight children compared with their healthy weight peers has also been documented [73]. Not surprisingly, there is great interest in better understanding the influence of excess fat mass on children's bone health. However, current studies are conflicting as to whether fat mass benefits or hinders bone accrual. This is likely due to, in part, the reliance on DXA-based studies of BMC and aBMD. Findings are also murky, as these studies did not account for the influence of muscle force when examining the fat-bone relationship.

In the context of mechanostat theory, fat mass represents a static load on the skeleton and as such will not directly influence bone strength [74]. However, overweight/obese children have greater muscle mass for height compared with their normal weight peers, seemingly, to compensate for the increased work needed to move around a greater body mass [75]. In turn, overweight children and adolescents are conferred greater absolute bone strength, adapted to their greater muscle mass, but not to their greater fat mass [62, 74]. This has been highlighted in several cross-sectional QCT-based studies in which positive associations between fat mass and BMD, bone (micro/macro) structure, or bone strength became either nonsignificant [76] or negative [77–79] after adjusting for surrogates of muscle force. Similarly, in a recent pQCT study, bone strength (section modulus) at the tibial shaft was significantly greater in obese (BMI > 97th percentile) adolescents compared with their normal weight peers (BMI ≤ 85th percentile), but when the greater muscle CSA, advanced maturation, and lower levels of physical activity of the obese adolescents were accounted for the bone strength advantage was no longer apparent [80]. The strong relation between muscle and bone is also evident in longitudinal studies: increases in tibial bone strength (by pQCT) during growth were closely tied to change in muscle CSA, and not fat mass, in girls and boys [62]. Thus, in overweight children the question becomes whether in the event of a fall, bones have sufficient strength to withstand the higher load associated with greater fat mass.

While absolute measures of body fat provide an indication of weight status, there is increasing interest in the influence of *regional* distribution of fat mass on bone health. In particular, fat within skeletal muscle and visceral adipose tissue may be considered pathogenic fat depots with negative implications for bone health. In young girls (9–12 years), higher skeletal muscle fat content (muscle density of the calf and thigh) was inversely associated with 2-year changes in tibial bone strength and BMD (by pQCT) [81]. These associations were independent of other factors that included muscle size, limb length, and maturity. Similarly, visceral adipose tissue was a negative predictor of QCT-derived mid-femur total and cortical bone area and moments of inertia in young women (15–25 years) [82], and abdominal fat (measured with DXA from the pelvis to the base of the skull) was negatively associated with 2-year change in cortical BMD at the tibial shaft in young girls (8–13 years) [83]. Although mechanisms that drive these relationships are unclear, the potentially harmful effects of excess visceral fat on BMD may be mediated by adipokines and pro-inflammatory cytokines [84]. The distribution of body fat changes with advancing maturity and differs between boys and girls [85]. As few studies address this, we perceive a need and an opportunity to further explore these relationships in longitudinal studies.

## *Physical Activity*

Physical activity plays a central role to ensure optimal bone accrual during growth. Evidence to support this is irrefutable and the osteogenic effect of weight-bearing exercise in children and adolescents is summarized in several excellent reviews [86–91]. In particular, pre- and peri-puberty may be the most opportune time for girls and boys to reap the skeletal benefits of physical activity. Exercise-related gains in bone strength in pre- and peri-pubertal children are most often due to adaptations in bone structure (e.g., increases in cortical thickness) rather than bone mass [90]. We know less about bone structural adaptations to exercise in older adolescents, and in light of the well-documented decline in physical activity in this age group [92] future studies that target this population would be invaluable.

Moving forward, researchers might more closely consider the potentially deleterious and independent effects of sedentary behavior on bone strength development. Today's youth spend as much as 60 % of their waking hours being sedentary while they sit in school, watch TV, or play computer games [93]. The potential consequences of "not loading" the growing human skeleton are not well documented as few studies investigated this relationship [57, 94–96]. Only one study of children that evaluated this relationship used QCT-based imaging [57]. Sedentary time (by self-report questionnaire and accelerometry) was not a significant predictor of tibial bone strength, BMD or macro/micro-structure (by HR-pQCT) in adolescent and young adult males and females. However, levels of physical activity were relatively high in this population. Further study would help to clarify and differentiate between the influence of physical activity versus sedentary behavior on bone, and whether these roles interrelate. For example, is there a threshold for sedentariness above which the consequences to growing bone are more detrimental? We also need to clarify how these complex relationships vary across skeletal sites and levels of maturity.

## Is Compromised Bone Strength a Risk Factor for Pediatric Fractures?

As noted in Chap. 1, prevention of pediatric fractures is of great importance particularly given the continued rise in the incidence of distal forearm fractures [97]. Although we currently have insufficient evidence to support the use of QCT-based bone outcomes to predict fracture risk in children [98], deficits in bone strength have been associated with fractures in children in several case-control studies [28, 29, 99]. Compromised bone quality in both the cortical and trabecular compartments may underpin lower bone strength in children with fractures, as smaller bone cross-sectional area [28, 43, 99], lower total and cortical BMD [29, 99, 100], thinner and more porous cortices [28, 29, 101] as well as fewer and thinner trabecule [29, 101] have all been identified as potential risk factors for forearm fracture in otherwise healthy children and adolescents.

Many fractures sustained during growth occur during regular physical activity, but it appears that the etiology of distal forearm fractures during growth differs according to trauma type [28, 29]. Specifically, deficits in cortical and trabecular BMD and structure result in a weaker bone that is unable to sustain loads associated with low- or mild-energy fractures (e.g., a fall from standing height) whereas fractures due to moderate energy trauma (e.g., fall from a bicycle) appear to occur in the context of normal or healthy bone strength (Fig. 11.4). However, recent evidence suggests that in boys, others modifiable factors may also come into play [29]. Poor balance, low levels of physical activity and excess body fat may all contribute to greater forearm fracture risk in young boys [29]. Prospective studies are needed to

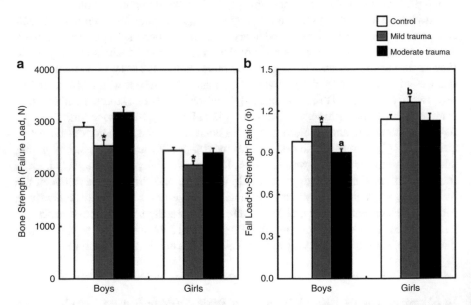

Fig. 11.4 (a) Bone strength (failure load [N, newtons]) and (b) fall load-to-strength ratio (factor of risk [Φ]) of the distal radius as measured with HR-pQCT in nonfracture controls and boys and girls with a history of either a mild- or moderate-trauma distal forearm fracture. The load-to-strength ratio is calculated as the ratio of the estimated load applied to the outstretched hand during a fall from standing height to failure load derived from finite element analysis of the HR-pQCT scan. Bars represent mean ± SE adjusted for bone age. *$p < 0.05$; (a) $p = 0.075$; (b) $p = 0.060$ compared with the respective nonfracture control group, using Dunnett adjustment for multiple comparisons. Reproduced from Farr et al. [28] with permission from Elsevier

confirm these relationships and to better characterize the ability of pQCT and HR-pQCT to assess fracture risk during growth. In addition, as young adults with a history of fracture demonstrate lower BMD and bone strength compared with their peers who did not sustain a fracture [102–105], there is a need to determine whether risk factors for forearm fractures in girls and boys track across adolescence and into adulthood.

## How Do Childhood Chronic Disease and Medications Affect Bone Accrual?

Myriad childhood chronic diseases and their therapies pose threats to musculoskeletal development. The impact may be immediate, resulting in fragility fractures during childhood [106–109], or delayed, due to suboptimal peak bone mass and consequent fractures in adulthood [110, 111]. Improved survival among children with diseases such as malignancies and cystic fibrosis has turned our attention to the prevention and treatment of skeletal comorbidities. Common threats to bone development in children and adolescents across multiple chronic diseases are summarized in Table 4.1. Numerous DXA studies reported abnormal aBMD and BMC in these disorders; however, DXA-based imaging does not provide insight into discrete and site-specific alterations in trabecular and cortical BMD and cortical dimensions that is needed to understand the impact of each risk factor on bone strength and to identify therapeutic targets. To date, the majority of QCT studies in this area focused on children and adolescents with inflammatory disorders who were treated with glucocorticoids, and/or children with muscle deficits. We focus on these key risk factors in this section, and highlight lessons learned from QCT studies.

Glucocorticoids (GCs) are highly effective and widely prescribed for the treatment of numerous childhood diseases; however, they have adverse effects on osteoblast, osteocyte, osteoclast, and muscle cell metabolism. It is well established that administration of GCs results in significant reductions in bone formation due to decreased generation of osteoblasts, impaired osteoblast function, and decreased osteoblast lifespan [112, 113]. GCs also increase osteocyte apoptosis [113]. GC therapy results in an early and transient increase in bone resorption due to enhanced osteoclastogenesis and osteoclast survival, followed by decreased osteoclast differentiation and function [114]. The growing skeleton is uniquely vulnerable to the effects of GCs on bone formation. GC effects on osteocytes and muscle mass may further compromise bone formation through decreased biomechanical loading and impaired signal transduction.

Many prior DXA studies of children treated with GCs were confounded by (a) the negative effects of GCs and the underlying disease on growth, resulting in underestimates of aBMD for age [115], and (b) the impact of the underlying inflammatory disease on bone. Inflammatory cytokines, such as tumor necrosis factor (TNF)-α, have direct adverse effects on osteoblast and muscle cells that are strikingly similar to GC effects [116, 117], with one exception: TNF-α results in prolonged and *persistent* increases in bone resorption while prolonged GC result in decreased bone resorption [118]. While studies of GC- and inflammation-induced osteoporosis in adults have almost exclusively focused on trabecular bone, studies in children must consider the impact on cortical bone accrual. Based on preclinical data, one would hypothesize that GC therapy and inflammation in children and adolescents would result in decreased trabecular BMD and impaired periosteal expansion as a consequence of decreased bone formation, while inflammation would also result in increased endocortical dimensions due to accelerated endosteal resorption. A series of pQCT studies examined trabecular and cortical BMD, cortical structure, and muscle CSA in children and young adults treated with GCs in childhood for inflammatory diseases, including nephrotic syndrome [119–121], inflammatory bowel disease [115, 122–126], systemic lupus erythematosus [127], and juvenile idiopathic arthritis [128–131]. Table 11.1 summarizes associations between bone and muscle outcomes in these clinical populations.

Persistent inflammation and elevated cytokine levels characterize childhood diseases treated with chronic GC such as inflammatory bowel disease and juvenile idiopathic arthritis. In contrast, steroid sensitive nephrotic syndrome (SSNS) responds promptly and completely to GC therapy, and the nephrotic state is quiescent during high-dose therapy. Unfortunately, SSNS relapses in the majority of children when the GC dose is reduced, resulting in protracted and repeated courses of therapy. Although relapses are associated with transiently increased cytokines levels, these abnormalities promptly resolve with GC therapy and disease remission [132]. Therefore, SSNS serves as a clinical model, with minimal systemic inflammation, to examine the independent effects of GC on BMD and structure during growth.

In this clinical model, pQCT imaging in children and adolescents with SSNS demonstrated significantly lower trabecular BMD and higher cortical BMD at the distal and shaft sites of the tibia, respectively, compared with healthy children [121]. Further, bone formation and resorption biomarkers were significantly and inversely associated with cortical BMD in SSNS and controls and were significantly lower in the 34 SSNS participants taking GCs at the time of the study compared with controls. The authors attributed the elevated cortical BMD to lower bone formation and greater secondary mineralization [121], a hypothesis that was supported by findings from a longitudinal follow-up study [133]: greater GC dose, lesser increases in tibia length and lesser increases in cortical area were significantly and independently associated with greater increases in cortical BMD in SSNS. Subsequently, other studies confirmed an association between GC therapy and increased cortical BMD in children with other chronic diseases [125, 127, 134]. Of note, posteroanterior spine aBMD did not differ between SSNS participants and controls, likely due to the superimposed lower trabecular BMD in the vertebral body and higher cortical BMD in the cortical shell and spinous processes [121]. These data highlight the utility of pQCT to capture GC effects that are not evident with DXA.

The clinical model of SSNS also provides the opportunity to examine how the muscle-bone relationship is affected by chronic disease and GC therapy. Compared with their healthy peers, children with SSNS had elevated BMI and lower extremity

**Table 11.1** QCT studies in children and adolescents with chronic inflammatory diseases treated with glucocorticoids (GC)

| Author | Disease (n); measurement site, study design | Trabecular BMD | Cortical BMD | Cortical structure | Muscle CSA |
|---|---|---|---|---|---|
| Wetzsteon et al. [121] | SSNS (55): tibia pQCT, cross-sectional | Decreased | Increased | Increased periosteal circumference in association with increased muscle and fat area | Greater than reference participants, associated with GC-induced gains in fat CSA |
| Tsampalieros et al. [133] | SSNS (56): tibia pQCT, longitudinal | Decreased | Increased; positively associated with GC dose | Greater increases in tibia length were associated with decreases in periosteal circumference Z-scores | Greater than reference participants, associated with GC-induced gains in fat CSA |
| Dubner et al. [123] | Crohn's disease (78): tibia pQCT, longitudinal incident cohort | Decreased at diagnosis, improved partially during the first 6 months of therapy | Normal at diagnosis, increased with GC therapy | Increased endosteal circumference at diagnosis. endosteal circumference improved with therapy but periosteal circumference lagged | Decreased at diagnosis, improved partially with therapy |
| Tsampalieros et al. [124] | Crohn's disease (55): tibia pQCT, longitudinal incident cohort | Persistent deficits at 3–4 years despite little clinical disease activity | Decreased in association with improvements in cortical area | Periosteal circumference comparable to controls at 3–4 years; endosteal circumference remained increased | Persistent deficits at 3–4 years |

(continued)

**Table 11.1** (continued)

| Author | Disease (n); measurement site, study design | Trabecular BMD | Cortical BMD | Cortical structure | Muscle CSA |
|---|---|---|---|---|---|
| Werkstetter et al. [125] | Crohn's disease and ulcerative colitis (102); radius pQCT, longitudinal mixed incident/prevalent cohort | Decreased | Increased | Preserved cortical area adjusted for height. The lack of adjustment for age potentially resulted in the comparison of pubertal inflammatory bowel disease participants with prepubertal controls, masking cortical deficits | Decreased muscle CSA |
| Burnham et al. [129] | Juvenile idiopathic arthritis (JIA, 101): tibia pQCT, cross-sectional | Decreased | Increased | Decreased periosteal circumference in polyarticular JIA and spondyloarthritis | Decreased in polyarticular JIA and spondyloarthritis |
| Stagi et al. [127] | Systemic lupus erythematosus (56); radius pQCT, cross-sectional | Decreased; negatively associated with GC dose | Increased; positively associated with GC dose | Decreased cortical bone area; no information on periosteal or endosteal circumference provided. | No different from controls; negatively associated with GC dose |

fat CSA (by pQCT), consistent with GC effects. In turn, similar to overweight and obese healthy children, children with SSNS had greater muscle CSA [135], which was associated with greater periosteal circumference at the tibial shaft. However, when these relationships were explored in the follow-up study, gains in tibia length were associated with declines in periosteal circumference Z-scores in children treated with GC for SSNS. These data suggest that the greater muscle mass (secondary to greater fat mass) in children treated with GC for SSNS promoted bone accrual, but GCs prevented normal gains in periosteal circumference during linear growth. Although GCs are known to impair muscle mass and function, a subsequent analysis in these SSNS patients demonstrated normal muscle strength relative to muscle CSA, assessed using ankle dynamometry measures of peak torque relative to pQCT calf muscle CSA [136].

Crohn's disease (CD) is an autoimmune condition of the gastrointestinal tract characterized by chronic inflammation and defective innate immune regulation of the gut microbiome. TNF-α plays a pivotal role in CD pathogenesis and the majority of children are treated with GC at diagnosis. Findings from an incident cohort study of children and adolescents with CD indicate that deficits in trabecular BMD at the distal tibia and cortical CSA (due to greater endosteal circumference) and muscle CSA at the tibial shaft are apparent at diagnosis when compared with healthy children [123, 124]. Following initiation of CD therapy, trabecular BMD and muscle CSA improved in this incident cohort, but periosteal dimensions failed to expand commensurate with linear growth. Periosteal circumference was significantly lower than that of healthy children 6 and 12 months after initiation of therapy. Although the Pediatric Crohn Disease Activity Index score indicated minimal active disease in 85 % of participants 3–4 years after diagnosis, significant deficits in trabecular BMD, cortical CSA (due to marginally lower periosteal circumference and significantly greater endosteal circumference, Fig. 11.5) and muscle CSA persisted. Further, greater GC doses and disease activity scores were significantly and independently associated with failure to accrue cortical area relative to tibia length, and these adverse effects were more pronounced with greater linear growth. As detailed in Table 11.1, studies in juvenile idiopathic arthritis, inflammatory bowel disease (CD, and ulcerative colitis) and juvenile onset systemic lupus erythematosus demonstrated similar patterns, with decreased trabecular BMD, increased cortical BMD, decreased cortical dimensions, and decreased muscle CSA.

The potential to reverse GC-induced deficits during growth was illustrated in a recent longitudinal study of children and adolescents enrolled following completion of maintenance dexamethasone therapy for acute lymphoblastic leukemia [137]. Studies following completion of chemotherapy in children in remissions provide an excellent model for recovery since the underlying indication for the GC therapy no longer has an impact of bone health. The study demonstrated rapid increases in trabecular BMD and cortical area Z-scores; the increases were most pronounced during the early months off therapy. The dramatic cortical bone accrual was associated with transient reductions in cortical BMD (Fig. 11.6), potentially related to the time necessary to fully mineralize new bone.

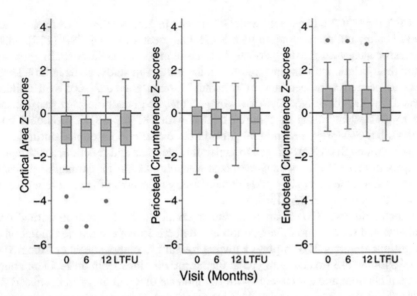

**Fig. 11.5** Cortical dimension Z-scores in children and adolescents with Crohn disease at diagnosis, 6 and 12 months after diagnosis, and the time of the long-term follow-up (LTFU) visit a median of 42 months after diagnosis. At diagnosis, cortical CSA was significantly reduced and endosteal circumference significantly increased, compared with reference participants. At the time of the final visit, these deficits were less pronounced but remained abnormal, compared with reference participants despite little clinical evidence of disease activity. Reproduced from Tsampalieros et al. [124] with permission from The Endocrine Society

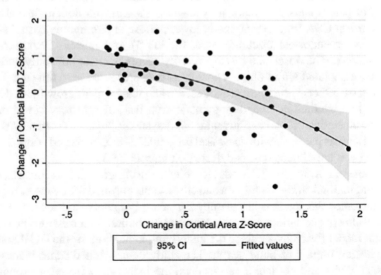

**Fig. 11.6** Change in cortical BMD Z-score is shown relative to the change in cortical CSA Z-score over a 1-year interval following completion of dexamethasone therapy for childhood acute lymphoblastic leukemia. Increases in cortical CSA Z-scores were significantly associated with declines in cortical BMD Z-scores, independent of the interval since completing therapy. Reproduced from Mostoufi-Moab et al. [139] with permission from the Endocrine Society

A consistent positive association between cortical bone and muscle CSA was evident in the cross-sectional studies summarized in Table 11.1. However, these relations may not be causal in nature; that is, the bone deficits may not be secondary to, or adapted to the muscle status. Rather, the underlying disease processes and treatments may have direct adverse effects on both bone and muscle development, as described above. For example, following initiation of therapy for CD, muscle CSA improved while periosteal circumference faltered [123]. Similarly, chronic kidney disease was associated with significant reductions in tibia cortical section modulus and calf muscle CSA; [134] however, following treatment with renal transplantation, muscle CSA (by pQCT), and muscle mass (by DXA) recovered completely while cortical bone CSA (by pQCT) and whole body BMC (by DXA) did not [115]. These patterns may be due to negative effects of GCs on bone accrual while treatment of the underlying disease may promote recovery of muscle. An alternative explanation is that both CD and chronic kidney disease result in abnormalities in muscle function that are not captured by pQCT or DXA measures [120, 136]. Finally, GCs and cytokine effects on osteocytes may disrupt the functional muscle bone unit.

Taken together, these studies suggest that both GCs and inflammation are associated with decreased trabecular BMD and periosteal circumference, consistent decreased bone formation. The increased endosteal circumference Z-scores in the incident CD cohort at diagnosis suggests that inflammation is associated with endocortical resorption secondary to inflammatory cytokines. Finally, the consistent observation of increased cortical BMD in multiple diseases treated with GCs (including renal transplantation [134]) suggests greater secondary bone mineralization in the setting of decreased new bone formation secondary to poor linear growth, decreased cortical modeling (due to less periosteal bone formation) and decreased intracortical remodeling. These deficits are largely reversible; however, persistent low-grade inflammation in chronic inflammatory diseases prohibits complete recovery of trabecular BMD and cortical area even when the disease is well controlled [124, 129].

Last, studies comparing DXA and pQCT results in childhood chronic diseases can be used to inform our interpretation of DXA results. For example, changes in lumbar spine aBMD Z-scores in pediatric kidney transplant recipients captured GC and parathyroid hormone effects that were also detected using pQCT measures of trabecular BMD [138]. Similarly, changes in DXA whole body BMC Z-scores were highly correlated with changes in cortical area Z-scores, but not cortical BMD Z-scores. This suggests that whole body BMC may provide an indication of the effects of GCs or chronic disease on cortical bone dimensions, but not on cortical BMD.

## Where Do We Go from Here?

It is clear that in the 8 years since the first edition of this book, we have accumulated a wealth of knowledge from QCT-based imaging studies of the pediatric skeleton. In moving beyond traditional 2D measures of bone mass we are gaining a better understanding of bone's complex structure and how sex- and maturity-related differences in BMD and bone macro- and microstructure influence bone strength during growth. We have also learned how childhood chronic diseases and their therapies impact discrete components of bone strength and have identified risk factors for impaired bone accrual. However, we still have a lot to learn. Additional longitudinal studies that utilize QCT-based imaging are needed to more accurately describe changes in BMD, bone structure, and strength across the critical period of adolescent growth and into young adulthood. Importantly, there are no longitudinal studies that relate QCT measures of bone strength to future fracture events in children and adolescents.

Before we embark on such investigations, however, we must first come to consensus on several important issues. First, we must develop standardized scan acquisition and analysis protocols [98]. Currently, protocols for reference line placement, measurement sites, and scan analysis vary widely across centers. Second, calibration differences within each modality (QCT, pQCT, and HR-pQCT) and between scanners at different sites have not been well characterized and are necessary before existing reference data can be used more broadly. Third, there is a need for prospective cohort studies in healthy children and children with chronic diseases in order to establish the short and long-term fracture implications of deficits in trabecular and cortical outcomes. Fourth, there is work to be done to describe relations between surrogate measures of bone strength (e.g. BSI and $SSI_p$) in healthy children and those with chronic diseases. Validation of these surrogate outcomes in childhood chronic diseases should guide randomized clinical trials to prevent and reverse these processes. For example, diseases characterized by decreased bone formation require anabolic interventions, while those characterized by excess resorption may benefit from anti-resorptive therapies or from biologic medications that target inflammatory cytokines. Last, additional studies comparing changes in QCT and DXA-based measures of BMC and aBMD should be used to aid the interpretation of DXA results in clinical practice and multicenter clinical trials.

## Summary Points

- QCT-based imaging permits evaluation of BMD, bone macro- and microstructure and bone strength in the growing skeleton.
- Adolescence is a critical period for bone strength acquisition, with boys demonstrating a bone strength advantage compared with girls as early as prepuberty.
- At distal sites of long bones, gains in trabecular bone volume during growth are more closely related to thickening of individual trabecular rather than an increase in the number of trabeculae, and rapid changes at the metaphyseal cortex may lead to a period of transient bone fragility during the period of peak linear growth.
- At shaft sites of long bones, boys experience more periosteal apposition than girls resulting in a larger bone size and greater bone bending strength.
- Gains in bone strength in boys and girls during growth are more closely tied to change in muscle mass, and not fat mass.

- Well-designed longitudinal studies that utilize QCT-based imaging are needed to accurately describe bone strength acquisition during adolescent growth and to relate these processes to short- and long-term fracture risk in healthy children and those with chronic disease.
- QCT-based studies have provided substantial insight into the impact of chronic diseases on skeletal modeling and the bone-muscle unit. Specific risk factors for abnormal trabecular and cortical BMD, and for cortical thinning on the periosteal and endosteal surface have been identified.
- Future randomized clinical trials are needed to prevent and treat bone deficits in childhood chronic diseases and QCT outcomes will serve as important surrogates for bone strength.

# References

1. Järvinen TL, Sievänen H, Jokihaara J, Einhorn TA. Revival of bone strength: the bottom line. J Bone Miner Res. 2005;20:717–20.
2. Einhorn TA. Bone strength: the bottom line. Calcif Tissue Int. 1992;51:333–9.
3. Manske S, Macdonald H, Nishiyama K, Boyd S, McKay H. Clinical tools to evaluate bone strength. Clinic Rev Bone Miner Metab. 2010;8:1–13.
4. Bouxsein ML. Determinants of skeletal fragility. Best Pract Res Clin Rheumatol. 2005;19:897–911.
5. Johnell O, Kanis JA, Oden A, Johansson H, De Laet C, Delmas P, et al. Predictive value of BMD for hip and other fractures. J Bone Miner Res. 2005;20:1185–94.
6. Bailey DA, McKay HA, Mirwald RL, Crocker PR, Faulkner RA. A six-year longitudinal study of the relationship of physical activity to bone mineral accrual in growing children: The University of Saskatchewan Bone Mineral Accrual Study. J Bone Miner Res. 1999;14:1672–9.
7. Lloyd T, Rollings N, Andon MB, Demers LM, Eggli DF, Kieselhorst K, et al. Determinants of bone density in young women. I. Relationships among pubertal development, total body bone mass, and total body bone density in premenarcheal females. J Clin Endocrinol Metab. 1992;75:383–7.
8. Mølgaard C, Thomsen BL, Michaelsen KF. Whole body bone mineral accretion in healthy children and adolescents. Arch Dis Child. 1999;81:10–5.
9. Theintz G, Buchs B, Rizzoli R, Slosman D, Clavien H, Sizonenko PC, et al. Longitudinal monitoring of bone mass accumulation in healthy adolescents: evidence for a marked reduction after 16 years of age at the levels of lumbar spine and femoral neck in female subjects. J Clin Endocrinol Metab. 1992;75:1060–5.
10. Kirmani S, Christen D, van Lenthe GH, Fischer PR, Bouxsein ML, Mccready LK, et al. Bone structure at the distal radius during adolescent growth. J Bone Miner Res. 2009;24:1033–42.
11. Nishiyama KK, Macdonald HM, Moore SA, Fung T, Boyd SK, McKay HA. Cortical porosity is higher in boys compared with girls at the distal radius and distal tibia during pubertal growth: an HR-pQCT study. J Bone Miner Res. 2012;27:273–82.
12. Schoenau E, Neu CM, Rauch F, Manz F. The development of bone strength at the proximal radius during childhood and adolescence. J Clin Endocrinol Metab. 2001;86:613–8.
13. Macdonald H, Kontulainen S, Petit M, Janssen P, McKay H. Bone strength and its determinants in pre- and early pubertal boys and girls. Bone. 2006;39:598–608.
14. Leonard MB, Elmi A, Mostoufi-Moab S, Shults J, Burnham JM, Thayu M, et al. Effects of sex, race, and puberty on cortical bone and the functional muscle bone unit in children, adolescents, and young adults. J Clin Endocrinol Metab. 2010;95:1681–9.

15. Macdonald HM, Kontulainen SA, Mackelvie-O'Brien KJ, Petit MA, Janssen P, Khan KM, et al. Maturity- and sex-related changes in tibial bone geometry, strength and bone-muscle strength indices during growth: a 20-month pQCT study. Bone. 2005;36:1003–11.
16. Gabel L, Nettlefold L, Brasher PM, Moore S, Ahamed Y, Macdonald HM, et al. Re-examining the surfaces of bone in boys and girls during adolescent growth: a 12-year mixed longitudinal pQCT study. J Bone Miner Res 2015;30:2158–67.
17. Seeman E. Pathogenesis of bone fragility in women and men. Lancet. 2002;359:1841–50.
18. MacNeil JA, Boyd SK. Bone strength at the distal radius can be estimated from high-resolution peripheral quantitative computed tomography and the finite element method. Bone. 2008;42:1203–13.
19. Crawford RP, Cann CE, Keaveny TM. Finite element models predict in vitro vertebral body compressive strength better than quantitative computed tomography. Bone. 2003;33:744–50.
20. Martin R. Determinants of the mechanical properties of bones. J Biomech. 1991;24:79.
21. Neu CM, Manz F, Rauch F, Merkel A, Schoenau E. Bone densities and bone size at the distal radius in healthy children and adolescents: a study using peripheral quantitative computed tomography. Bone. 2001;28:227–32.
22. Wang Q, Wang X-F, Iuliano-Burns S, Ghasem-Zadeh A, Zebaze R, Seeman E. Rapid growth produces transient cortical weakness: a risk factor for metaphyseal fractures during puberty. J Bone Miner Res. 2010;25:1521–6.
23. Mora S, Goodman WG, Loro ML, Roe TF, Sayre J, Gilsanz V. Age-related changes in cortical and cancellous vertebral bone density in girls: assessment with quantitative CT. Am J Roentgenol. 1994;162:405–9.
24. Loro ML, Sayre J, Roe TF, Goran MI, Kaufman FR, Gilsanz V. Early identification of children predisposed to low peak bone mass and osteoporosis later in life. J Clin Endocrinol Metab. 2000;85:3908–18.
25. Augat P, Schorlemmer S. The role of cortical bone and its microstructure in bone strength. Age Ageing. 2006;35 Suppl 2:ii27–31.
26. Parfitt AM. The two faces of growth: benefits and risks to bone integrity. Osteoporosis Int. 1994;4:382–98.
27. Rauch F, Neu C, Manz F, Schoenau E. The development of metaphyseal cortex—implications for distal radius fractures during growth. J Bone Miner Res. 2001;16:1547–55.
28. Farr JN, Amin S, Melton LJ, Kirmani S, Mccready LK, Atkinson EJ, et al. Bone strength and structural deficits in children and adolescents with a distal forearm fracture resulting from mild trauma. J Bone Miner Res. 2014;29:590–9.
29. Määttä M, Macdonald HM, Mulpuri K, McKay HA. Deficits in distal radius bone strength, density and microstructure are associated with forearm fractures in girls: an HR-pQCT study. Osteoporosis Int. 2015;26:1163–74.
30. Chevalley T, Bonjour J-P, Ferrari S, Rizzoli R. Deleterious effect of late menarche on distal tibia microstructure in healthy 20-year-old and premenopausal middle-aged women. J Bone Miner Res. 2009;24:144–52.
31. Garn SM, Frisancho AR, Sandusky ST, McCann MB. Confirmation of the sex difference in continuing subperiosteal apposition. Am J Phys Anthropol. 1972;36:377–80.
32. Frisancho AR, Garn SM, Ascoli W. Subperiosteal and endosteal bone apposition during adolescence. Hum Biol. 1970;42:639–64.
33. Neu CM, Rauch F, Manz F, Schoenau E. Modeling of cross-sectional bone size, mass and geometry at the proximal radius: a study of normal bone development using peripheral quantitative computed tomography. Osteoporosis Int. 2001;12:538–47.
34. Gilsanz V, Kovanlikaya A, Costin G, Roe TF, Sayre J, Kaufman F. Differential effect of gender on the sizes of the bones in the axial and appendicular skeletons. J Clin Endocrinol Metab. 1997;82:1603–7.
35. Rauch F. Bone accrual in children: adding substance to surfaces. Pediatrics. 2007;119 Suppl 2:S137–40.
36. Kim B-T, Mosekilde L, Duan Y, Zhang X-Z, Tornvig L, Thomsen JS, et al. The structural and hormonal basis of sex differences in peak appendicular bone strength in rats. J Bone Miner Res. 2003;18:150–5.

37. Seeman E. Periosteal bone formation—a neglected determinant of bone strength. N Engl J Med. 2003;349:320–3.
38. Rauch F. Bone growth in length and width: the Yin and Yang of bone stability. J Musculoskelet Neuronal Interact. 2005;5:194–201.
39. Xu L, Nicholson P, Wang Q, Alen M, Cheng S. Bone and muscle development during puberty in girls: a seven-year longitudinal study. J Bone Miner Res. 2009;24:1693–8.
40. Wang Q, Alén M, Nicholson P, Lyytikäinen A, Suuriniemi M, Helkala E, et al. Growth patterns at distal radius and tibial shaft in pubertal girls: a 2-year longitudinal study. J Bone Miner Res. 2005;20:954–61.
41. Kontulainen SA, Macdonald HM, Khan KM, McKay HA. Examining bone surfaces across puberty: a 20-month pQCT trial. J Bone Miner Res. 2005;20:1202–7.
42. Gilsanz V, Skaggs DL, Kovanlikaya A, Sayre J, Loro ML, Kaufman F, et al. Differential effect of race on the axial and appendicular skeletons of children. J Clin Endocrinol Metab. 1998;83:1420–7.
43. Skaggs DL, Loro ML, Pitukcheewanont P, Tolo V, Gilsanz V. Increased body weight and decreased radial cross-sectional dimensions in girls with forearm fractures. J Bone Miner Res. 2001;16:1337–42.
44. Kontulainen SA, Macdonald HM, McKay HA. Change in cortical bone density and its distribution differs between boys and girls during puberty. J Clin Endocrinol Metab. 2006;91:2555–61.
45. Pocock NA, Eisman JA, Hopper JL, Yeates MG, Sambrook PN, Eberl S. Genetic determinants of bone mass in adults. A twin study. J Clin Invest. 1987;80:706–10.
46. Wang X, Kammerer CM, Wheeler VW, Patrick AL, Bunker CH, Zmuda JM. Pleiotropy and heterogeneity in the expression of bone strength-related phenotypes in extended pedigrees. J Bone Miner Res. 2007;22:1766–72.
47. Havill LM, Mahaney MC, Binkley LT, Specker BL. Effects of genes, sex, age, and activity on BMC, bone size, and areal and volumetric BMD. J Bone Miner Res. 2007;22:737–46.
48. Xu X-H, Dong S-S, Guo Y, Yang T-L, Lei S-F, Papasian CJ, et al. Molecular genetic studies of gene identification for osteoporosis: the 2009 update. Endocr Rev. 2010;31:447–505.
49. Ralston SH. Genetics of osteoporosis. Ann N Y Acad Sci. 2010;1192:181–9.
50. Rauch F, Schoenau E. The developing bone: slave or master of its cells and molecules? Pediatr Res. 2001;50:309–14.
51. Frost HM. Bone "mass" and the "mechanostat": a proposal. Anat Rec. 1987;219:1–9.
52. Macdonald HM, Hoy CL, McKay HA. Bone acquisition in adolescence. In: Marcus R, Feldman D, Dempster DW, Luckey M, Cauley JA, editors. Osteoporosis. 4th ed. San Diego, CA: Academic; 2013.
53. Bass SL, Eser P, Daly R. The effect of exercise and nutrition on the mechanostat. J Musculoskelet Neuronal Interact. 2005;5:239–54.
54. Burr DB. Muscle strength, bone mass, and age-related bone loss. J Bone Miner Res. 1997;12:1547–51.
55. Schönau E. The development of the skeletal system in children and the influence of muscular strength. Horm Res. 1998;49:27–31.
56. Schoenau E, Neu CM, Beck B, Manz F, Rauch F. Bone mineral content per muscle cross-sectional area as an index of the functional muscle-bone unit. J Bone Miner Res. 2002;17:1095–101.
57. Gabel L, McKay HA, Nettlefold L, Race D, Macdonald HM. Bone architecture and strength in the growing skeleton: the role of sedentary time. Med Sci Sports Exerc. 2014;47:363–72.
58. Wetzsteon RJ, Zemel BS, Shults J, Howard KM, Kibe LW, Leonard MB. Mechanical loads and cortical bone geometry in healthy children and young adults. Bone. 2011;48:1103–8.
59. Ashby RL, Adams JE, Roberts SA, Mughal MZ, Ward KA. The muscle-bone unit of peripheral and central skeletal sites in children and young adults. Osteoporosis Int. 2011;22:121–32.
60. Binkley TL, Specker BL. Muscle-bone relationships in the lower leg of healthy pre-pubertal females and males. J Musculoskelet Neuronal Interact. 2008;8:239–43.
61. Farr JN, Laddu DR, Blew RM, Lee VR, Going SB. Effects of physical activity and muscle quality on bone development in girls. Med Sci Sports Exerc. 2013;45:2332–40.

62. Wetzsteon RJ, Petit MA, Macdonald HM, Hughes JM, Beck TJ, McKay HA. Bone struc-ture and volumetric BMD in overweight children: a longitudinal study. J Bone Miner Res. 2008;23:1946–53.
63. Jackowski SA, Faulkner RA, Farthing JP, Kontulainen SA, Beck TJ, Baxter-Jones ADG. Peak lean tissue mass accrual precedes changes in bone strength indices at the proximal femur during the pubertal growth spurt. Bone. 2009;44:1186–90.
64. Daly RM, Stenevi-Lundgren S, Linden C, Karlsson MK. Muscle determinants of bone mass, geometry and strength in prepubertal girls. Med Sci Sports Exerc. 2008;40:1135–41.
65. Greene DA, Naughton GA. Calcium and vitamin-D supplementation on bone structural prop-erties in peripubertal female identical twins: a randomised controlled trial. Osteoporos Int. 2011;22:489–98.
66. Moyer-Mileur LJ, Xie B, Ball SD, Pratt T. Bone mass and density response to a 12-month trial of calcium and vitamin D supplement in preadolescent girls. J Musculoskelet Neuronal Interact. 2003;3:63–70.
67. Moon RJ, Harvey NC, Davies JH, Cooper C. Vitamin D and skeletal health in infancy and childhood. Osteoporosis Int. 2014;25:2673–84.
68. Mansbach JM, Ginde AA, Camargo CA. Serum 25-hydroxyvitamin D levels among US chil-dren aged 1 to 11 years: do children need more vitamin D? Pediatrics. 2009;124:1404–10.
69. Ginde AA, Liu MC, Camargo CA. Demographic differences and trends of vitamin D insuf-ficiency in the US population, 1988-2004. Arch Intern Med. 2009;169:626–32.
70. Lehtonen-Veromaa MKM, Möttönen TT, Nuotio IO, Irjala KMA, Leino AE, Viikari JSA. Vitamin D and attainment of peak bone mass among peripubertal Finnish girls: a 3-y prospective study. Am J Clin Nutr. 2002;76:1446–53.
71. Ward KA, Das G, Roberts SA, Berry JL, Adams JE, Rawer R, et al. A randomized, controlled trial of vitamin D supplementation upon musculoskeletal health in postmenarchal females. J Clin Endocrinol Metab. 2010;95:4643–51.
72. Ogden CL, Carroll MD, Kit BK, Flegal KM. Prevalence of childhood and adult obesity in the United States, 2011-2012. JAMA. 2014;311:806–14.
73. Goulding A, Taylor RW, Jones IE, McAuley KA, Manning PJ, Williams SM. Overweight and obese children have low bone mass and area for their weight. Int J Obes Relat Metab Disord. 2000;24:627–32.
74. Petit MA, Beck TJ, Shults J, Zemel BS, Foster BJ, Leonard MB. Proximal femur bone geom-etry is appropriately adapted to lean mass in overweight children and adolescents. Bone. 2005;36:568–76.
75. Leonard MB, Shults J, Wilson BA, Tershakovec AM, Zemel BS. Obesity during child-hood and adolescence augments bone mass and bone dimensions. Am J Clin Nutr. 2004;80:514–23.
76. Hoy CL, Macdonald HM, McKay HA. How does bone quality differ between healthy-weight and overweight adolescents and young adults? Clin Orthop Relat Res. 2013;471:1214–25.
77. Ducher G, Bass SL, Naughton GA, Eser P, Telford RD, Daly RM. Overweight children have a greater proportion of fat mass relative to muscle mass in the upper limbs than in the lower limbs: implications for bone strength at the distal forearm. Am J Clin Nutr. 2009;90:1104–11.
78. Farr JN, Chen Z, Lisse JR, Lohman TG, Going SB. Relationship of total body fat mass to weight-bearing bone volumetric density, geometry, and strength in young girls. Bone. 2010;46:977–84.
79. Fricke O, Sumnik Z, Tutlewski B, Stabrey A, Remer T, Schoenau E. Local body composition is associated with gender differences of bone development at the forearm in puberty. Horm Res. 2008;70:105–11.
80. Leonard MB, Zemel BS, Wrotniak BH, Klieger SB, Shults J, Stallings VA, et al. Tibia and radius bone geometry and volumetric density in obese compared to non-obese adolescents. Bone. 2014;73:69–76.

81. Laddu DR, Farr JN, Lee VR, Blew RM, Stump C, Houtkooper L, et al. Muscle density predicts changes in bone density and strength: a prospective study in girls. J Musculoskelet Neuronal Interact. 2014;14:195–204.
82. Gilsanz V, Chalfant J, Mo AO, Lee DC, Dorey FJ, Mittelman SD. Reciprocal relations of subcutaneous and visceral fat to bone structure and strength. J Clin Endocrinol Metab. 2009;94:3387–93.
83. Laddu DR, Farr JN, Laudermilk MJ, Lee VR, Blew RM, Stump C, et al. Longitudinal relationships between whole body and central adiposity on weight-bearing bone geometry, density, and bone strength: a pQCT study in young girls. Arch Osteoporos. 2013;8:156.
84. Russell M, Mendes N, Miller KK, Rosen CJ, Lee H, Klibanski A, et al. Visceral fat is a negative predictor of bone density measures in obese adolescent girls. J Clin Endocrinol Metab. 2010;95:1247–55.
85. Zemel BS. Quantitative computed tomography and computed tomography in children. Curr Osteoporos Rep. 2011;9:284–90.
86. McKay H, Smith E. Winning the battle against childhood physical inactivity: the key to bone strength? J Bone Miner Res. 2008;23:980–5.
87. Hind K, Burrows M. Weight-bearing exercise and bone mineral accrual in children and adolescents: a review of controlled trials. Bone. 2007;40:14–27.
88. Gunter KB, Almstedt HC, Janz KF. Physical activity in childhood may be the key to optimizing lifespan skeletal health. Exerc Sport Sci Rev. 2012;40:13–21.
89. Nikander R, Sievänen H, Heinonen A, Daly RM, Uusi-Rasi K, Kannus P. Targeted exercise against osteoporosis: a systematic review and meta-analysis for optimising bone strength throughout life. BMC Med. 2010;8:47.
90. Tan VPS, Macdonald HM, Kim S, Nettlefold L, Gabel L, Ashe MC, et al. Influence of physical activity on bone strength in children and adolescents: a systematic review and narrative synthesis. J Bone Miner Res. 2014;29:2161–81.
91. Burt LA, Ducher G, Naughton GA, Courteix D, Greene DA. Gymnastics participation is associated with skeletal benefits in the distal forearm: a 6-month study using peripheral Quantitative Computed Tomography. J Musculoskelet Neuronal Interact. 2013;13:395–404.
92. Dumith SC, Gigante DP, Domingues MR, Kohl HW. Physical activity change during adolescence: a systematic review and a pooled analysis. Int J Epidemiol. 2011;40:685–98.
93. Colley RC, Garriguet D, Janssen I, Craig CL, Clarke J, Tremblay MS. Physical activity of Canadian children and youth: accelerometer results from the 2007 to 2009 Canadian Health Measures Survey. Health Rep. 2011;22:15–23.
94. Chastin SF, Mandrichenko O, Skelton DA. The frequency of osteogenic activities and the pattern of intermittence between periods of physical activity and sedentary behaviour affects bone mineral content: the cross-sectional NHANES study. BMC Public Health. 2014;14:4.
95. Vicente-Rodriguez G, Ortega FB, Rey-López JP, España-Romero V, Blay VA, Blay G, et al. Extracurricular physical activity participation modifies the association between high TV watching and low bone mass. Bone. 2009;45:925–30.
96. Gracia-Marco L, Rey-López JP, Santaliestra-Pasías AM, Jiménez-Pavón D, Díaz LE, Moreno LA, et al. Sedentary behaviours and its association with bone mass in adolescents: the HELENA cross-sectional study. BMC Public Health. 2012;12:971.
97. Khosla S, Melton LJ, Dekutoski MB, Achenbach SJ, Oberg AL, Riggs BL. Incidence of childhood distal forearm fractures over 30 years: a population-based study. JAMA. 2003;290:1479–85.
98. Adams JE, Engelke K, Zemel BS, Ward KA. Quantitative computer tomography in children and adolescents: the 2013 ISCD Pediatric Official Positions. J Clin Densitom. 2014;17:258–74.
99. Kalkwarf HJ, Laor T, Bean JA. Fracture risk in children with a forearm injury is associated with volumetric bone density and cortical area (by peripheral QCT) and areal bone density (by DXA). Osteoporosis Int. 2011;22:607–16.
100. Cheng S, Xu L, Nicholson PHF, Tylavsky F, Lyytikäinen A, Wang Q, et al. Low volumetric BMD is linked to upper-limb fracture in pubertal girls and persists into adulthood: a seven-year cohort study. Bone. 2009;45:480–6.

101. Bala Y, Bui QM, Wang X-F, Iuliano S, Wang Q, Ghasem-Zadeh A, et al. Trabecular and cortical microstructure and fragility of the distal radius in women. J Bone Miner Res. 2015;30:621–9.
102. Darelid A, Ohlsson C, Rudäng R, Kindblom JM, Mellström D, Lorentzon M. Trabecular volumetric bone mineral density is associated with previous fracture during childhood and adolescence in males: the GOOD study. J Bone Miner Res. 2010;25:537–44.
103. Farr JN, Khosla S, Achenbach SJ, Atkinson EJ, Kirmani S, Mccready LK, et al. Diminished bone strength is observed in adult women and men who sustained a mild trauma distal forearm fracture during childhood. J Bone Miner Res. 2014;29:2193–202.
104. Chevalley T, Bonjour JP, van Rietbergen B, Ferrari S, Rizzoli R. Fractures during childhood and adolescence in healthy boys: relation with bone mass, microstructure, and strength. J Clin Endocrinol Metab. 2011;96:3134–42.
105. Chevalley T, Bonjour JP, van Rietbergen B, Rizzoli R, Ferrari S. Fractures in healthy females followed from childhood to early adulthood are associated with later menarcheal age and with impaired bone microstructure at peak bone mass. J Clin Endocrinol Metab. 2012;97:4174–81.
106. Semeao EJ, Stallings VA, Peck SN, Piccoli DA. Vertebral compression fractures in pediatric patients with Crohn's disease. Gastroenterology. 1997;112:1710–3.
107. Halton J, Gaboury I, Grant R, Alos N, Cummings EA, Matzinger M, et al. Advanced vertebral fracture among newly diagnosed children with acute lymphoblastic leukemia: results of the Canadian Steroid-Associated Osteoporosis in the Pediatric Population (STOPP) research program. J Bone Miner Res. 2009;24:1326–34.
108. Rodd C, Lang B, Ramsay T, Alos N, Huber AM, Cabral DA, et al. Incident vertebral fractures among children with rheumatic disorders 12 months after glucocorticoid initiation: a national observational study. Arthritis Care Res. 2012;64:122–31.
109. Helenius I, Remes V, Salminen S, Valta H, Mäkitie O, Holmberg C, et al. Incidence and predictors of fractures in children after solid organ transplantation: a 5-year prospective, population-based study. J Bone Miner Res. 2006;21:380–7.
110. Burnham JM, Shults J, Weinstein R, Lewis JD, Leonard MB. Childhood onset arthritis is associated with an increased risk of fracture: a population based study using the General Practice Research Database. Ann Rheum Dis. 2006;65:1074–9.
111. Rossini M, Del Marco A, Dal Santo F, Gatti D, Braggion C, James G, et al. Prevalence and correlates of vertebral fractures in adults with cystic fibrosis. Bone. 2004;35:771–6.
112. Canalis E, Delany AM. Mechanisms of glucocorticoid action in bone. Ann N Y Acad Sci. 2002;966:73–81.
113. Weinstein RS, Jilka RL, Parfitt AM, Manolagas SC. Inhibition of osteoblastogenesis and promotion of apoptosis of osteoblasts and osteocytes by glucocorticoids. Potential mechanisms of their deleterious effects on bone. J Clin Invest. 1998;102:274–82.
114. Kim HJ, Zhao H, Kitaura H, Bhattacharyya S, Brewer JA, Muglia LJ, et al. Glucocorticoids and the osteoclast. Ann N Y Acad Sci. 2007;1116:335–9.
115. Tsampalieros A, Berkenstock MK, Zemel BS, Griffin L, Shults J, Burnham JM, et al. Changes in trabecular bone density in incident pediatric Crohn's disease: a comparison of imaging methods. Osteoporosis Int. 2014;25:1875–83.
116. Osta B, Benedetti G, Miossec P. Classical and paradoxical effects of TNF-alpha on bone homeostasis. Frontiers Immunol. 2014;5:48.
117. Rall LC, Roubenoff R. Rheumatoid cachexia: metabolic abnormalities, mechanisms and interventions. Rheumatology (Oxford). 2004;43:1219–23.
118. Kitaura H, Kimura K, Ishida M, Kohara H, Yoshimatsu M, Takano-Yamamoto T. Immunological reaction in TNF-alpha-mediated osteoclast formation and bone resorption in vitro and in vivo. Clin Dev Immunol. 2013;2013:181849.
119. Hegarty J, Mughal MZ, Adams J, Webb NJ. Reduced bone mineral density in adults treated with high-dose corticosteroids for childhood nephrotic syndrome. Kidney Int. 2005;68:2304–9.
120. Tsampalieros A, Kalkwarf HJ, Wetzsteon RJ, Shults J, Zemel BS, Foster BJ, et al. Changes in bone structure and the muscle-bone unit in children with chronic kidney disease. Kidney Int. 2013;83:495–502.

121. Wetzsteon RJ, Shults J, Zemel BS, Gupta PU, Burnham JM, Herskovitz RM, et al. Divergent effects of glucocorticoids on cortical and trabecular compartment BMD in childhood nephrotic syndrome. J Bone Miner Res. 2009;24:503–13.
122. Bechtold S, Alberer M, Arenz T, Putzker S, Filipiak-Pittroff B, Schwarz HP, et al. Reduced muscle mass and bone size in pediatric patients with inflammatory bowel disease. Inflamm Bowel Dis. 2010;16:216–25.
123. Dubner SE, Shults J, Baldassano RN, Zemel BS, Thayu M, Burnham JM, et al. Longitudinal assessment of bone density and structure in an incident cohort of children with Crohn's disease. Gastroenterology. 2009;136:123–30.
124. Tsampalieros A, Lam CK, Spencer JC, Thayu M, Shults J, Zemel BS, et al. Long-term inflammation and glucocorticoid therapy impair skeletal modeling during growth in childhood Crohn disease. J Clin Endocrinol Metab. 2013;98:3438–45.
125. Werkstetter KJ, Pozza SB, Filipiak-Pittroff B, Schatz SB, Prell C, Bufler P, et al. Long-term development of bone geometry and muscle in pediatric inflammatory bowel disease. Am J Gastroenterol. 2011;106:988–98.
126. Werkstetter KJ, Schatz SB, Alberer M, Filipiak-Pittroff B, Koletzko S. Influence of exclusive enteral nutrition therapy on bone density and geometry in newly diagnosed pediatric Crohn's disease patients. Ann Nutr Metab. 2013;63:10–6.
127. Stagi S, Cavalli L, Bertini F, Matucci Cerinic M, Luisa Brandi M, Falcini F. Cross-sectional and longitudinal evaluation of bone mass and quality in children and young adults with juvenile onset systemic lupus erythematosus (JSLE): role of bone mass determinants analyzed by DXA, PQCT and QUS. Lupus. 2014;23:57–68.
128. Felin EMO, Prahalad S, Askew EW, Moyer-Mileur LJ. Musculoskeletal abnormalities of the tibia in juvenile rheumatoid arthritis. Arthritis Rheum. 2007;56:984–94.
129. Burnham JM, Shults J, Dubner SE, Sembhi H, Zemel BS, Leonard MB. Bone density, structure, and strength in juvenile idiopathic arthritis: importance of disease severity and muscle deficits. Arthritis Rheum. 2008;58:2518–27.
130. Roth J, Linge M, Tzaribachev N, Schweizer R, Kuemmerle-Deschner J. Musculoskeletal abnormalities in juvenile idiopathic arthritis—a 4-year longitudinal study. Rheumatology (Oxford). 2007;46:1180–4.
131. Roth J, Palm C, Scheunemann I, Ranke MB, Schweizer R, Dannecker GE. Musculoskeletal abnormalities of the forearm in patients with juvenile idiopathic arthritis relate mainly to bone geometry. Arthritis Rheum. 2004;50:1277–85.
132. Daniel V, Trautmann Y, Konrad M, Nayir A, Scharer K. T-lymphocyte populations, cytokines and other growth factors in serum and urine of children with idiopathic nephrotic syndrome. Clin Nephrol. 1997;47:289–97.
133. Tsampalieros A, Gupta P, Denburg MR, Shults J, Zemel BS, Mostoufi-Moab S, et al. Glucocorticoid effects on changes in bone mineral density and cortical structure in childhood nephrotic syndrome. J Bone Miner Res. 2013;28:480–8.
134. Terpstra AM, Kalkwarf HJ, Shults J, Zemel BS, Wetzsteon RJ, Foster BJ, et al. Bone density and cortical structure after pediatric renal transplantation. J Am Soc Nephrol. 2012;23:715–26.
135. Foster BJ, Shults J, Zemel BS, Leonard MB. Interactions between growth and body composition in children treated with high-dose chronic glucocorticoids. Am J Clin Nutr. 2004;80:1334–41.
136. Lee DY, Wetzsteon RJ, Zemel BS, Shults J, Organ JM, Foster BJ, et al. Muscle torque relative to cross-sectional area and the functional muscle-bone unit in children and adolescents with chronic disease. J Bone Miner Res. 2015;30:575–83.
137. Mostoufi-Moab S, Brodsky J, Isaacoff EJ, Tsampalieros A, Ginsberg JP, Zemel B, et al. Longitudinal assessment of bone density and structure in childhood survivors of acute lymphoblastic leukemia without cranial radiation. J Clin Endocrinol Metab. 2012;97:3584–92.
138. Tsampalieros A, Griffin L, Terpstra AM, Kalkwarf HJ, Shults J, Foster BJ, et al. Changes in DXA and quantitative CT measures of musculoskeletal outcomes following pediatric renal transplantation. Am J Transplant. 2014;14:124–32.
139. Mostoufi-Moab S, Ginsberg JP, Bunin N, Zemel B, Shults J, Leonard MB. Bone density and structure in long-term survivors of pediatric allogeneic hematopoietic stem cell transplantation. J Bone Miner Res. 2012;27:760–9.

# Chapter 12
# Evaluation of Fracture Without Known Trauma: Use of DXA in Differential Diagnosis

M. Zulf Mughal, Amanda T. Whitaker, and Aenor J. Sawyer

## Outline

1. Nonaccidental injury and osteogenesis imperfecta.
2. Fractures in children with disabilities.
3. Fractures in children with syndrome of congenital insensitivity to pain.

## Concern for Nonaccidental Injury

The possibility of physical child abuse or nonaccidental injury (NAI) has to be considered whenever an infant or child presents with multiple fractures at different skeletal sites and in various stages of healing. However, clinicians also have a duty to exclude accidental injury as well as an underlying medical disorder associated with diminished bone strength that can lead to fractures during routine day-to-day handling, when dealing with a child with an unexplained fracture(s). Such children may have also suffered other forms of abuse from their caregivers, such as neglect, emotional abuse, or sexual abuse. Skeletal injuries due to NAI may arise from

M.Z. Mughal, M.B.Ch.B., F.R.C.P. (✉)
Department of Paediatric Endocrinology, Royal Manchester Children's Hospital,
Oxford Road, Manchester M20 3TF, UK
e-mail: zulf.mughal@cmft.nhs.uk

A.T. Whitaker, M.D.
Department of Orthopaedic Surgery, Boston Children's Hospital,
300 Longwood Avenue, Hunwell 2, Boston, MA 02115, USA
e-mail: amanda.t.whitaker@gmail.com

A.J. Sawyer, M.D., M.S.
Director, UCSF Skeletal Health Service, Assistant Clinical Professor,
Department of Orthopaedic Surgery, University of California, San Francisco

© Springer International Publishing Switzerland 2016
E.B. Fung et al. (eds.), *Bone Health Assessment in Pediatrics*,
DOI 10.1007/978-3-319-30412-0_12

deliberately inflected injuries or from neglect, for example when a pre-mobile child is left unsupervised in a hazardous environment. Pediatric disorders such as osteogenesis imperfecta (OI), pan-hypopituitarism, cortical hyperostosis (Caffey Disease), and Ehlers-Danlos syndrome have all been associated with bone fragility and may present with multiple fractures.

Osteogenesis imperfecta is the most common bone disorder considered in the differential diagnosis of a young child with unexplained fractures, however. This section deals with the role of bone densitometry in discriminating between healthy infants and children (with possible NAI) from those with osteogenesis imperfecta.

## Fractures Due to Nonaccidental Injury

Nonaccidental skeletal injuries are common and cause fractures in infants. In one study, up to 82 % of long bone fractures in infants less than 1 year of age were considered to be due to NAI [1]. Unexplained fractures in a non-ambulatory child, especially if the fractures are multiple and of differing ages, are highly suspicious of inflicted injury. Suspicion of NAI is also aroused when the history of an injury provided by parents or caregivers, is not consistent with physical findings; when there is variation in the histories of the injury given to health professionals; when there is delay in seeking medical attention; frequent visits to the emergency room or primary care physician; and when the given mechanism of injury is not consistent with development of the child or the past medical or social history of the child. The affected infant or child may also have other features of physical, emotional, or sexual abuse.

Pre-mobile children and infants <2 years of age are less prone to accidental injury, and thus in this group unexplained fractures are more likely to have occurred as result of inflicted injuries. The incidence of fractures in those less than 12 months old is 4.55/1000 and 17/1000 in those 13–24 months old [2]. Nonaccidental trauma is the leading cause of fractures in infants due to their nonmobile status [3]. Children who present with a single episode of nonaccidental trauma are at a 10 % risk of death, whereas those with repeat nonaccidental trauma are at a 25 % risk of death [4]. Therefore, any suspicion of nonaccidental fractures should lead to a multidisciplinary assessment with social services and other child protection agencies. In the majority of cases, the diagnosis of NAI can be reached through a careful appraisal of detailed histories obtained from caretakers, a thorough clinical examination, and review of high quality radiographic skeletal survey, undertaken in accordance with standards published by the American College of Radiology [5] or The Royal College of Radiologists and The Royal College of Paediatrics and Child Health in the UK [6]. Such radiographs should be reviewed by an experienced paediatric radiologist familiar with imaging typically associated with NAI compared to rare skeletal dysplasias. The radiologist has an important role in identifying the number, age, and interpreting the severity of fractures. In addition to the skeletal survey, bone scintigraphy with technetium-99 m-labeled bisphosphonate may help to disclose injuries that are not readily visible on the radiographic skeletal survey, including periosteal injuries, fresh rib fractures, and bony injuries in a complex area such as the pelvis [7]. In addition to the radiographic evaluation, thorough physical examinations by a paediatrician and paediatric orthopaedic surgeon are essential.

Although virtually any fracture can result from a nonaccidental injury, certain fractures are considered to be more suggestive of abuse. These include metaphyseal fractures (Fig. 12.1a, b), posterior rib fractures (Fig. 12.2a, b), physeal separations, vertebral compression fractures, scapular fractures, spinous process fractures, sternal fractures, complex skull fractures, and any long bone fracture especially transverse femur fractures (Fig. 12.3) [8, 9]. Transverse femur fractures are suggestive of a high energy direct blow to the femur or tibia. Metaphyseal fractures are suggestive of a high force twisting or wringing action to the extremity. Vertebral compression fractures can be from shaking, dropping or forceful sitting. Posterior rib fractures are indication of anterior–posterior compression of the rib-cage (resulting in stress of the posterior rib, where it articulates with the transverse process of vertebral body), or of being hit on the back. One retrospective review associates 82 % of posterior rib fractures with nonaccidental trauma [10]. A useful reference source is *Diagnostic Imaging of Child Abuse*, 3rd Edition, edited by Kleinman [11].

Other associations with nonaccidental trauma include children with head trauma, interhemispheric extra-axial hemorrhage, shear-type brain injury, and small bowel hematoma or laceration. These are often associated with shaking, direct head

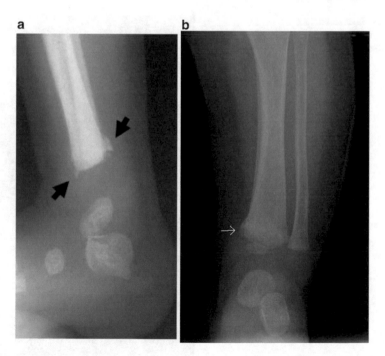

**Fig. 12.1**  (**a**) Radiograph of an infant's lower leg, showing metaphyseal fractures of the distal tibia (*arrows*). (**b**) Metaphyseal fracture of the left distal tibia in a 2-month-old (*arrow*)

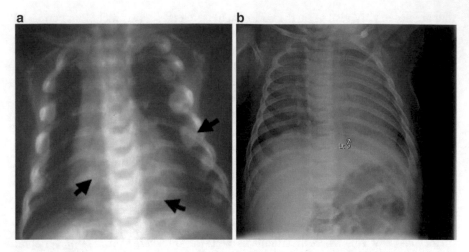

**Fig. 12.2** (**a**) Radiograph of an infant's chest, showing posterior and lateral rib fractures (*arrows*). (**b**) Posterior 9th rib fracture in a 2-month-old (*arrow*)

**Fig. 12.3** Transverse left femoral fracturein a 5-month-old

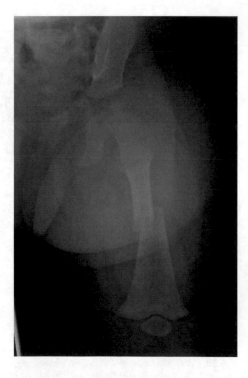

trauma, and trauma to the abdomen. The history cannot always corroborate the injury, so the provider must be aware. In children with unwitnessed head trauma, 22 % have been related to nonaccidental trauma with a skeletal survey [12]. A head CT is recommended in children less than 12 months old with a single, proximal, extremity fracture and a history of a nonaccidental trauma workup [13].

In older children, neurological and psychological conditions are often present in nonaccidental trauma victims [14]. This is a vulnerable population that often is non-ambulatory and any fracture should be concerning. Also, children with neurologic and psychiatric disorders can have metabolic bone diseases that predispose them to fractures. Poor nutrition, lack of sunlight exposure, medications, and lack of ambulation or physical activity decrease bone mineral density in this population [15]. Therefore, their fractures are multifactorial. Bone density decreases after immobilization and leads to an increased risk after surgical procedures to fractures in the immobilized extremity. Fractures in children with neuromuscular conditions are often spiral fractures from a twist or a fall out of their wheelchair. Concerning patterns are transverse fractures, metaphyseal fractures, and physeal separations as to the mechanism of the injury and the child's inability to inflict the injury up on themselves.

Rickets secondary to vitamin D deficiency can predispose children to fractures. Radiographs may show widening of the physis, cupping of the metaphysis with diffuse osteopenia and bowing deformities of the lower extremities [16]. Children who are exclusively breastfed are pre-disposed to vitamin D deficiency [17]. While biochemical vitamin D deficiency may be found in children with multiple fractures, this deficiency is common in the pediatric population as well [18, 19]. Therefore, though biochemical vitamin D deficiency may be associated in a case of NAI, it should not presumed to be the cause of suspicious fractures in children, especially those that are non-ambulatory.

# Osteogenesis Imperfecta

Osteogenesis imperfecta (OI) is a heterogeneous group of connective tissue disorders characterized be increased propensity to fractures throughout life. Other clinical features of OI include short stature, dentinogenesis imperfecta, fragile skin with increased tendency to bruising, a blue or gray scleral color, joint laxity, joint dislocations and pre-senile deafness. The clinical course of OI is extremely variable, ranging from stillbirth due to multiple intrauterine fractures to a lifelong absence of fractures. OI is the most common bone condition that has to be considered in the differential diagnosis of an infant with unexplained fractures.

In 1979, using clinical, radiographic and genetic criteria, Sillence and colleagues [20] classified OI into four major types (I–IV). However, the numbers of OI types have increased with the discovery of new genetic defects. Currently, 16 genes have been identified in the Online Medelian Inheritance in Man (OMIM) database. In 90 % of cases, OI is caused by heterozygous mutations in the *COL1A1* and *COL1A2* genes that encode for the pro-alpha-1(I) and pro-alpha-2(I) chains of type I collagen. These forms of OI are inherited as an autosomal- dominant trait; however, up to 25 % of children with OI have new mutations. Recurrence of OI without an affected parent may occur due to gonadal mosaicism mutations in one of the parents.

OI type I, (*the mild nondeforming form with blue sclera*) is the mildest form of the disease. The majority of patients with type1 OI have mutations in *COL1A1* allele leading to approximately 50 % reduction or haploinsufficiency in the synthesis of type 1 procollagen. Fractures usually start during pre-school years, when the child becomes increasingly ambulant and tend to decrease after puberty. Intrauterine long-bone fractures, fractures before walking age, and skeletal deformities, such as bowing, are rare. The majority of OI types II to IV arise from mutations in *COL1A1* and *COL1A2* genes that lead to the production of structurally abnormal collagen. OI type II, (*the perinatal lethal form*), is the most severe form of the disease. Affected individuals have multiple intrauterine fractures with crumpled femora and beaded ribs. Most patients die in utero or shortly after birth due to respiratory failure. Patients with OI type III, (*the severe deforming type*), have limb deformities from numerous fractures occurring in utero and characteristic triangular facies and yellowish opalescent teeth (i.e., dentinogenesis imperfecta). Patients with OI type IV, (*the moderately deforming type*), usually have white sclerae, and most (but not all) patients have dentinogenis imperfecta. The severity of bone disease in subjects with OI type IV can be variable; some have fractures in utero leading to deformities, whereas others suffer only a few fractures throughout their life. OI type V accounts for around 5 % of cases and is inherited in an autosomal dominant manner. It is caused by heterozygous mutation in the gene, which encodes interferon-induced transmembrane protein 5 (IFITM5). These patients have distinctive features: hyperplastic callus formation, a dense metaphyseal band adjacent to the growth plate during infancy and progressive calcification of the interosseous membranes in forearms and legs. They are also prone to radial head dislocation. Patients with OI type 5 have white sclera and dentinogenesis imperfecta is not present.

Autosomal recessive forms of OI account for around 10 % of cases, and are caused by deficiencies in proteins responsible for posttranslational modification, folding and chaperoning of type I collagen. Mutations in some of these genes CRTAP, PPIB & LEPRE1, SERPINF1, SERPINH1, SP7, WNT1, PLS3, BMP1, PLOD2, CREB3L1, TMEM38B and FKBP10 account for some of the causes of OI type II to IV [21].

Radiographic features in milder types of OI may be nonspecific but include slender (gracile) bones with thin cortices and osteopenia. Wormian bones measuring $6 \times 4$ mm or larger in size and more than 10 in number around the lambdoid suture on skull radiographs are suggestive of OI. Rib and metaphyseal fractures, which are seen in infants with NAI, may also occur in OI, but are less common in those with milder forms of the disease (types I & IV).

In a child with unexplained fracture(s), the clinical diagnosis of OI is based on obtaining the relevant the family history (fragility fractures, joint dislocations, dentinogenesis imperfect), undertaking a clinical examination looking for the signs and symptoms of the disease (blue-gray sclera, characteristic triangular facies, dentinogenesis imperfect, limb deformities and joint hypermobility) and looking for characteristic radiographic features (Wormian bones in the skull vault, osteopenia and gracile looking long-bones). Unfortunately, bluish-gray sclerae are not uncommon in healthy infants and therefore this finding is not particularly useful in the first 6-months of life. Dentinogenesis imperfecta, which is more likely to affect primary than permanent dentition, is usually not present in a child with OI type I, and some forms of OI type IV. Joint hypermobility is not uncommon in otherwise healthy infants and toddlers. Wormian bones are only present in around 30 % of cases of OI type I [22]. Osteopenia and gracile appearance of long-bones, which are subjective radiographic features of OI, may not be evident on radiographs of children with milder forms of OI (types I & IV). In summary, the diagnosis of OI is relatively straightforward in a child with a positive family history who has typical clinical and radiological features of the disease. Milder forms of OI, especially type IV with normal sclera and absence of dentinogenesis imperfecta, can be difficult to diagnose clinically, especially if classical radiological features of the disease are absent and no other family members are affected. Unexplained fractures in infants with such forms of OI may be confused with NAI. In such cases, genetic testing should be considered. Marlow et al studied skin fibroblasts of 262 samples that had been submitted to their laboratory in whom NAI was suspected, but OI was also considered or could not be excluded [23]. Skin fibroblast cells in 11 (4.2 %) infants had abnormalities consistent with OI and in 11 others the diagnosis could not be excluded. Therefore, clinical evaluation did not identify some children with mild forms of OI. Genetic testing is justified in these children as failure to diagnose OI may lead to prolonged separation of the child from his/her parents, and in some case they may be put up for adoption. In such cases, Pepin & Byers recommend sequence of *COL1A1* (OI type I or IV), *COL1A2* (OI type IV), and IFITM5 (OI type V) genes simultaneously. If a causative mutation is not identified, and the infant with unexplained fractures does not have clinical features of OI, no additional gene testing is indicated. However, such analysis may uncover variants of unknown significance, which may or may not be pathogenic. If the variant is identified in one of the asymptomatic parents then it is likely to be nonpathogenic. If the variant segregates with a bone phenotype then it may be pathogenic and further studies, such as protein studies, may be required [24].

## The Role of Bone Densitometry in the Assessment of an Infant with Multiple Unexplained Fractures

As mentioned previously, milder phenotypes of OI, especially type IV, may be difficult to differentiate from NAI. In cases where parents deny harming their child, it is not uncommon for the parents and their legal representatives to inquire as to whether measurement of bone mineral density will help in differentiating normal children who have been victims of NAI from those with milder forms of OI, as 30–40 % of bone mineral density must be lost in order to have radiographic changes [25].

DXA measurements of bone mineral density (BMD) in older children and adults with OI have provided conflicting results. Paterson and Mole [26] found areal BMD (aBMD) to be within the reference range in most adults with type I or type IV OI. In contrast, others [27–30] reported that aBMD in children with OI was significantly lower than that of age-matched controls. In a cross-sectional study, Rauch et al found that after adjustment for age, sex, and height Z-scores, the mean LS aBMD Z-scores of children with OI type 1 with mean age was 7.5 years (confirmed by genetic testing) was −4.0 [31].

Lund et al. [32] measured whole body and lumbar spine bone area (BA), bone mineral content (BMC), and aBMD in 63 subjects with both mild and severe types of OI. Their study cohort included 24 children (17 males), aged 5–18 years, of whom 15 were classified as having OI type I or OI type IV. The authors used the approach of Mølgaard et al. [33] to determine whether (a) the subject's height was appropriate for age (looking for "short bones"), (b) the bone area was appropriate for height (looking for "narrow bones"), and (c) the BMC was appropriate for bone area (looking for "light bones"). They compared these findings with quantitative and qualitative defects in type 1 collagen produced by subjects' cultured skin fibroblasts. Mean aBMD for age in both children and adults was low in patients with OI type III or IV and/or a qualitative collagen defect. Reduced BMC for age in OI children was due to reduced height (short bones) and reduced BMC for BA (light bones). In contrast, their BA for height was normal (normal bone width). Forty percent of all subjects studied and 75 % of those with either OI type I, a quantitative collagen defect, or both had aBMD for age values within the reference range. The fact that OI subjects suffered recurrent fractures despite normal or only slightly low aBMD for age suggests that impaired skeletal mineralization alone was not the only cause of bone fragility. The authors concluded that DXA has limited value in the assessment of recurrent fractures because aBMD in OI can be normal and because there are few pediatric reference data for children under the age of 2 years, the period when fractures due to NAI are most prevalent.

Very few studies have measured BMD in young infants with the milder forms of OI (i.e., type I and type IV) that would be considered in the differential diagnosis of fractures due to NAI. One small study of 14 children with OI by Miller and Hangartner recommended that the investigation of the infant with unexplained fractures should include assessment of BMD by quantitative computed tomography (QCT) [34]. However, few centers have QCT scanners capable of measuring volumetric BMD in infants, and there is a paucity of age and gender reference data to allow calculation of Z-scores. Larger studies are needed to confirm the authors' preliminary findings.

Bishop and colleagues [35] compared aBMD of the lumbar spine (LS) by DXA in infants with fractures due to OI and those whose fractures were thought to have occurred nonaccidentally. They found that LS aBMD of infants less than 6 months of age in both groups were within the reference range and were not significantly different. There was considerable overlap in BMD between subjects with and without OI who were up to 2 years of age. In follow-up examinations, however, the increment in LS aBMD in OI infants was significantly lower ($27/cm^2/year$) than that of non-OI infants ($115/cm^2/year$). The authors concluded that a single BMD measurement was not helpful in differentiating between infants whose fractures resulted from OI versus NAI. Longitudinal aBMD measurements, however, may be helpful in discriminating between normal infants and those with milder OI phenotypes.

In summary, for the majority of infants with unexplained fractures, the diagnosis of NAI or OI can be reached with a detailed clinical history, a thorough clinical examination by a clinician experienced in bone disorders, and a skeletal survey interpreted by an experienced pediatric radiologist. DXA measurements do not help to distinguish healthy infants who have been victims of abuse from those with milder types of OI. Thus, in an infant with unexplained fractures, measurement of BMD cannot be used to diagnosed or exclude OI. Since up to 5 % of children evaluated for NAI may have OI, genetic testing may be justified to exclude OI in infants with unexplained fractures [24].

## Fractures in Children with Disabilities

Postnatal skeletal development is modulated by the mechanical forces to which it is subjected to, which primarily arise from muscle contraction. The skeleton of a healthy growing child continuously adapts to increasing mechanical loading from bigger and stronger muscles by increasing bone mass and altering bone geometry. By contrast, non-ambulant children such as those with cerebral palsy, muscle weakness, spasticity, and lack of normal load bearing activities result in reduced periosteal bone expansion. This leads to development of slender long bones of abnormal shape, which have increased propensity to fracture due to altered mechanics. In muscle disorders such as Duchenne muscular dystrophy, progressive reduction in the mechanical loading and exposure to glucocorticoid therapy result in accelerated bone loss, as well as failure to accrue bone mass. Concern for skeletal fragility resulting from muscle disuse in children and adolescents often leads to investigations of skeletal status. Cognitive impairment, spastic movements, inability to lie still and seizures pose unique challenges for obtaining accurate densitometry measurements.

## Cerebral Palsy

Cerebral palsy (CP) is a term used to describe a group of non-progressive disorders of movement and posture, resulting from an insult to the developing brain. It is one of the commonest chronic disabling childhood conditions, which is often associated with other comorbidities: cognitive impairment, behavioral problems, hearing and visual problems, feeding difficulties, poor growth, recurrent respiratory infections and epilepsy. Secondary musculoskeletal problems include joint contractures, kyphoscoliosis, hip subluxation, long bone deformity, and propensity to low trauma fractures of limb bones. Fractures in children and adolescents with CP tend to be more common in lower limb bones, especially around the knee [36–38]. They are more common in non-ambulant children and adolescents, who have severe forms of CP defined as level IV or V according to the Gross Motor Function Classification System (GMFCS) [39]. Such fractures often occur during normal activities such as dressing, handling and transferring. However, the cause of fracture may not be clear; the lack of a clear history of the injury causing the fracture due to difficulties in communication and delay in seeking medical attention for a fracture sometimes leads to suspicion of child abuse [40]. The prevalence of fragility fractures in non-ambulant children and adolescents with CP has been reported to be between 6 and 12 % [37, 38], and an annual incidence of 4 % [41].

In severely disabled children with CP, whole body, hip, or spine assessment of BMD by DXA can be challenging due to joint contractures, hip dysplasia, scoliosis or use of metal fixation devices. As mentioned previously, the majority of fractures in non-ambulant children and adolescents in CP occur in lower limb bones, especially in the distal femur [37–40]. Harcke and colleagues have described the technique for measuring areal bone mineral density (aBMD) at the distal femoral region, the most common fracture site in children with CP [42, 43]. Almost all children, even those with significant contractures can be comfortably placed in the position to obtain an accurate distal femur scan. An example of correct positioning and analysis for the distal femur measurement is found in Figs. 12.4 and 12.5. The lateral distal femur (LDF) scans are divided into three rectangular sub-regions, representing metaphyseal bone (LDF Region 1), the transition zone from the metaphysis to the diaphysis (LDF Region 2), and diaphyseal bone (LDF Region 3). Zemel et al have published LDF reference data based on over 800 children and adolescents, for the Hologic Discovery/Delphi DXA machines [44]. More details on how to perform this scan in patients with disabilities can be found in Chap. 9. In children with chronic immobilization, the 2013 Pediatric Official Positions of the International Society for Clinical Densitometry recommends assessment of BMD at the LDF site, which is the most common fracture site in children with CP [45]. Henderson and colleagues studied the relation between LDF aBMD Z-scores and fracture history in a cross-sectional study of 619 children aged 6–18 years with muscular dystrophy ($n = 112$) or moderate to severe cerebral palsy ($n = 507$), cared for at eight canters in the USA [46]. There was a strong correlation between fracture history and LDF aBMD Z-scores; 35–42 % of those with aBMD Z-scores less than −5 had fractured compared with 13–15 % of those with aBMD Z-scores greater than −1. Each 1.0 decrease in LDF aBMD Z-scores increased the fracture risk by 6–15 %. Systemically administered bisphosphonates have been used to treat children with CP. Cross-sectional studies have shown an increase in the aBMD of the lateral distal femoral metaphyseal region (LDF region 1) following treatment with cyclical intravenous pamidronate therapy in non-ambulant children with CP [47, 48]. The observed increase in aBMD in region 1 of the LDF had virtually returned back to baseline 2 years after the treatment was discontinued [48].

In summary, non-ambulant children with CP are prone to fragility fractures. Such fractures predominantly occur in lower limb bones. Normative data are available for estimation of aBMD at the LDF site in children with CP, using Hologic Discovery/Delphi densitometers.

**Fig. 12.4** Example of analysis of lateral distal femur scan by DXA, 3 regions of interest include LDF Region 1: metaphyseal bone, LDF Region 2: the transition zone from the metaphysis to the diaphysis, and LDF Region 3: diaphyseal bone

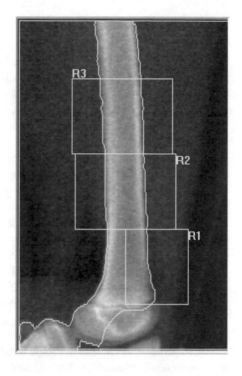

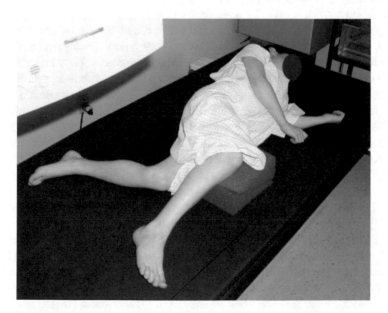

**Fig. 12.5** Correct positioning of a patient for lateral distal femur measurement

## Duchenne Muscular Dystrophy

Duchenne muscular dystrophy (DMD) is an X-linked recessive disorder due to mutations in the dystrophin gene, which affects 1 in 3600–6000 live male births [49]. The symptoms of DMD tend to manifest around 3 years of age. Affected boys present with delay in walking, abnormal gait, reduced ability to run or rise from the floor (Gowers' sign). Muscle weakness continues to progress so that affected boys are wheelchair bound by early teen years. DMD is associated with low BMD and increased risk of long-bone fractures. Currently, the standard of care for DMD boys includes treatment with glucocorticosteroids (prednisolone or deflazacort), which are administered in order to improve or preserve muscle strength, with the goal of prolonging the period of independent walking. Glucocorticoid therapy may also help to slow the progression of scoliosis, deterioration in cardiopulmonary function, delay the need for noninvasive ventilatory support and increase survival rate of DMD boys [50]. However, glucocorticoids increase the fracture risk, both in long bones and vertebrae, which in turn accelerate the loss of ambulation in affected boys.

In a longitudinal study, Larson & Henderson [51] measured aBMD of LS and proximal femur in 41 glucocorticoid naïve boys with DMD while they were ambulatory, and again when they were no longer walking. During the ambulatory phase, the proximal femoral aBMD was reduced even when gait was minimally affected (mean Z score −1.6) and then progressively fell to mean SDS of almost −4, when boys became non-ambulant. Loss of ambulation was also associated with a decline in LS aBMD. Bianchi et al. [52] measured total body and LS aBMD by DXA in 32 ambulant boys with DMD; 22 were on long term glucocorticoid therapy and 10 were glucocorticoid naïve. These investigators found that trunk and lower limb aBMD, derived from total body scans, were more reduced compared to the upper extremities. It was further shown that corticosteroid-treated boys had even lower aBMD values, especially at the LS. Crabtree et al. [53] undertook longitudinal measurements of the projected bone area (BA), bone mineral content (BMC) and lean body mass (LBM), at the lumbar spine and subcranial skeleton, in 25 ambulant boys with DMD on an intermittent glucocorticoid (10 days on 10 days off) regimen. At baseline the total body less head (TBLH) bone area (BA) for height and TBLH BMC for lean body mass (LBM) were significantly reduced, suggesting that reduced mechanical load from diminished muscle function had resulted in narrower, lighter bones. After 30 months of glucocorticoid therapy there was a significant increase in TBLH BA for height (wider bones) but a significant reduction of TBLH BMC for area (lighter bones). The authors suggested that periosteal bone envelopes had become bigger as an adaptive response to bone loss, secondary to the disease and glucocorticoid therapy. At the lumbar spine, the baseline BMC for BA was low but appropriate for reduced LBM. At follow-up, there were no significant changes in BA but small increases in BMC both for BA and LBM, suggesting lack of detrimental effect on bone, at this site, after 30 months of glucocorticoid therapy.

In summary, progressive muscle weakness in boys with DMD is associated with declines in BMD as measured by DXA and increased propensity to long-bone fractures. Treatment with glucocorticoids prolongs ambulation but is associated with increased risk of vertebral and long-bone fractures.

## Fractures in Children with Congenital Insensitivity to Pain

Congenital insensitivity to pain (CIP) is a rare autosomal-recessive disorder associated with lack of perception to pain. However, other sensory modalities including touch, proprioception, itch, tickle, pressure, temperature discrimination and vibration are preserved. CIP is caused by loss-of-function alterations in the transmembrane voltage-gated sodium channel, Na(v)1.7, encoded by the SCN9A gene [54]. Children with CIP lack protective behavior to noxious stimuli which predisposes them to fractures, burns and self-mutilation, e.g. biting leading to lacerations/amputations of lips & tongue. A limp, inability to walk or a swollen leg may be the only clinical sign of a fracture of the femur/tibia a child with CIP (Fig. 12.6). In a previously undiagnosed child with CIP, lack of a clear history of an injury causing the fracture or soft tissue injury may lead to consideration of nonaccidental injury. In one of author's experience (MZM), bone mineral density (whole body, lumbar spine & distal radius) in a child with CIP due to a homozygous mutation in SCN9A gene, who had suffered recurrent long-bone fractures, was normal. Besides fractures, other skeletal manifestations of CIP include limb-length discrepancies due to physeal fractures, joint dislocations, heterotopic ossification, and avascular necrosis.

**Fig. 12.6** Late presentation of left distal femoral fracture, with exuberant callus formation, in a boy with congenital insensitivity to pain with anhidrosis

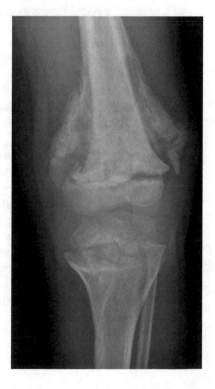

Ultimately, these children may go on to develop Charcot joints [55]. More recently, CIP due to dysfunction of the Na(v)1.9, caused by heterozygous by gain-of-function mutations the SCN11A gene has also been described [56]. In addition to congenital insensitivity to pain, children with this mutation also suffer from hypotonia and gastrointestinal motility disturbances. Congenital insensitivity to pain with anhidrosis (CIPA) is a rare autosomal-recessive disorder characterized by absence of reaction to painful stimuli, recurrent episodes of unexplained fever, absence of sweating and mental retardation. CIPA is caused by homozygous or compound heterozygous loss-of-function mutations in the TRKA (NTRK1) gene, which encodes a high-affinity tyrosine kinase receptor for nerve growth factor (neurotrophic tyrosine kinase) [57].

## Summary Points

- Red flags for nonaccidental injury (NAI) include: unexplained multiple fractures in non-ambulatory infants, physical findings inconsistent with the history provided by the caregiver or the development of the child, delay in seeking medical attention, and other signs of physical, emotional or sexual abuse.
- A skeletal survey is the most useful radiographic study in cases of suspected NAI. Nonaccidental injury should be considered in non-ambulatory children with multiple fractures and a thorough radiographic, physical and social investigation completed.
- Characteristic fracture patterns, such as transverse long bone fractures, physeal separations, metaphyseal fractures, and posterior rib fractures, and multiple fractures or fractures in different stages of healing warrant a skeletal survey and head CT as risk of death is high in NAI cases.
- In young children with unexplained fractures, bone mineral density measurement by DXA is not conclusive in differentiating between NAI and mild forms of osteogenesis imperfecta.
- Osteogenesis imperfecta is the most common genetic disorder of bone fragility and should be considered in the diagnosis of an infant with unexplained fractures and suspected NAI.
- Milder forms of OI may be difficult to diagnose clinically, especially in the absence of classical radiographic features of the disease and/or affected family members. In such cases, genetic testing is warranted.
- Non-ambulant children with neurologic conditions are prone to fragility fractures, which may arise during normal activities. The lack of a clear history of the injury causing the fracture due to difficulties in communication and delay in seeking medical attention for a fracture sometimes leads to suspicion of child abuse.

# References

1. Leventhal JM, Thomas SA, Rosenfield NS, Markowitz RI. Fractures in young children. Distinguishing child abuse from unintentional injuries. Am J Dis Child. 1993;147(1):87–92.
2. Hansoti B, Beattie TF. Limb fractures and nonaccidental injury in children less than 24 months of age. Eur J Emerg Med. 2008;15(2):63–6.
3. Kemp AM, Dunstan F, Harrison S, Morris S, Mass M, Rolfe K et al. Patterns of skeletal fractures in child abuse: systematic review. BMJ 2008;337;a1518.
4. Deans KJ, et al. Mortality increases with recurrent episodes of nonaccidental trauma in children. J Trauma Acute Care Surg. 2013;75(1):161–5.
5. American College of Radiology. ACR practice guideline for skeletal surveys in children. 2006. http://www.acr.org/secondarymainmenucategories/quality_safety/guidelines/pediatric/skeletal_surveys.aspx.
6. The Royal College of Radiologists and Royal College of Paediatrics and Child Health. Standards for radiological investigations of suspected non-accidental injury. London: RCR/RCPCH; 2008.
7. Conway JJ, Collins M, Tanz RR, Radkowski MA, Anandappa E, Hernandez R, Freeman EL. The role of bone scintigraphy in detecting child abuse. Semin Nucl Med. 1993;23:321–33.
8. Murphy R, et al. Transverse fractures of the femoral shaft are a better predictor of nonaccidental trauma in young children than spiral fractures are. J Bone Joint Surg Am. 2015;97(2):106–11.
9. Kocher MS, Kasser JR. Orthopaedic aspects of child abuse. J Am Acad Orthop Surg. 2000;8(1):10–20.
10. Bulloch B, et al. Cause and clinical characteristics of rib fractures in infants. Pediatrics. 2000;105(4), E48.
11. In: Kleinman PK, editor. Diagnostic imaging of child abuse: third edition. Cambridge University Press. 2015. ISBN: 9781107010536. 978-1-107-01053-6.
12. Rangel EL, et al. Eliminating disparity in evaluation for abuse in infants with head injury: use of a screening guideline. J Pediatr Surg. 2009;44(6):1229–34. discussion 1234–5.
13. Wilson PM, et al. Utility of head computed tomography in children with a single extremity fracture. J Pediatr. 2014;164(6):1274–9.
14. Loder RT, Feinberg JR. Orthopaedic injuries in children with nonaccidental trauma: demographics and incidence from the 2000 kids' inpatient database. J Pediatr Orthop. 2007;27(4):421–6.
15. Henderson RC, Lin PP, Greene WB. Bone-mineral density in children and adolescents who have spastic cerebral palsy. J Bone Joint Surg Am. 1995;77(11):1671–81.
16. Tortolani PJ, McCarthy EF, Sponseller PD. Bone mineral density deficiency in children. J Am Acad Orthop Surg. 2002;10(1):57–66.
17. Clarke NM, Page JE. Vitamin D deficiency: a paediatric orthopaedic perspective. Curr Opin Pediatr. 2012;24(1):46–9.
18. Schilling S, et al. Vitamin D status in abused and nonabused children younger than 2 years old with fractures. Pediatrics. 2011;127(5):835–41.
19. Shorr RM, Chesney RW. Rickets: part II. Pediatr Radiol. 2013;43:152–72.
20. Sillence D, Senn A, Danks D. Genetic heterogeneity in osteogenesis imperfecta. J Med Genet. 1979;16:101–6.
21. Biggin A, Munns CF. Osteogenesis imperfecta: diagnosis and treatment. Curr Osteoporos Rep. 2014;12(3):279–88.
22. Semler O, Cheung MS, Glorieux FH, Rauch F. Wormian bones in osteogenesis imperfecta: correlation to clinical findings and genotype. Am J Med Genet A. 2010;152A(7):1681–7.
23. Marlowe A, Pepin MG, Byers PH. Testing for osteogenesis imperfecta in cases of suspected non-accidental injury. J Med Gen. 2002;39:382–6.
24. Pepin MG, Byers PH. What every clinical geneticist should know about testing for osteogenesis imperfecta in suspected child abuse cases. Am J Med Genet C Semin Med Genet. 2015. doi:10.1002/ajmg.c.31459.

25. Johnston Jr CC, Epstein S. Clinical, biochemical, radiographic, epidemiologic, and economic features of osteoporosis. Orthop Clin North Am. 1981;12(3):559–69.
26. Paterson CR, Mole PA. Bone density in osteogenesis imperfecta may well be normal. Postgrad Med J. 1994;70:104–7.
27. Davie M, Haddaway M. Bone mineral content and density in healthy subjects and in osteogenesis imperfecta. Arch Dis Child. 1994;70:331–4.
28. Glorieux F, Lanoue G, Chabot G, Travers R. Bone mineral density in osteogenesis imperfecta. J Bone Min Res. 1994;9:225.
29. Zionts LE, Nash JP, Rude R, Ross T, Stott NS. Bone mineral density in children with mild osteogenesis imperfecta. J Bone Joint Surg Br. 1995;77B:143–7.
30. Cepollaro C, Gonnelli S, Pondrelli C, Montagnani A, Martini S, Bruni D, Gennari C. Osteogenesis imperfecta: bone turnover, bone density, and ultrasound parameters. Calcif Tissue Int. 1999;65:129–32.
31. Rauch F, Lalic L, Roughley P, Glorieux FH. Relationship between genotype and skeletal phenotype in children and adolescents with osteogenesis imperfecta. J Bone Miner Res. 2010;25(6):1367–74.
32. Lund AM, Mølgaard C, Muller J, Skovby F. Bone mineral content and collagen defects in osteogenesis imperfecta. Acta Pædiatr. 1999;88:1083–8.
33. Mølgaard C, Thomsen BL, Prentice A, Cole TJ, Michaelsen KF. Whole body bone mineral content in healthy children and adolescents. Arch Dis Child. 1997;76:9–15.
34. Miller ME, Hangartner TN. Bone density measurements by computed tomography in osteogenesis imperfecta-type 1. Osteoporos Int. 1999;9:427–32.
35. Bishop NJ, Plotkin H, Lanoue G, Chabot G, Glorieux FH. When is a fracture child abuse? Bone. 23(5):F198 (abstract).
36. Brunner R, Doderlein L. Pathological fractures in patients with cerebral palsy. J Pediatr Orthop B. 1996;5:232–8.
37. Leet AI, Mesfin A, Pichard C, Launay F, Brintzenhofeszoc K, Levey EB, Sponseller DP. Fractures in children with cerebral palsy. J Pediatr Orthop. 2006;26:624–7.
38. Presedo A, Dabney KW, Miller F. Fractures in patients with cerebral palsy. J Pediatr Orthop. 2007;27:147–53.
39. Mughal MZ. Fractures in children with cerebral palsy. Curr Osteoporos Rep. 2014;12(3):313–8.
40. Lingham S, Joester J. Spontaneous fractures in children and adolescents with cerebral palsy. BMJ. 1994;309:265.
41. Mergler S, Evenhuis HM, Boot AM, De Man SA, Bindels-De Heus KG, Huijbers WA, Penning C. Epidemiology of low bone mineral density and fractures in children with severe cerebral palsy: a systematic review. Dev Med Child Neurol. 2009;51:773–8.
42. Harcke HT, Taylor A, Bachrach S, Miller F, Henderson RC. Lateral femoral scan: an alternative method for assessing bone mineral density in children with cerebral palsy. Pediatr Radiol. 1998;28:241–6.
43. Henderson RC, Lark RK, Newman JE, Kecskemthy H, Fung EB, Renner JB, Harcke HT. Pediatric reference data for dual X-ray absorptiometric measures of normal bone density in the distal femur. Am J Radiol. 2002;178:439–43.
44. Zemel BS, Stallings VA, Leonard MB, Paulhamus DR, Kecskemethy HH, Harcke HT, Henderson RC. Revised pediatric reference data for the lateral distal femur measured by Hologic Discovery/Delphi dual-energy X-ray absorptiometry. J Clin Densitom. 2009;12(2):207–18.
45. Bianchi ML, Leonard MB, Bechtold S, Högler W, Mughal MZ, Schönau E, Sylvester FA, Vogiatzi M, van den Heuvel-Eibrink MM, Ward L. Bone health in children and adolescents with chronic diseases that may affect the skeleton: the 2013 ISCD Pediatric Official Positions. J Clin Densitom. 2014;17(2):281–94.
46. Henderson RC, Berglund LM, May R, Zemel BS, Grossberg RI, Johnson J, Plotkin H, Stevenson RD, Szalay E, Wong B, Kecskemethy HH, Harcke HT. The relationship between fractures and DXA measures of BMD in the distal femur of children and adolescents with cerebral palsy or muscular dystrophy. J Bone Miner Res. 2010;25(3):520–6.

47. Henderson RC, Lark RK, Kecskemethy HH, Miller F, Harcke HT, Bachrach SJ. Bisphosphonates to treat osteopenia in children with quadriplegic cerebral palsy: a randomized, placebo-controlled clinical trial. J Pediatr. 2002;141:644–65.
48. Bachrach SJ, Kecskemethy HH, Harcke HT, Lark RK, Miller F, Henderson RC. Pamidronate treatment and posttreatment bone density in children with spastic quadriplegic cerebral palsy. J Clin Densitom. 2006;9:167–74.
49. Bushby K, Finkel R, Birnkrant DJ, Case LE, Clemens PR, Cripe L, Kaul A, Kinnett K, McDonald C, Pandya S, Poysky J, Shapiro F, Tomezsko J, Constantin C, DMD Care Considerations Working Group. Diagnosis and management of Duchenne muscular dystrophy, part 1: diagnosis, and pharmacological and psychosocial management. Lancet Neurol. 2010;9(1):77–93.
50. Moxley 3rd RT, Pandya S. Weekend high-dosage prednisone: a new option for treatment of Duchenne muscular dystrophy. Neurology. 2011;77(5):416–7.
51. Larson CM, Henderson RC. Bone mineral density and fractures in boys with Duchenne muscular dystrophy. J Pediatr Orthop. 2000;20:71–4.
52. Bianchi ML, Mazzanti A, Galbiati E, Saraifoger S, Dubini A, Cornelio F, Morandi L. Bone mineral density and bone metabolism in Duchenne muscular dystrophy. Osteoporos Int. 2003;14:761–7.
53. Crabtree NJ, Roper H, McMurchie H, Shaw NJ. Regional changes in bone area and bone mineral content in boys with Duchenne muscular dystrophy receiving corticosteroid therapy. J Pediatr. 2010;156(3):450–5.
54. Cox JJ, Reimann F, Nicholas AK, et al. An SCN9A channelopathy causes congenital inability to experience pain. Nature. 2006;444:894–8.
55. Bar-On E, Weigl D, Parvari R, et al. Congenital insensitivity to pain: orthopaedic manifestations. J Bone Joint Surg (Br). 2002;84:252–7.
56. Leipold E, Liebmann L, Korenke GC, et al. A de novo gain-of-function mutation in SCN11A causes loss of pain perception. Nat Genet. 2013;45:1399–404.
57. Mardy S, Miura Y, Endo F, Matsuda I, Sztriha L, Frossard P, et al. Congenital insensitivity to pain with anhidrosis: novel mutations in the TRKA (NTRK1) gene encoding a high-affinity receptor for nerve growth factor. Am J Hum Genet. 1999;64:1570–9.

# Chapter 13
# What's Next in the Field of Bone Health in Pediatrics? Research Considerations

Sharmila Majumdar, Tony M. Keavney, Luis Del Rio, Oliver Semler, and Renaud Winzenrieth

## Introduction

The first 12 chapters of this 2nd edition have provided a thorough overview of the current uses of dual-energy X-ray absorptiometry (DXA) in children and adolescents. The purpose of this final chapter is to offer a glimpse into future research areas in which significant advances in bone densitometry are likely to be forthcoming over the next 5–10 years. These novel research techniques will likely improve our understanding of pediatric bone metabolism.

As has been described in detail in the previous chapters, there continues to be a shortage of data on the relationship between BMC or aBMD and fracture risk in the

S. Majumdar, Ph.D. (✉)
Radiology and Biomedical Imaging, University of California San Francisco,
1700 4th Street, 203 D Byers Hall, San Francisco, CA 94502, USA
e-mail: sharmila.majumdar@ucsf.edu

T.M. Keavney, Ph.D.
Mechanical Engineering and Bioengineering, University of California,
5140 Etcheverry Hall, MC 1740, Berkeley, CA 94720-1740, USA
e-mail: tonykeaveny@berkeley.edu

L. Del Rio, M.D., C.C.D.
Department of Bone Densitometry, Hospital Sant Joan De Deu,
Londres 6, Passeig De Sant Joan De Deu, 2, Esplugues de Llobregat, Barcelona 08029, Spain
e-mail: ldelrio@cetir.es

O. Semler, M.D.
Department of Rare Skeletal Disease, Children's Hospital, University of Cologne,
Kerpenerstr. 62, Cologne 50931, Germany
e-mail: joerg.semler@ukkoeln.de

R. Winzenrieth, Ph.D.
Research and Development Department, Medimaps SASU,
5 Avenue Henri Becquerel, Merignac, France
e-mail: rwinzenrieth@medimapsgroup.com

© Springer International Publishing Switzerland 2016
E.B. Fung et al. (eds.), *Bone Health Assessment in Pediatrics*,
DOI 10.1007/978-3-319-30412-0_13

very young. The incidence and type of pediatric fractures vary according to sex, age, and skeletal region. From childhood to adolescence, there is an increased fracture rate, with the highest incidence coinciding with the peak of height velocity. Although theories have been postulated regarding the relationship between fractures and the practice of high-risk activities, an explanation for this higher rate of fractures in the peri-pubertal period can be justified by the imbalance between the growth rates among the height and bone acquisition. A more accurate accounting of bone strength would be useful in pediatrics particularly for those with chronic conditions.

Though aBMD by DXA is a surrogate variable for bone strength, it does not capture all parameters determining bone fracture risk. Biomechanical bone strength depends largely on bone mineral density but other factors also participate such as bone geometry, thickness of the cortical bone and microarchitecture of the trabecular bone [1]. aBMD measurements report the integrated bone mineral density (cortical + trabecular) and it is not possible to discern if a disease or therapeutic treatment predominantly affects a type of bone or the other. There is increasing information on bone microarchitecture in pediatric populations obtained in peripheral regions with pQCT [2, 3], but for the moment there is little information on the microstructural involvement in regions of the central skeleton in childhood in therapeutic interventions or illness.

Radiological techniques that potentially allow the evaluation of bone microarchitecture in the central and peripheral skeleton include Magnetic Resonance Imaging (MRI), Finite Element Analysis from High Resolution Peripheral Quantitative Computed Tomography (HRpQCT) and Trabecular Bone Score from DXA. Each technique has its own benefits and limitations in children and adolescents. The basis of MRI was discussed in chapter two, but will be expanded in this chapter to the current areas of research for the pediatric patient, and what we are to expect in the future. Finite Element Analysis (FEA) from Computed Tomography scans has been in development for over two decades in academia, but is now in use in some specialized institutions as a "virtual stress test." Trabecular Bone Score (TBS) is now commonly used as an additional predictor of fracture in adults. Given the increased availability of the software for all of these new tools, it is anticipated that these will be used more frequently in the coming years. The utility of these powerful tools will be described in detail herein, and their potential use for pediatric applications.

## *Magnetic Resonance Imaging (MRI)*

Magnetic resonance imaging (MRI) is a noninvasive three-dimensional imaging technique that does not require the use of ionizing radiation and thus is an attractive modality for acquiring high-resolution images of cortical and trabecular bone in vivo. Unlike X-ray imaging, MRI uses the stimulation and subsequent emission of nonionizing electromagnetic radiation of low energy ($10^{-8}$–$10^{-6}$ eV) by biological tissue. Soft tissue consists of approximately 60–80 % of water and the nucleus imaged in MRI is the hydrogen nucleus (proton).

For MR imaging, the subject is placed in a magnet, the main magnetic field provides a strong, constant static magnetic field (B0) that can be up to several thousand times stronger than the earth's magnetic field, and today ranges from 1.5 to 7 T for human whole body imaging. In MRI the protons being imaged interact with the main magnetic field and are aligned to the main magnetic field, the MR signal is produced by applying a radiofrequency (rf) pulse (using a transmit coil) which creates a perturbation, after which the response of the nuclei then produce an electromagnetic signal that can be detected by rf (receiver) coils. After an initial perturbation, the nuclei tend to return to their equilibrium position, and in doing so interact with the surrounding environment and with each other giving rise to different contrast in the acquired MR images. Details of MR imaging methods and contrast may be studied from these references [4].

In conventional MRI, there is low abundance of hydrogen nuclei in mineralized bone, furthermore due to the solid nature of the tissue, the protons in bone have a very short T2 relaxation characteristic [5]. This leads to a total loss of signal, or negative signal from bone. Bone marrow on the other hand consists of more mobile and a higher abundance of protons and thus produces the high signal intensity in MR images. Trabecular and cortical bone in conventional MRI are thus dark, and the structure is revealed against the high intensity marrow and other soft tissues.

## Trabecular Bone MRI

The main challenge for the accurate depiction of the trabecular microstructure as needed for morphological analysis is the need for high spatial resolution achieved by the modality. The spatial resolution currently achievable with MRI in a clinically feasible scan time is in the order of the trabecular thickness (100–150 μm) or above. Representative images depicting trabecular bone structure in the radius, tibia, and femur are shown in Fig. 13.1a–c.

## Cortical Bone MRI

Cortical bone MRI, especially for the estimation of cortical thickness for the proximal femur, may ensure greater accuracy since the image plane can be oriented perpendicular to the neck [6]. Using advanced MRI methods with ultra short echo times (UTE), the bone water content in the microscopic pores of the haversian and the lacunocanalicular systems of cortical bone can be quantified. They contain approximately 20 % water by volume [7, 8]. A smaller water fraction is also bound to collagen and the matrix substrate and imbedded in the crystal structure of the mineral [9]. These micro pores maybe difficult to visualize due to their size compared to the spatial resolution of the images, but the quantification of bone water using MRI could potentially provide a surrogate measure of bone porosity without resolving these individual small pores.

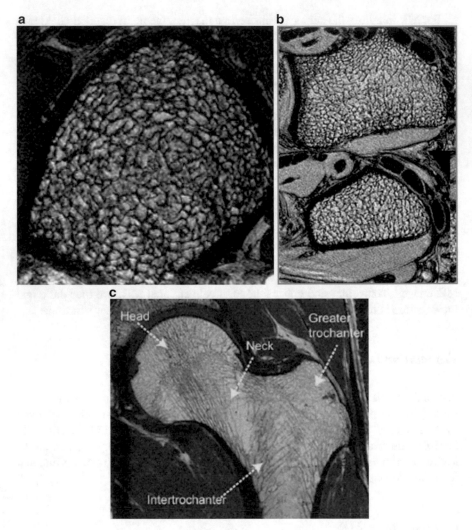

**Fig. 13.1** High-resolution MR image showing bright bone marrow, dark cortical bone, and trabecular bone (**a**) Tibia (**b**) radius and (**c**) Proximal femur

## Image Analysis

Image analysis of trabecular bone images in MRI involves the selection of initial separate regions of interest consisting of trabecular bone and cortical bone, followed by corrections of spatial signal homogeneity corrections, if needed, and image separation into a bone and a marrow phase. Following this, a number of characteristics of the trabecular and cortical bone structures may be derived. If the MRI images are generated from longitudinal studies over time, the subsequent images may require serial image registration [10]. Image analysis techniques to segment both the inner and outer cortical boundary from their surroundings are commonly semi-automatic. A software algorithm featuring a deformable contour (snake) to conform to the strongest gradient edges in the neighborhood of the manually placed cortical bone region of interest has been used [11]. Another method used for image analysis is the distance transform method [12] where the measurements of cortical thickness are further improved by fitting a sphere into the segmented cortical shell. Thickness measurements from MR data have been compared with HR-pQCT, and while significant correlations were found, the values for the MRI measures were higher [13].

For the assessment of structural information of trabecular bone, three classes of parameters can be defined including scale, topology, and orientation [14, 15]. Scale describes the amount of bone in a region of interest (ROI) and the thickness of the trabeculae or the spacing between the trabeculae. Investigating the plate- or rod-like structure of the network assesses the bone topology. And finally the anisotropic character of the structure defines its orientation. Early assessments of trabecular bone applying the principles of stereology are based on scale [16]. In MRI, trabecular thickness can be obtained from the mean intercept length (MIL) of parallel test lines across the ROI averaged over multiple angles [17, 18]. From MIL and BV/TV measurements, trabecular thickness (TbTh), trabecular spacing (TbSp), and trabecular number (TbN) can be obtained [19]. These measures are usually called "apparent" parameters because of the limited spatial in vivo resolution of MRI. These measurements are usually conducted on a slice-by-slice basis. Other approaches have been proposed such as 3D wavelets analysis [20], fuzzy distance transform [21] have also been proposed.

Describing bone structure through bone topology is useful for osteoporotic bone loss which results in a fenestration of trabecular plates and a conversion from plate to a more rod like bone structure [16, 22–24]. Methods for assessing trabecular bone connectivity and digital topological analysis (DTA) have also been suggested [25, 26]. The technique was successfully applied to trabecular bone topology [27, 28] and enhanced the prediction of mechanical properties and bone strength [29]. A more recent technique provides a complete assessment of scale, topology, and anisotropy using geodesic topological analysis (GTA) [30].

## Applications

The developments over the past few years have made quantitative MRI of bone clinically practical [27, 31–41]. A substantial improvement in fracture discrimination by including structural information in addition to bone mineral density (BMD) has been well established [36–38]. The effect of salmon calcitonin on bone structure was investigated using MRI at the distal radius and calcaneous of 91 postmenopausal women over a period of 2 years [42]. The treatment group showed improved trabecular structure compared to the placebo group but no significant change in BMD was detected. Topological changes of the trabecular bone network after menopause and the protective effect of estradiol were reported by Wehrli and colleagues in 2008 [43]. The effect of testosterone replacement on trabecular architecture in hypogonadal men was investigated in the distal tibial metaphysis of 10 severely testosterone-deficient hypogonadal men [32]. A subvolume of each MR image was converted to a finite element model. No significant changes in estimated elastic moduli and morphological parameters were detected in the eugonadal group over 24 months but a significant increase in four estimated elastic moduli was found in hypogonadal men. These increases were accompanied by significant increases in trabecular plate thickness.

In a pediatric population of 40, 6–12-year-old subjects, high-resolution magnetic resonance images were collected immediately above the growth plate in the distal femur [44]. Measures of trabecular bone microarchitecture [i.e., apparent trabecular bone volume to total volume (appBV/TV), trabecular number (appTb.N), and trabecular separation (appTb.Sp)] showed strong correlations with the distance from the growth plate reflecting the spatial heterogeneity of trabecular bone (Fig. 13.2) [45]. Gender differences were not found in MRI-based measures of trabecular bone microarchitecture, consistent with the BMD measures by DXA at the distal femur [45]. MR derived measures were moderately to strongly related to aBMD and BMC. In a separate study, Modlesky et al observed children with cerebral palsy had

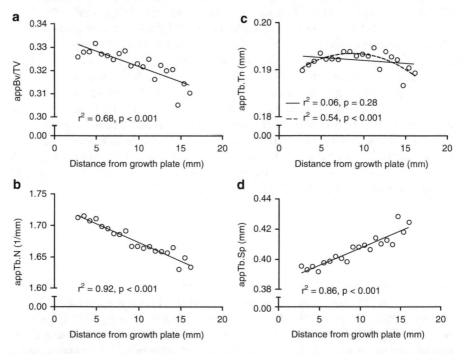

**Fig. 13.2** The pattern of trabecular bone microarchitecture in the distal femur of typically developing children and its effect on processing of magnetic resonance images, Christopher M. Modlesky, Daniel G. Whitney, Patrick T. Carter, Brianne M. Allerton, Joshua T. Kirby, Freeman Miller, Bone 2014

a 30 % lower appBV/TV, a 21 % lower appTb.N, a 12 % lower appTb.Th and a 48 % higher appTb.Sp in the distal femur than controls ($n = 10$/group; $p < 0.001$) [46]. The short-term reliability of the trabecular bone microarchitecture measures was very good, with coefficients of variation ranging from 2.0 to 3.0 % in children with CP ($n = 6$) and 1.8–3.5 % in controls ($n = 6$).

In a study investigating the cortical thickness of 41 postmenopausal osteopenic women and 22 postmenopausal osteoporotic women with spine fractures, significant changes in the cortical thickness between the two groups were found underlying the importance of morphologic measurements of the cortical bone structure [11]. In 2009, images of the distal radius and the distal tibia of 49 postmenopausal osteopenic women (age $56 \pm 3.7$) were acquired with both HR-pQCT and MRI [47]. It was found that the amount of cortical porosity did not vary greatly between subjects but the type of cortical pore containing marrow versus not containing marrow, varied highly between subjects. Additionally, the number of cortical pores containing marrow did not depend on the amount of porosity and there was no relationship between cortical pore size and the presence of bone marrow. The data suggest that cortical pore spaces contain different components and that there may be more than one mechanism for the development of cortical porosity and more than one type of bone fluid present in cortical pores. However, this approach only captures relatively large cortical pores, which can be visualized within the resolution limits of MRI.

In a recent study measurements in vivo revealed that the bone water content was increased 65 % in the postmenopausal group compared to the premenopausal group [41]. Patients with renal osteodystrophy had 135 % higher bone water content than the premenopausal group whereas conventional BMD measurements showed an opposite behavior, with much smaller group differences.

In a study with non-Hispanic white adolescent females ($N = 24$; 18–19 years of age), two bone-specific retrospective physical activity loading tools were used, the Bone Loading History Questionnaire (BLHQ) and the Bone-Specific Physical Activity Questionnaire (BPAQ), along with a 7 day physical activity recall to assess energy expenditure. Hip BLHQ scores were correlated with mid-tibia cortical volume assessed by MRI ($r = 0.43$; $p = 0.03$) [48]. Adjusted hip and spine BLHQ scores were correlated with all mid-tibia cortical measures ($r = 0.50$–$0.58$; $p < 0.05$) and distal radius apparent trabecular number ($r = 0.46$–$0.53$; $p < 0.05$). BPAQ scores were correlated with all mid-tibia cortical ($r = 0.41$–$0.51$; $p < 0.05$). These data demonstrated that greater load-specific physical activity scores, but not energy expenditure, are indicative of greater mid-tibia cortical bone quality.

## Conclusion

MR imaging is a noninvasive method for three-dimensional imaging of both trabecular and cortical bone, and can be used for assessing skeletal growth, metabolic diseases, and other bone-related diseases in a pediatric population. The added advantage of being nonionizing and the potential for characterizing muscle, bone marrow as well as body fat makes this an exciting tool for the pediatric musculo-skeletal system.

## *Finite Element Analysis*

Finite element analysis of patient computed tomography (CT) scans has been in development in academia for over 25 years [49–55] and is now becoming available clinically for assessing fracture risk and monitoring treatment. This analysis technique combines medical image processing of CT scans, bone biomechanics, and the engineering finite element analysis technique [56] to provide a "virtual stress test" [53] of a bone under a prescribed set of external forces. The primary outcome of the analysis is an estimate of the breaking strength, in units of force (i.e. Newtons) of a patient's whole bone or portion thereof, e.g. a vertebral body, proximal femur, or distal radius or tibia.

When analyzing a CT scan with finite element analysis, measures of volumetric bone mineral density (BMD, in $mg/cm^3$) can also be provided, as well as measures of DXA-equivalent areal BMD (in $g/cm^2$) and the associated T-scores [53, 57–61]. By combining measures of both BMD and bone strength, the overall analysis provides a comprehensive noninvasive assessment of bone competence, and can be applied as an "add-on" analysis to previously taken clinical CT scans that are originally ordered for some other nonbone indication, such as a gastroenterology exam [58].

In a research setting, finite element analysis has been used in a number of clinical studies to longitudinally monitor changes in bone strength in response to various therapeutic treatments. By altering the finite element structural models in a controlled fashion, for example, by virtually removing an outer layer of bone or by averaging out the spatial distribution of bone mineral density within the boundaries of the bone—the analysis can also provide measures of bone strength associated with changes in just the cortical bone, the trabecular bone, or the external bone geometry, all of which can provide unique insight into changes related to growth, aging, disease, and treatment [62–64].

This review summarizes some of the key principles involved in finite element analysis of bones from CT scans of live people and its application to pediatric patients. For more detail on the overall approach, the reader is referred to several reviews [53, 54, 57, 65, 66].

## Resolution Effects: The Different Types of Finite Element Analyses

In general, there are three different types of finite element models that can be generated from CT scans, depending on the spatial resolution of the CT scan that is used as input to the analysis. Starting at the highest spatial resolution, using images from a highly specialized "micro-CT" scanner as input, one can generate finite element models having a spatial resolution as low as 20 μm [67]. Such high-resolution models can only be generated for small specimens of cadaver bone and thus this type of finite element analysis is not applicable to clinical studies on live people (and will not be reviewed further in this chapter). However, one relevant result to the current discussion is that the models can predict strength very well, with $R^2$ values of at least 0.85 at both the hip and spine [68, 69]. Since those models do not contain any features at a resolution of less than about 20 µm, variations in any patient-specific factors at that scale or below—for example, bone tissue material properties, collagen cross-linking, damage, or geometric features of lacunae or the remodeling space—do not appear to play any appreciable role in the overall whole-bone strength. That is, at least for these cadaver studies. Clearly, certain disease states or perhaps other factors may alter these lower-scale properties and affect overall bone strength. But it appears otherwise that typical patient-specific variations in these low-scale features may have little influence on overall whole-bone strength.

At a slightly lower resolution, models having a resolution on the order of 100 µm can be generated from "high-resolution peripheral quantitative CT" (HR-pQCT) scanners [65]. These are also specialized types of CT scanners but they are clinically available at some medical centers. While these types of finite element models can include patient-specific descriptions of the trabecular microarchitecture, cortical thickness, and even cortical vascular porosity, because of constraints on the size of a body part that can be scanned, the input scans can only be obtained for the extremities in live humans, most commonly at the distal radius and tibia. Because of the relatively low radiation exposure associated with HR-pQCT scans, these types of finite element analyses have now been used in a number of clinical research studies in pediatric research applications.

At the lowest level of resolution, one can generate finite element models from clinical CT scanners, having a spatial resolution on the order of 1 mm. These models typically cannot provide explicit descriptions of the trabecular microarchitecture, nor of the cortical porosity, and do not have sufficient resolution to accurately capture the cortices where they are thin (<0.5 mm), such as in the vertebral body and in portions of the proximal femur [70]. Even so, because these types of finite element models can be generated for any part of the body—particularly the hip and spine—and because they capture both the three-dimensional shape of a whole bone and its internal spatial distribution of bone mineral density, and because they have been in development for so long [51], they have found the most widespread use so far in research studies in adults and are the only types of finite element models currently approved by FDA for clinical diagnostic purposes. However, partly because of concerns about radiation exposure associated with clinical CT scanning of the hip or spine regions in growing children, these types of finite element analyses have not been utilized much in pediatric research applications.

In all three types of finite element analyses, the same general "voxel-conversion" technique is typically used to generate a patient-specific model of a whole bone, or portion thereof, from the CT scan. In this technique, the attenuation of the input CT scan is calibrated into units of bone mineral density and then each image voxel (i.e. 3D equivalent of a pixel) is converted directly into a box-shaped finite element, perhaps with some resampling if the desired size of the finite element differs from the image voxels. The images are then registered into a common coordinate system to enable virtual forces to be applied in a standardized fashion. Finally, mechanical properties of the bone tissue are assigned to the individual finite elements based on

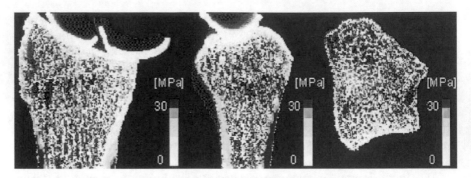

**Fig. 13.3** Example of patient-specific finite element models generated by the commonly used voxel-conversion technique. A model of the distal radius generated from a HR-pQCT scan, the colors depicting different levels of stress within the bone tissue. Taken with permission from: Pistoia W. et al. Estimation of distal radius failure load with micro-finite element analysis models based on three-dimensional peripheral quantitative computed tomography images. *Bone*, 30:842–8, 2002

the calibrated BMD values of the individual voxels. Precisely how this last step is done depends on the spatial resolution of the CT scan and what assumptions are made about the mechanical behavior of the bone tissue, and what relation is used to map the calibrated BMD for each finite element into mechanical properties, all of which can differ at different anatomic sites and with different software implementations of the finite element analysis. The result is a "voxel-based" finite element model (Fig. 13.3), which can be generated in a highly automated fashion due to the direct approach of converting image voxels into finite elements. While more complex methods can be used to process the images and create the finite elements [71], this voxel-conversion approach is currently the most widely used approach for patient-specific analysis and is discussed further below for use with HR-pQCT and clinical CT scans.

## Finite Element Analysis Utilizing HR-pQCT Scans

HR-pQCT scans are typically acquired for the peripheral skeleton, for example, the distal radius and/or tibia. These images currently have a spatial resolution of about 80 µm. In the process of converting image voxels to finite elements, the bone is virtually separated from the marrow space, resulting in a finite element model that contains only bone elements. Thus, the microstructure and pore spaces are explicitly captured with this approach (Fig. 13.4), although the resolution is not ideal since individual trabeculae have a thickness on the order of the element size and thus substantial volume-averaging can occur at all bone-marrow interfaces. Despite this limitation, a number of cadaver studies have demonstrated that the technique can provide good correlations ($R^2 = 0.66$–$0.97$) between its predicted strength of the

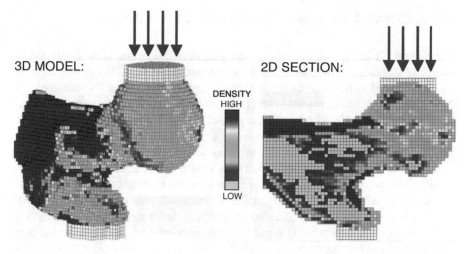

**Fig. 13.4** Example of a patient specific finite element models generated by the commonly used voxel-conversion technique. A model of the proximal femur generated from a clinical CT scan, the colors depicting the local values of BMD of each voxel. Taken from, with permission: Keaveny TM, McClung MR, Xiaohai W, Kopperdahl DL, Mitlak BH, Krohn K: Femoral strength in osteoporotic women treated with teriparatide or alendronate. *Bone*, 50:165–70, 2012

distal radius during a simulated fall on the outstretched hand and the strength as measured by direct mechanical testing [55, 72–75], and these correlations are typically higher than those provided by any BMD measures [66].

Clinical validation studies show more mixed results, especially when compared to BMD as measured by DXA [66]. In a series of studies that assessed distal radius fractures in postmenopausal women, the odds ratios for finite element analysis and DXA-BMD (at the wrist) were both statistically significant but were similar to each other [74, 76, 77]. When assessing any type of osteoporotic (prevalent) fracture, odds ratios for finite element analysis and DXA-BMD (at the wrist) again were both statistically significant but were either similar to each other or trending (but not statistically significant) higher for finite element analysis [78–80]. Some results suggest that the finite element analysis performs slightly better when used at the distal tibia, and there may be advantages to developing predictive algorithms that combine together various different outcomes from the finite element analysis [74, 80]. No prospective incident-fracture outcome validation studies have yet been reported and thus this represents an important topic for future research. Due in part to the limited availability of HR-pQCT scanners, and since this analysis technique cannot be used to assess changes at the hip or spine in live humans, these types of finite element models have so far found relatively limited use in clinical research studies in adults for assessing treatment effects [81–87]. Even so, the technique does provide unique insight into biomechanical consequences of any treatment-related changes in bone microstructure and has been validated for assessing treatment-related changes in strength in a large animal model [88].

## Finite Element Analysis Utilizing Clinical CT Scans

For clinical CT scans, central sites can be imaged and the sites of most interest for assessment of osteoporosis are the proximal femur and vertebral body, which can be rapidly scanned with minimal motion artifact using contemporary CT scanners. The typical resolution of the resulting images is about 1–2 mm. Thus, in these types of finite element analyses, the bone tissue and marrow are volume-averaged at that scale, so that the models do not include any explicit descriptions of the microstructure or porosity. Instead, the porosity of the bone is represented by intra-bone variations in the levels of bone mineral density throughout the bone, and any real presence of blood or marrow is accounted for by calibrating the attenuation values to units of attenuation-equivalent BMD. Despite these limitations, this type of finite element analysis has also been well validated in cadaver studies and clinical studies. For example, cadaver experiments from multiple research groups have consistently shown good predictions of experimentally measured femoral strength ($R^2 = 0.75$–$0.96$) [50, 89–96] and vertebral strength ($R^2 = 0.75$–$0.96$) [49, 97–101].

Clinical validation studies have consistently shown that prevalent vertebral fractures [51, 64, 102–104] and new (incident) vertebral [61, 97] and hip [60, 61, 105] fractures, in women and men, are highly associated with finite element-estimated strength and almost always more so than DXA-measured BMD. Prospective fracture-outcome studies have also demonstrated that finite element analysis-derived measures of vertebral and hip strength provide additional diagnostic information beyond BMD by identifying patients without osteoporosis who have "fragile bone strength," that is, low levels of vertebral or hip strength that place them at a high a risk of a new vertebral or hip fracture as a patient with BMD-defined osteoporosis [58, 61]. Because clinical CT scanners are so widely available, and because of the keen interest in evaluating therapeutic-related changes in bone strength at the hip and spine in older adults, these types of finite element models have been quite widely used in clinical research studies in adults to assess longitudinal changes in bone strength in response to various osteoporosis therapeutic treatments [63, 103, 106–118].

Since the same CT scans used for finite element analysis can also be used to measure a DXA-equivalent BMD T-score at the hip, [53, 57–61], and a vertebral trabecular BMD at the spine [61, 119, 120], these types of quantitative analysis of CT scans provide measures of both BMD and bone strength, resulting in a more comprehensive clinical assessment of bone quality than one based on BMD alone.

## Pediatric Applications

In general, finite element analysis has been applied to a wide variety of pediatric applications, ranging from injury criteria for trauma and motor vehicle accidents, to surgical planning, to the study of etiological factors in various topics related to growth and development. Examples of patient-specific analyses (Table 13.1) as applied to the biomechanics of growth and development include studies on athletes,

**Table 13.1** Some literature studies from 2013 to 2015 that have utilized some form of computed tomography (CT) or other medical imaging to generate patient-specific finite element models for pediatric applications

| Study | General topic | Number subjects | Age range (years) | Type of input image | Analysis site |
|---|---|---|---|---|---|
| Ackerman [123] | G&D: athletes | 175 | 14–25 | HR-pQCT | Distal radius Distal tibia |
| Caouette [124] | Surgical planning | 1 | 7 | X-rays | Tibia |
| Chevalley [125] | G&D: genetics | 176 | 14–17[a] | HR-pQCT | Distal tibia |
| Faje [122] | G&D: anorexia | 44 | 14–22 | HR-pQCT | Distal radius |
| Farr [121] | G&D: obesity | 198 | 8–15 | HR-pQCT | Distal radius Distal tibia |
| Farr [126] | G&D: fracture etiology | 223 | 8–15 | HR-pQCT | Distal radius Distal tibia |
| Gabel [127] | G&D: activity levels | 328 | 9–20 | HR-pQCT | Distal tibia |
| Li [128] | G&D: reference values | 15 | 0–3 Months | QCT | Femur |
| Singhal [129] | G&D: hormones | 50 | 14–21[b] | HR-pQCT | Distal radius |

*G&D* growth and development, *HR-pQCT* high-resolution peripheral quantitative CT, *QCT* quantitative CT
[a]Estimated from the reported mean (±SD) of 15.2±0.5 years
[b]Age range was reported for their full cohort of $n=85$; finite element analysis was only performed on $n=50$

anorexia, genetics, hormonal influences, activity levels, and fracture etiology. Mostly, HR-pQCT is the scanning method of choice, although some patient-specific analyses have utilized X-rays (multiplanar) and clinical (quantitative) CT scans.

These finite element studies have provided unique insight into fracture etiology. For example, in a study of 198 boys and girls ages 8–15 [121], results suggested that fat mass may have a different adaptive influence on whole-bone strength at weight-bearing (e.g. distal tibia) compared to non-weight-bearing (e.g. distal radius) sites. This in turn leads to relatively weak bones at the distal radius in relation to body mass in obese children—which would explain why obese children are at higher risk of fall-related wrist fractures. In a study of anorexia involving 44 adolescent girls [122], distal radius bone strength from finite element analysis was significantly lower in girls with anorexia than in a group of control girls without anorexia, even after controlling for distal radius BMD as measured by DXA. The underlying mechanisms were due in part to alterations of both the cortical and trabecular microarchitecture, including a lower cortical area.

Given the relative novelty of patient-specific finite element analysis for pediatric applications, and the continuing improvement of CT scanning technology in terms of delivering higher quality images at lower radiation doses, it is expected that much new insight will be gained as patient-specific finite element analysis is expanded for pediatric applications.

## *Trabecular Bone Score*

For the last 10 years, a new technique appears able to evaluate bone texture at the spine using conventional DXA acquisitions: the Trabecular Bone Score (TBS) [130–132]. Although widely used in adults, TBS (TBS iNsight, Medimaps SASU, Mérignac, France) could be a promising tool to assess bone microarchitectural texture in pediatrics. TBS demonstrates several advantages over other microstructure assessment tools (CT, HR-pQCT, or MRI). Among them, TBS requires no additional acquisition time or radiation exposure since it is calculated using the same DXA acquisition as used for areal Bone Mineral Density (aBMD). It is evaluated at axial skeleton (PA spine) and it is an easy-to-use tool since it is fully automatic and integrated in the standard DXA workflow.

## TBS: Mathematical Framework

TBS is a texture parameter related to the fractional Brownian motion (fBm) approach [133]. It is an estimator of the generalized Hurst exponent (Hq) which characterizes what type of process the fBm is. Hq is related to the global behavior of the spatial data (for instance, from the pixel distribution contained in a X-ray image) [134]. Several techniques exist to evaluate Hq [134, 135]. Among them, the variogram is one of the most popular approaches based on variance for the evaluation of the average trend [136]. Hq is calculated at the slope of an interpolated straight line in the log–log system of the variogram [136, 137]. TBS uses a custom version of the variogram approach (Fig. 13.5). Although TBS seems to be an estimator of Hq [136, 137], it is not one, owing to some "black box" differences (patented method and industrial secrets).

A part of TBS algorithm has been originally described by Pothuaud et al. [130] and subsequently enhanced to obtain the actual version of the algorithm [131, 132]. TBS has been designed to analyze images provided by DXA devices. It is evaluated directly from the raw data of the device sensor (i.e. DXA sensor). It characterizes the rate of variation in the gray levels of the 2D projection image and is expressed without units (see Fig. 13.6). Basically, it takes into account gray level amplitudes, the number of these amplitudes and their distributions over the DXA image.

DXA image texture is linked to the texture of the projected bone but also to the acquisition "noise" which is mainly due to the soft tissues above and under the bone in the region of interest. This noise negatively impacts TBS [132], that is, the thicker the soft tissue, the greater the "noise," which lessens TBS. To overcome this effect, a soft tissue correction based on subject's body mass index (BMI), has been implemented and validated for adults.

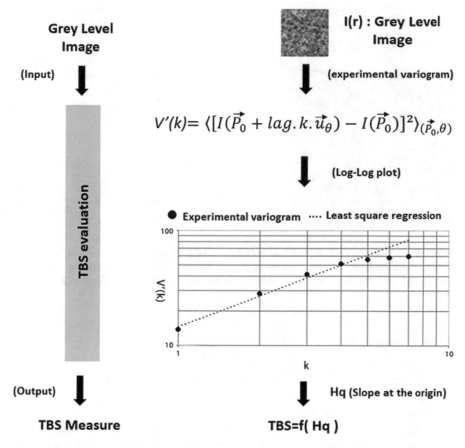

**Fig. 13.5** Explanation of the variogram approach. The generalized Hurst exponent (Hq) is computed, from a gray-level image, as the slope of an interpolated straight line in the log–log system of the variogram. The Trabecular Bone Score (TBS) is derived from Hq

## TBS: A Parameter Evaluating Bone Micro-architectural Texture

TBS is calculated from PA lumbar spine DXA images only. Using such imaging techniques, it is not possible to directly measure classical 3D bone microarchitecture parameters. However, gray level variations—as evaluated on 2D DXA projected images—reflect global variations in X-ray absorption properties in the corresponding 3D tissue microarchitecture. TBS is an indirect evaluation of the 3D structure; i.e. TBS correlates with some 3D bone microarchitecture parameters such as bone volume fraction, trabecular bone number, trabecular separation, connectivity density, and Structure Model Index at vertebrae [131, 132] but also at the radius [138–140] or at iliac crests [141].

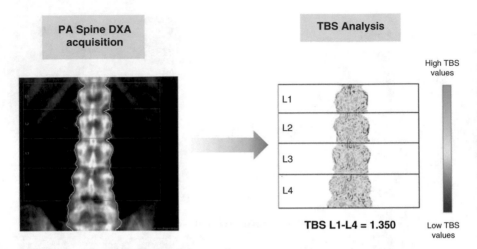

**Fig. 13.6** Example of TBS computation from a PA spine DXA acquisition. A TBS value is calculated for each bone pixel of the considered Region of Interest (L1-L4) and provided as a TBS map. The average TBS value of the selected Region of Interest is also provided. TBS is reported without units

## TBS: Clinical Use

TBS can be evaluated using all available DXA images acquired on Hologic (Delphi™, Discovery™, Horizon™ or QDR4500™ series; Bedford, MA, USA) or GE-Lunar DXA devices (Prodigy™ or iDXA™ series; Madison, WI, USA). TBS is calculated using the same region of interest (ROI) as the aBMD measurement: if a vertebra is excluded from the aBMD evaluation (ex: presence of a fracture), the same vertebra is automatically excluded from the TBS analysis. A TBS value is calculated for each bone pixel of the considered ROI. A TBS value is provided by vertebra composing the ROI (average of the pixel TBS values) as well as the TBS value for the entire ROI (average of the vertebrae TBS values, as presented in Fig. 13.6). TBS is reported without unit. TBS is embedded into TBS iNsight™ software (Medimaps SASU, Mérignac, France) a CE marked and FDA 510 k cleared tool used for clinical purposes in adults.

## TBS: Clinical Validation in Adults

To date, more than 100 articles have been published examining the information gleaned from TBS in adults with osteoporosis [142, 148]. The findings suggest that: (1) TBS is able to predict osteoporotic fracture (osteoporotic hip fractures or major osteoporotic fractures) as well as the aBMD but independently of aBMD and Clinical Risk Factors (CRF) [143–147]; (2) TBS in combination with aBMD improves fracture prediction [143–145]; (3) TBS is an independent CRF [146]; (4) TBS can assess the fracture risk in some causes of secondary osteoporosis [40]: diabetes [149–151], glucocorticoid induced osteoporosis [152, 153] or hyperparathyroidism [154, 155]; (5) TBS is not impacted by lumbar spine osteoarthritis [156, 157]; and (6) TBS exhibits a different response upon treatment types [158–160]. Recommendations generated by several international scientific societies have suggested that TBS be included in clinical practice for adults only [148, 161, 162].

## TBS: From Adult to Pediatric Application

From a technical point of view, TBS has been optimized for use in adults. More particularly, soft tissue effects on TBS have been evaluated and compensated based on BMI of a patient as a surrogate for tissue thickness. This approach is not appropriate for use in growing children because of changes in body composition, bones, or muscles during growth which vary by individual. In addition, these body modifications are gender-dependent and are neither linear nor uniform with aging. It is therefore important to assess TBS without the adult soft tissue compensation, and simply report a raw TBS value given no dedicated soft tissue correction algorithms yet exist for children. Future strategies could apply a correction using theoretical tissue thickness effect on TBS (using cx vivo data for instance) instead of BMI.

## TBS: Clinical Studies in the Pediatric Field

Although widely characterized, used and understood in adults, TBS is at its beginnings in children. Sparse data have been published or presented [163–170] and some of these studies have used the TBS software version dedicated for adults [163, 164]. Consequently, results and conclusions obtained in these two studies have to be interpreted with caution and will not be discussed here.

Other studies [165–170] have used either raw TBS data [165–167] or raw TBS data with a tissue correction based on spine tissue thickness [168–170]. Positive relationships between TBS and the Tanner stage have been observed in both girls [165, 170] and boys [144]. Similarly, positive correlations have been observed between TBS and aBMD or estimates of volumetric BMD or the Bone Mineral Content (BMC) [165–170]. These results are consistent with TBS normative data previously presented [167]. However, it seems that the strength of this association is gender-dependent [165, 167] and also age-dependent [167]. Few data exist in infants [166]. Using a cohort of 109 and 143 healthy male and female infants (aged between birth to 2 years old), the authors [166] observed "U shaped" age-related TBS curves (a decrease followed by an increase) which could be explained by the reorganization of the trabecular structure; trabeculae changed from a radial orientation to a vertical/horizontal orientation [171] in response to changes in the mechanical loading of the spine. Vertebrae are altered with development from a bedrest phase (with small amount of mechanical loading) followed by sitting and then standing phases where weight load is applied. These preliminary reference raw data [166, 167] are a first step. However, as with pediatric norms for aBMD, different factors of the growing skeleton influencing the results have to be investigated and compensated for. Especially, it is important to determine if parameters that influence DXA measurements for aBMD also affect the TBS score. For example, aBMD measurements are influenced by height and gender of patients. Tall children tend to have a higher aBMD compared to small children regardless of their volumetric ("true") bone mineral density. Reference values for aBMD are adjusted for the hormonal and pubertal status of the individual. In male adolescents an increase of testosterone during puberty leads to an increase of muscle mass which is the most important predictor of bone mass in boys. In pubertal girls the increased estrogen levels inhibit remodeling processes on the endosteal surface resulting in an increased bone mass endosteal compared to boys. These gender-dependent changes during puberty may influence the TBS results and have to be considered. Another difference between children and adults is the presence of growth plates in children. There is very limited knowledge about the influence of the increased amount of cartilage on DXA measurements and this has to be reflected in the interpretation of TBS measurements in children and adolescents.

TBS has been examined in children suffering from Duchenne muscular dystrophy [169]. Both aBMD and TBS increased in the subjects during growth with a weak correlation between aBMD and TBS changes ($r^2=0.26$). Despite these gains with growth, aBMD and TBS values remained below normal values for age (when compared with reference data for age [167]). Further, TBS seemed to be associated with the total fat mass while aBMD was not.

## TBS: Interpretation Limitations

Caution is necessary when interpreting TBS in children. It is important to take into account specificity of the growing bone, including: (1) overall vertebra shape modification including vertebral body shape modification [172–174]; (2) modification of the trabeculae orientation from radial to vertical/horizontal orientations [171]; (3) structure mineralization from mineralized cartilage to mineralized bone matrix [171, 175, 176].

## Overall Vertebra Shape

Individual vertebral dimensions (width, height, and depth) increase over time [172–174]. However, these modifications are not uniform in all three dimensions and vary by gender [172–174]. As with aBMD, TBS is evaluated from a 2D projection of the vertebra. TBS takes into account the size of the bone area (i.e. the number of bone pixels in the ROI) but not the depth dimension. An approach based on estimates of three-dimensional TBS using a cylindrical model [177] or a cube model [178] may prove to be appropriate.

## Modification of the Trabeculae Structure

The orientation of the trabecular structure, into the vertebrae, is modified during growth changing from a radial pattern at birth [171] to a vertical/horizontal directional pattern commonly observed in adults. This pattern modification occurs during the first months of life. Consequently, TBS has to be interpreted as a reflection of the structure orientation modifications in these first months rather than the overall quality of the structure which can be observed after (orientation of the microstructure in steady state).

## Structure Mineralization

Concomitant with modification of the trabecular structure, mineralized cartilage is replaced by a mineralized bone [171]. This process of bone mineralization continues during growth [171]. However, mineralization is not uniform over the vertebrae and not constant in terms of mineralization velocity [171, 175, 176]. Altogether, these processes impact TBS by generating gray-level nonuniformity distribution which is superimposed to gray-level variations linked to the bone structure itself (i.e. the trabecular bone can be view as a structure coupled with a mineral distribution). So, a part of the TBS value is linked to the bone mineralization. However, preliminary studies showed that this impact accounts for 0–15 % (~60 % mineralization increase) of the overall TBS value when homogenous modification is considered.

## Future Clinical Directions

When interpreting results of bone density measurements in children, the cumulative information of aBMD measurements provided by conventional DXA scans is not sufficient to analyze bone quality. Until now, additional investigations using HR-pQCT or pQCT have been needed to assess bone structure and to calculate the strength-strain-index and detailed parameters of bone architecture.

Primary and secondary osteoporosis may have differing effects on cortical and trabecular bone. Even if the cortical bone (which has the strongest influence on aBMD measurements) is in the normal range, a reduction of trabecular bone can provide important information about the skeletal status and can offer important diagnostic perspectives. Based on the underlying pathophysiology of a specific disease, bone architecture may be altered in general or changed only in one part of the bone (cancellous bone, cortical bone). In most secondary skeletal diseases, several factors contribute to the altered bone structure leading to an increased fragility. For example in children with Duchenne muscular dystrophy (DMD), a progressive loss of muscle function and immobilization leads to a reduced trabecular bone mass. Additionally, the frequent use of glucocorticoids impairs osteoblastic function resulting in reduced cortical bone. To optimize treatment, it would be helpful to know if reductions in aBMD are caused by the immobility or the effects of drug therapy. Here TBS might be a helpful tool to personalize therapeutic regimes.

In patients with primary osteoporosis such as osteogenesis imperfecta, treatment with bisphosphonates is commonly evaluated by examining changes in aBMD. This anti-resorptive agent reduces the activity of osteoclasts, reduces skeletal pain and contributes to increased mobility which has an anabolic effect on bone. To differentiate between the influence of these factors, it would be extremely helpful to incorporate information about the bone texture in this specific case. Indeed, skeletal pain is often caused by micro fractures in the trabecular bone and TBS might allow to measure changes of bone stability in the trabecular parts without invasive bone biopsies.

Currently it is unclear if TBS will be helpful in distinguishing between osteoporosis (clinical bone fragility) and reduced mineralization in children. At the moment a reduced aBMD is regarded as osteoporosis but a mineralization defect (like in adults with osteomalacia or children with rickets) can result in the same aBMD values. Assessing trabecular structure with TBS might help to distinguish between these pathophysiological conditions and improve the choice of therapy.

TBS is a promising tool which could become, as the aBMD, a valuable tool for the evaluation of the skeleton during childhood. Additional studies are warranted to develop pediatric norms and to explore its value in predicting fragility fractures and monitoring therapy in the growing patient.

## Summary Points

- MRI is a noninvasive 3-D method for imaging both trabecular and cortical bone, which can be used for assessing skeletal growth, metabolic diseases, and other bone-related diseases in pediatrics.
- The advantage of MRI to DXA is that it has the potential for characterizing muscle, bone marrow, and body fat in both peripheral as well as axial sites, without ionizing radiation.
- Finite element analysis (FEA) was originally developed for use from clinical CT scans over 20 years ago to provide a "virtual stress test" of a bone under a prescribed set of external forces

- There are three different types of finite element models that can be generated from CT scanners (micro-CT, HRpQCT, clinical CT), from each model, validation studies performed in adults have consistently shown that vertebral and hip fractures are associated with FEA strength almost always more so than DXA-measured BMD.
- Given the relative novelty of patient-specific FEA for pediatric applications, and the continuing improvement of CT scanning technology, it is expected that new insight will be gained as patient-specific FEA is expanded for pediatric applications.
- Trabecular Bone Score (TBS) is a texture parameter, assessed from spine PA DXA scans, which correlate with bone microarchitectural parameters.
- Due to limitations of soft tissue correction algorithms for pediatric patients, TBS assessed in infants, children, and adolescents should be expressed as raw data, without soft tissue correction.
- Caution is necessary when interpreting TBS in pediatric patients. Multiple factors may alter TBS in children and adolescents including variability of soft tissue thickness with growth, poor uniformity of mineralization of vertebral bodies, microstructure orientation, and overall vertebral shape variability.
- While robust pediatric reference data must be created, TBS is a promising tool which could become a valuable tool for the evaluation of skeletal deficits during childhood.

# References

1. Rauch F, Tutlewski B, Fricke O, Rieger-Wettengl G, Schauseil-Zipf U, Herkenrath P, Neu CM, Schoenau E. Analysis of cancellous bone turnover by multiple slice analysis at distal radius: a study using peripheral quantitative computed tomography. J Clin Densitom. 2001;4(3):257–62.
2. Moxley 3rd RT, Pandya S. Weekend high-dosage prednisone: a new option for treatment of Duchenne muscular dystrophy. Neurology. 2011;77(5):416–7.
3. Viljakainen H, Korhonen T, Hytinantti T, et al. Maternal vitamin D status affects bone growth in early childhood—a prospective cohort study. Osteoporos Int. 2011;22:883–9.
4. Mansfield P, Morris PG. NMR imaging in biomedicine. New York: Academic Press; 1982.
5. Gatehouse PD, Bydder GM. Magnetic resonance imaging of short T2 components in tissue. Clin Radiol. 2003;58(1):1–19.
6. Gomberg BR, Saha PK, Wehrli FW. Method for cortical bone structural analysis from magnetic resonance images. Acad Radiol. 2005;12(10):1320–32.
7. Elliott SR, Robinson RA. The water content of bone. I. The mass of water, inorganic crystals, organic matrix, and CO2 space components in a unit volume of the dog bone. J Bone Joint Surg Am. 1957;39-A(1):167–88.
8. Mueller KH, Trias A, Ray RD. Bone density and compostiton. Age-related and pathological changes in water and mineral content. J Bone Joint Surg Am. 1966;48(1):140–8.
9. Timmins PA, Wall JC. Bone water. Calcif Tissue Res. 1977;23(1):1–5.
10. Newitt DC, Van Rietbergen B, Majumdar S. Processing and analysis of in vivo high-resolution MR images of trabecular bone for longitudinal studies: reproducibility of structural measures and micro-finite element analysis derived mechanical properties. Osteoporos Int. 2002;13:278–87.

11. Hyun B, Newitt DC, Majumdar S. Assessment of cortical bone structure using high-resolution magnetic resonance imaging. In: Proceedings 13th scientific meeting, international society for magnetic resonance in medicine, Miami; 2005.
12. Hildebrand T, Ruegsegger P. A new method for the model-independent assessment of thickness in three-dimensional images. J Microsc. 1997;185:67–75.
13. Kazakia GJ, et al. In vivo determination of bone structure in postmenopausal women: a comparison of HR-pQCT and high-field MR imaging. J Bone Miner Res. 2008;23(4):463–74.
14. Wehrli FW, et al. Quantitative MRI for the assessment of bone structure and function. NMR Biomed. 2006;19(7):731–64.
15. Wehrli FW. Structural and functional assessment of trabecular and cortical bone by micro magnetic resonance imaging. J Magn Reson Imaging. 2007;25(2):390–409.
16. Parfitt AM, et al. Relationships between surface, volume, and thickness of iliac trabecular bone in aging and in osteoporosis. Implications for the microanatomic and cellular mechanisms of bone loss. J Clin Invest. 1983;72(4):1396–409.
17. Chung HW, et al. Quantitative analysis of trabecular microstructure by 400 MHz nuclear magnetic resonance imaging. J Bone Miner Res. 1995;10(5):803–11.
18. Majumdar S, et al. Evaluation of technical factors affecting the quantification of trabecular bone structure using magnetic resonance imaging. Bone. 1995;17(4):417–30.
19. Majumdar S, et al. Correlation of trabecular bone structure with age, bone mineral density, and osteoporotic status: in vivo studies in the distal radius using high resolution magnetic resonance imaging. J Bone Miner Res. 1997;12(1):111–8.
20. Krug R, et al. Wavelet-based characterization of vertebral trabecular bone structure from magnetic resonance images at 3T compared with micro-computed tomographic measurements. Magn Reson Imaging. 2007;25(3):392–8.
21. Saha PK, Wehrli FW. Measurement of trabecular bone thickness in the limited resolution regime of in vivo MRI by fuzzy distance transform. IEEE Trans Med Imaging. 2004;23(1):53–62.
22. Amling M, et al. Architecture and distribution of cancellous bone yield vertebral fracture clues. A histomorphometric analysis of the complete spinal column from 40 autopsy specimens. Arch Orthop Trauma Surg. 1996;115(5):262–9.
23. Boyce RW, et al. Unbiased estimation of vertebral trabecular connectivity in calcium-restricted ovariectomized minipigs. Bone. 1995;16(6):637–42.
24. Kinney JH, Ladd AJ. The relationship between three-dimensional connectivity and the elastic properties of trabecular bone. J Bone Miner Res. 1998;13(5):839–45.
25. Saha PK, Chaudhuri BB. 3D digital topology under binary transformation with applications. Comput Vis Image Underst. 1996;63(3):418–29.
26. Gomberg BR, et al. Topological analysis of trabecular bone MR images. IEEE Trans Med Imaging. 2000;19(3):166–74.
27. Pothuaud L, et al. In vivo application of 3D-line skeleton graph analysis (LSGA) technique with high-resolution magnetic resonance imaging of trabecular bone structure. Osteoporos Int. 2004;15(5):411–9.
28. Pothuaud L, et al. Three-dimensional-line skeleton graph analysis of high-resolution magnetic resonance images: a validation study from 34-microm-resolution microcomputed tomography. J Bone Miner Res. 2002;17(10):1883–95.
29. Pothuaud L, et al. Combination of topological parameters and bone volume fraction better predicts the mechanical properties of trabecular bone. J Biomech. 2002;35(8):1091–9.
30. Carballido-Gamio J, et al. Geodesic topological analysis of trabecular bone microarchitecture from high-spatial resolution magnetic resonance images. Magn Reson Med. 2009;61(2): 448–56.
31. Benito M, et al. Deterioration of trabecular architecture in hypogonadal men. J Clin Endocrinol Metab. 2003;88(4):1497–502.
32. Benito M, et al. Effect of testosterone replacement on trabecular architecture in hypogonadal men. J Bone Miner Res. 2005;20(10):1785–91.

33. Link TM, et al. Changes in calcaneal trabecular bone structure after heart transplantation: an MR imaging study. Radiology. 2000;217(3):855–62.
34. Link TM, et al. In vivo high resolution MRI of the calcaneus: differences in trabecular structure in osteoporosis patients. J Bone Miner Res. 1998;13(7):1175–82.
35. Link TM, et al. Changes in calcaneal trabecular bone structure assessed with high-resolution MR imaging in patients with kidney transplantation. Osteoporos Int. 2002;13(2):119–29.
36. Majumdar S, et al. Trabecular bone architecture in the distal radius using magnetic resonance imaging in subjects with fractures of the proximal femur. Magnetic Resonance Science Center and Osteoporosis and Arthritis Research Group. Osteoporos Int. 1999;10(3):231–9.
37. Wehrli FW, et al. Digital topological analysis of in vivo magnetic resonance microimages of trabecular bone reveals structural implications of osteoporosis. J Bone Miner Res. 2001;16(8):1520–31.
38. Wehrli FW, et al. Cancellous bone volume and structure in the forearm: noninvasive assessment with MR microimaging and image processing. Radiology. 1998;206(2):347–57.
39. Wehrli FW, et al. Quantitative high-resolution magnetic resonance imaging reveals structural implications of renal osteodystrophy on trabecular and cortical bone. J Magn Reson Imaging. 2004;20(1):83–9.
40. Wehrli FW, et al. Role of magnetic resonance for assessing structure and function of trabecular bone. Top Magn Reson Imaging. 2002;13(5):335–55.
41. Techawiboonwong A, et al. Cortical bone water: in vivo quantification with ultrashort echo-time MR imaging. Radiology. 2008;248(3):824–33.
42. Chesnut 3rd CH, et al. Effects of salmon calcitonin on trabecular microarchitecture as determined by magnetic resonance imaging: results from the QUEST study. J Bone Miner Res. 2005;20(9):1548–61.
43. Wehrli FW, et al. In vivo magnetic resonance detects rapid remodeling changes in the topology of the trabecular bone network after menopause and the protective effect of estradiol. J Bone Miner Res. 2008;23(5):730–40.
44. Modlesky CM, et al. Evaluation of the femoral midshaft in children with cerebral palsy using magnetic resonance imaging. Osteoporos Int. 2009;20(4):609–15.
45. Modlesky CM, et al. Sex differences in trabecular bone microarchitecture are not detected in pre and early pubertal children using magnetic resonance imaging. Bone. 2011;49(5):1067–72.
46. Modlesky CM, Subramanian P, Miller F. Underdeveloped trabecular bone microarchitecture is detected in children with cerebral palsy using high-resolution magnetic resonance imaging. Osteoporos Int. 2008;19(2):169–76.
47. Goldenstein J, Kazakia G, Majumdar S. In vivo evaluation of the presence of bone marrow in cortical porosity in postmenopausal osteopenic women. Ann Biomed Eng. 2010;38(2):235–46.
48. Kindler JM, Ross HL, Laing EM, Modlesky CM, Pollock NK, Baile CA, Lewis RD. Load-specific physical activity scores are related to tibia bone architecture. Int J Sport Nutr Exerc Metab. 2014;25(2):136–44.
49. Crawford RP, Cann CE, Keaveny TM. Finite element models predict in vitro vertebral body compressive strength better than quantitative computed tomography. Bone. 2003;33(4):744–50.
50. Cody DD, et al. Femoral strength is better predicted by finite element models than QCT and DXA. J Biomech. 1999;32(10):1013–20.
51. Faulkner KG, Cann CE, Hasegawa BH. Effect of bone distribution on vertebral strength: assessment with patient-specific nonlinear finite element analysis. Radiology. 1991;179(3):669–74.
52. Keyak JH, et al. Automated 3-dimensional finite-element modeling of bone—a new method. J Biomed Eng. 1990;12(5):389–97.
53. Keaveny TM. Biomechanical computed tomography-noninvasive bone strength analysis using clinical computed tomography scans. Ann N Y Acad Sci. 2010;1192:57–65.
54. Zysset PK, et al. Finite element analysis for prediction of bone strength. Bonekey Rep. 2013;2:386.

55. Pistoia W, et al. Estimation of distal radius failure load with micro-finite element analysis models based on three-dimensional peripheral quantitative computed tomography images. Bone. 2002;30(6):842–8.
56. Reddy JN. An introduction to the finite element method. 3rd ed. New York, NY: McGraw-Hill Higher Education; 2006. p. 766.
57. Engelke K, et al. Advanced CT based in vivo methods for the assessment of bone density, structure, and strength. Curr Osteoporos Rep. 2013;11(3):246–55.
58. Weber NK, et al. Validation of a CT-derived method for osteoporosis screening in IBD patients undergoing contrast-enhanced CT enterography. Am J Gastroenterol. 2014;109(3): 401–8.
59. Khoo BC, et al. Comparison of QCT-derived and DXA-derived areal bone mineral density and T scores. Osteoporos Int. 2009;20(9):1539–45.
60. Keyak JH, et al. Male-female differences in the association between incident hip fracture and proximal femoral strength: a finite element analysis study. Bone. 2011;48(6):1239–45.
61. Kopperdahl DL, et al. Assessment of incident spine and hip fractures in women and men using finite element analysis of CT scans. J Bone Miner Res. 2014;29(3):570–80.
62. Keaveny TM, et al. Comparison of the effects of teriparatide and alendronate on parameters of total hip strength as assessed by finite element analysis: results from the Forteo and Alendronate comparison trial. J Bone Miner Res. 2007;22:S26.
63. Keaveny TM, et al. Femoral bone strength and its relation to cortical and trabecular changes after treatment with PTH, alendronate, and their combination as assessed by finite element analysis of quantitative CT scans. J Bone Miner Res. 2008;23(12):1974–82.
64. Melton 3rd LJ, et al. Relation of vertebral deformities to bone density, structure, and strength. J Bone Miner Res. 2010;25(9):1922–30.
65. Cheung AM, et al. High-resolution peripheral quantitative computed tomography for the assessment of bone strength and structure: a review by the Canadian Bone Strength Working Group. Curr Osteoporos Rep. 2013;11(2):136–46.
66. van Rietbergen B, Ito K. A survey of micro-finite element analysis for clinical assessment of bone strength: the first decade. J Biomech. 2015;48(5):832–41.
67. Bevill G, et al. The influence of boundary conditions and loading mode on high-resolution finite element-computed trabecular tissue properties. Bone. 2009;44(4):573–8.
68. Fields AJ, et al. Vertebral fragility and structural redundancy. J Bone Miner Res. 2012;27(10):2152–8.
69. Nawathe S, et al. Microstructural failure mechanisms in the human proximal femur for sideways fall loading. J Bone Miner Res. 2014;29(2):507–15.
70. Prevrhal S, et al. Accuracy of CT-based thickness measurement of thin structures: modeling of limited spatial resolution in all three dimensions. Med Phys. 2003;30(1):1–8.
71. Zadpoor AA, Weinans H. Patient-specific bone modeling and analysis: the role of integration and automation in clinical adoption. J Biomech. 2015;48(5):750–60.
72. Mueller TL, et al. Computational finite element bone mechanics accurately predicts mechanical competence in the human radius of an elderly population. Bone. 2011;48(6):1232–8.
73. Macneil JA, Boyd SK. Bone strength at the distal radius can be estimated from high-resolution peripheral quantitative computed tomography and the finite element method. Bone. 2008;42(6):1203–13.
74. Christen D, et al. Improved fracture risk assessment based on nonlinear micro-finite element simulations from HRpQCT images at the distal radius. J Bone Miner Res. 2013;28(12):2601–8.
75. Varga P, et al. HR-pQCT based FE analysis of the most distal radius section provides an improved prediction of Colles' fracture load in vitro. Bone. 2010;47(5):982–8.
76. Boutroy S, et al. Finite element analysis based on in vivo HR-pQCT images of the distal radius is associated with wrist fracture in postmenopausal women. J Bone Miner Res. 2008;23(3):392–9.
77. Melton 3rd LJ, et al. Assessing forearm fracture risk in postmenopausal women. Osteoporos Int. 2010;21(7):1161–9.

78. Vilayphiou N, et al. Finite element analysis performed on radius and tibia HR-pQCT images and fragility fractures at all sites in postmenopausal women. Bone. 2010;46(4):1030–7.
79. Vilayphiou N, et al. Finite element analysis performed on radius and tibia HR-pQCT images and fragility fractures at all sites in men. J Bone Miner Res. 2011;26(5):965–73.
80. Nishiyama KK, et al. Women with previous fragility fractures can be classified based on bone microarchitecture and finite element analysis measured with HR-pQCT. Osteoporos Int. 2013;24(5):1733–40.
81. Tsai JN, et al. Comparative effects of teriparatide, denosumab, and combination therapy on peripheral compartmental bone density, microarchitecture, and estimated strength: the DATA-HRpQCT Study. J Bone Miner Res. 2015;30(1):39–45.
82. Burghardt AJ, et al. A longitudinal HR-pQCT study of alendronate treatment in postmenopausal women with low bone density: relations among density, cortical and trabecular microarchitecture, biomechanics, and bone turnover. J Bone Miner Res. 2010;25(12):2558–71.
83. Hansen S, et al. Differing effects of PTH 1-34, PTH 1-84, and zoledronic acid on bone microarchitecture and estimated strength in postmenopausal women with osteoporosis: an 18-month open-labeled observational study using HR-pQCT. J Bone Miner Res. 2013;28(4):736–45.
84. Nishiyama KK, et al. Teriparatide increases strength of the peripheral skeleton in premenopausal women with idiopathic osteoporosis: a pilot HR-pQCT study. J Clin Endocrinol Metab. 2014;99(7):2418–25.
85. Cheung AM, et al. Effects of odanacatib on the radius and tibia of postmenopausal women: improvements in bone geometry, microarchitecture, and estimated bone strength. J Bone Miner Res. 2014;29(8):1786–94.
86. Leung KS, et al. Structural, densitometric and biomechanical evaluations of Chinese patients with long-term bisphosphonate treatment. Chin Med J (Engl). 2013;126(1):27–33.
87. Tang XL, et al. Alterations of bone geometry, density, microarchitecture, and biomechanical properties in systemic lupus erythematosus on long-term glucocorticoid: a case-control study using HR-pQCT. Osteoporos Int. 2013;24(6):1817–26.
88. Cabal A, et al. High-resolution peripheral quantitative computed tomography and finite element analysis of bone strength at the distal radius in ovariectomized adult rhesus monkey demonstrate efficacy of odanacatib and differentiation from alendronate. Bone. 2013;56(2):497–505.
89. Dall'Ara E, et al. A nonlinear QCT-based finite element model validation study for the human femur tested in two configurations in vitro. Bone. 2013;52(1):27–38.
90. Keyak JH. Improved prediction of proximal femoral fracture load using nonlinear finite element models. Med Eng Phys. 2001;23(3):165–73.
91. Keyak JH, et al. Prediction of femoral fracture load using automated finite element modeling. J Biomech. 1998;31(2):125–33.
92. Bessho M, et al. Prediction of strength and strain of the proximal femur by a CT-based finite element method. J Biomech. 2007;40(8):1745–53.
93. Koivumaki JE, et al. Ct-based finite element models can be used to estimate experimentally measured failure loads in the proximal femur. Bone. 2012;50(4):824–9.
94. Dragomir-Daescu D, et al. Robust QCT/FEA models of proximal femur stiffness and fracture load during a sideways fall on the hip. Ann Biomed Eng. 2011;39(2):742–55.
95. Duchemin L, et al. An anatomical subject-specific FE-model for hip fracture load prediction. Comput Methods Biomech Biomed Engin. 2008;11(2):105–11.
96. van den Munckhof S, Zadpoor AA. How accurately can we predict the fracture load of the proximal femur using finite element models? Clin Biomech (Bristol, Avon). 2014;29(4):373–80.
97. Wang X, et al. Prediction of new clinical vertebral fractures in elderly men using finite element analysis of CT scans. J Bone Miner Res. 2012;27(4):808–16.
98. Dall'Ara E, et al. A nonlinear finite element model validation study based on a novel experimental technique for inducing anterior wedge-shape fractures in human vertebral bodies in vitro. J Biomech. 2010;43(12):2374–80.

99. Martin H, et al. Noninvasive assessment of stiffness and failure load of human vertebrae from CT-data. Biomed Tech (Berl). 1998;43(4):82–8.
100. Buckley JM, Loo K, Motherway J. Comparison of quantitative computed tomography-based measures in predicting vertebral compressive strength. Bone. 2007;40(3):767–74.
101. Imai K, et al. Nonlinear finite element model predicts vertebral bone strength and fracture site. Spine. 2006;31(16):1789–94.
102. Melton LJ, et al. Structural determinants of vertebral fracture risk. J Bone Miner Res. 2007;22(12):1885–92.
103. Imai K, et al. Assessment of vertebral fracture risk and therapeutic effects of alendronate in postmenopausal women using a quantitative computed tomography-based nonlinear finite element method. Osteoporos Int. 2009;20(5):801–10.
104. Anderson DE, et al. The associations between QCT-based vertebral bone measurements and prevalent vertebral fractures depend on the spinal locations of both bone measurement and fracture. Osteoporos Int. 2014;25(2):559–66.
105. Orwoll ES, et al. Finite element analysis of the proximal femur and hip fracture risk in older men. J Bone Miner Res. 2009;24(3):475–83.
106. Chevalier Y, et al. Biomechanical effects of teriparatide in women with osteoporosis treated previously with alendronate and risedronate: results from quantitative computed tomography-based finite element analysis of the vertebral body. Bone. 2010;46(1):41–8.
107. Graeff C, et al. Improvements in vertebral body strength under teriparatide treatment assessed in vivo by finite element analysis: results from the EUROFORS study. J Bone Miner Res. 2009;24(10):1672–80.
108. Imai K. Vertebral fracture risk and alendronate effects on osteoporosis assessed by a computed tomography-based nonlinear finite element method. J Bone Miner Metab. 2011;29(6):645–51.
109. Gluer CC, et al. Comparative effects of teriparatide and risedronate in glucocorticoid-induced osteoporosis in men: 18-month results of the EuroGIOPs trial. J Bone Miner Res. 2013;28(6):1355–68.
110. Keaveny TM, et al. Effects of teriparatide and alendronate on vertebral strength as assessed by finite element modeling of QCT scans in women with osteoporosis. J Bone Miner Res. 2007;22(1):149–57.
111. Mawatari T, et al. Vertebral strength changes in rheumatoid arthritis patients treated with alendronate, as assessed by finite element analysis of clinical computed tomography scans: a prospective randomized clinical trial. Arthritis Rheum. 2008;58(11):3340–9.
112. Lewiecki EM, et al. Once-monthly oral ibandronate improves biomechanical determinants of bone strength in women with postmenopausal osteoporosis. J Clin Endocrinol Metab. 2009;94(1):171–80.
113. Keaveny TM, et al. Femoral strength in osteoporotic women treated with teriparatide or alendronate. Bone. 2012;50(1):165–70.
114. Brixen K, et al. Bone density, turnover, and estimated strength in postmenopausal women treated with odanacatib: a randomized trial. J Clin Endocrinol Metab. 2013;98(2):571–80.
115. Cosman F, et al. Hip and spine strength effects of adding versus switching to teriparatide in postmenopausal women with osteoporosis treated with prior alendronate or raloxifene. J Bone Miner Res. 2013;28(6):1328–36.
116. Keaveny TM, et al. Femoral and vertebral strength improvements in postmenopausal women with osteoporosis treated with denosumab. J Bone Miner Res. 2014;29(1):158–65.
117. Orwoll ES, et al. Evaluation of teriparatide treatment in adults with osteogenesis imperfecta. J Clin Invest. 2014;124(2):491–8.
118. Kleerekoper M, et al. Assessing the effects of teriparatide treatment on bone mineral density, bone microarchitecture, and bone strength. J Bone Joint Surg Am. 2014;96(11):e90.
119. Engelke K, et al. Clinical use of quantitative computed tomography and peripheral quantitative computed tomography in the management of osteoporosis in adults: the 2007 ISCD Official Positions. J Clin Densitom. 2008;11(1):123–62.
120. American College of Radiology. Practice parameter for the performance of quantitative computed tomography (QCT) bone densitometry. Amended. 2014;39:1–14.

121. Farr JN, et al. Body composition during childhood and adolescence: relations to bone strength and microstructure. J Clin Endocrinol Metab. 2014;99(12):4641–8.
122. Faje AT, et al. Adolescent girls with anorexia nervosa have impaired cortical and trabecular microarchitecture and lower estimated bone strength at the distal radius. J Clin Endocrinol Metab. 2013;98(5):1923–9.
123. Ackerman KE, et al. Fractures in relation to menstrual status and bone parameters in young athletes. Med Sci Sports Exerc. 2015;47(8):1577–86.
124. Caouette C, et al. Biomechanical analysis of fracture risk associated with tibia deformity in children with osteogenesis imperfecta: a finite element analysis. J Musculoskelet Neuronal Interact. 2014;14(2):205–12.
125. Chevalley T, et al. Tracking of environmental determinants of bone structure and strength development in healthy boys: an eight-year follow up study on the positive interaction between physical activity and protein intake from prepuberty to mid-late adolescence. J Bone Miner Res. 2014;29(10):2182–92.
126. Farr JN, et al. Bone strength and structural deficits in children and adolescents with a distal forearm fracture resulting from mild trauma. J Bone Miner Res. 2014;29(3):590–9.
127. Gabel L, et al. Bone architecture and strength in the growing skeleton: the role of sedentary time. Med Sci Sports Exerc. 2015;47(2):363–72.
128. Li X, et al. Developing CT based computational models of pediatric femurs. J Biomech. 2015;48(10):2034–40.
129. Singhal V, et al. Irisin levels are lower in young amenorrheic athletes compared with eumenorrheic athletes and non-athletes and are associated with bone density and strength estimates. PLoS One. 2014;9(6):e100218.
130. Pothuaud L, Carceller P, et al. Correlations between grey-level variations in 2D projection images (TBS) and 3D microarchitecture: applications in the study of human trabecular bone microarchitecture. Bone. 2008;42:775–87.
131. Hans D, Barthe N, et al. Correlations between TBS, measured using antero-posterior DXA acquisition, and 3D parameters of bone micro-architecture: an experimental study on human cadavre vertebrae. J Clin Densitom. 2011;14(3):302–11.
132. Winzenrieth R, Michelet F, et al. Three-dimensional (3D) microarchitecture correlations with 2D projection image gray-level variations assessed by trabecular bone score using high-resolution computed tomographic acquisitions: effects of resolution and noise. J Clin Densitom. 2013;16(3):287–96.
133. Mandelbrot B, Van Ness J, et al. Fractional Brownian motions, fractional noises and applications. SIAM Rev. 1968;10:422–37.
134. Coeurjolly J-F. Simulation and identification of the fractional Brownian motion: a bibliographical and comparative study. J Statist Soft. 2000;5:1–53.
135. Bardet J-M, Lang G, et al. Semi-parametric estimation of the long-range dependence parameter: a survey. In: Doukhan P, Oppenheim G, Taqqu MS, editors. Theory and applications of long-range dependence. Boston: Birkhäuser; 2003. p. 557–77.
136. Olea RA. Fundamentals of semivariogram estimation, modeling, and usage. In: Yarus JM, Chambers RL, editors. Stochastic modeling and geostatistics, vol. 3. Tulsa, OK: AAPG Computer Applications in Geology; 1994. p. 27–35.
137. Kelkar M, Shibli S. Description of reservoir properties using fractals. In: Yarus JM, Chambers RL, editors. Stochastic modeling and geostatistics, vol. 3. Tulsa OK: AAPG Publication; 1994. p. 261.
138. Silva BC, Boutroy S, et al. Trabecular bone score (TBS)—a novel method to evaluate bone microarchitectural texture in patients with primary hyperparathyroidism. J Clin Endocrinol Metab. 2013;98(5):1963–70.
139. Popp AW, Buffat H, et al. Microstructural parameters of bone evaluated using HR-pQCT correlate with the DXA-derived cortical index and the trabecular bone score in a cohort of randomly selected premenopausal women. PLoS One. 2014;9(2):e88946.
140. Kocijan R, Muschitz C, et al. Bone structure assessed by HR-pQCT, TBS and DXL in adult patients with different types of osteogenesis imperfecta. Osteoporos Int. 2015. [Epub ahead of print].

141. Muschitz C, Kocijan R, et al. TBS reflects trabecular microarchitecture in remeno-pausal women and men with idiopathic osteoporosis and low-traumatic fractures. Bone. 2015;79:259–66.
142. Silva BC, Leslie WD, et al. Trabecular bone score: a noninvasive analytical method based upon the DXA image. J Bone Miner Res. 2014;29:518–30.
143. Hans D, Goertzen AL, et al. Bone microarchitecture assessed by TBS predicts osteo-porotic fractures independent of bone density: the Manitoba study. J Bone Miner Res. 2011;26(11):2762–9.
144. Briot K, Paternotte S, et al. Added value of trabecular bone score to bone mineral density for prediction of osteoporotic fractures in postmenopausal women: the OPUS study. Bone. 2013;57(1):232–6.
145. Iki M, Tamaki J, et al. Trabecular bone score (TBS) predicts vertebral fractures in Japanese women over 10 years independently of bone density and prevalent vertebral deformity: the Japanese population-based osteoporosis (JPOS) cohort study. J Bone Miner Res. 2014;29(2):399–407.
146. Leslie WD, Krieg MA, et al. Clinical factors associated with trabecular bone score. J Clin Densitom. 2013;16(3):374–9.
147. Boutroy S, Hans D, et al. Trabecular bone score improves fracture risk prediction in non-osteoporotic women: the OFELY study. Osteoporos Int. 2013;24(1):77–85.
148. Harvey NC, Glüer CC, et al. Trabecular bone score (TBS) as a new complementary approach for osteoporosis evaluation in clinical practice. Bone. 2015;78:216–24.
149. Dhaliwal R, Cibula D, Ghosh C, Weinstock RS, Moses AM. Bone quality assessment in type 2 diabetes mellitus. Osteoporos Int. 2014;25(7):1969–73.
150. Leslie WD, Aubry-Rozier B, Lamy O, Hans D, Manitoba Bone Density Program. TBS (tra-becular bone score) and diabetes-related fracture risk. J Clin Endocrinol Metab. 2013;98(2):602–9.
151. Kim JH, Choi HJ, Ku EJ, Kim KM, Kim SW, Cho NH, Shin CS. Trabecular bone score as an indicator for skeletal deterioration in diabetes. J Clin Endocrinol Metab. 2015;100(2):475–82.
152. Paggiosi MA, Peel NF, et al. The impact of glucocorticoid therapy on trabecular bone score in older women. Osteoporos Int. 2015;26(6):1773–80.
153. Leib E, Winzenrieth R. Bone status in glucocorticoid treated men and women. Osteoporos Int. 2015;8. Epub ahead of print.
154. Eller-Vainicher C, Filopanti M, et al. Bone quality, as measured by trabecular bone score, in patients with primary hyperparathyroidism. Eur J Endocrinol. 2013;169:155–62.
155. Romagnoli E, Cipriani C, et al. "Trabecular Bone Score" (TBS): an indirect measure of bone micro-architecture in postmenopausal patients with primary hyperparathyroidism. Bone. 2013;53:154–9.
156. Dufour R, Winzenrieth R, et al. Generation and validation of a normative, age-specific refer-ence curve for lumbar spine trabecular bone score (TBS) in French women. Osteoporos Int. 2013;24:2837–46.
157. Kolta S, Briot K, et al. TBS result is not affected by lumbar spine osteoarthritis. Osteoporos Int. 2014;25:1759–64.
158. Popp AW, Guler S, et al. Effects of zoledronate versus placebo on spine bone mineral density and microarchitecture assessed by the trabecular bone score in postmenopausal women with osteoporosis: a three-year study. J Bone Miner Res. 2013;28(3):449–54.
159. Senn C, Günther B, et al. Comparative effects of teriparatide and ibandronate on spine bone mineral density (BMD) and microarchitecture (TBS) in postmenopausal women with osteo-porosis: a 2-year open-label study. Osteoporos Int. 2014;25(7):1945–51.
160. Di Gregorio S, Del Rio L, et al. Comparison between different bone treatments on areal bone mineral density (aBMD) and bone microarchitectural texture as assessed by the trabecular bone score (TBS). Bone. 2015;75:138–43.
161. Silva BC, Broy SB, et al. Fracture risk prediction by non-BMD DXA measures: the 2015 ISCD Official Positions part 2: trabecular bone score. J Clin Densitom. 2015;18(3):309–30.

162. http://www.dv-osteologie.org/dvo_leitlinien/osteoporose-leitlinie-2014.
163. Donaldson AA, Feldman HA, et al. Spinal bone texture assessed by trabecular bone score in adolescent girls with anorexia nervosa. J Clin Endocrinol Metab. 2015;100(9):3436–42.
164. Heiniö L, Nikander R, et al. Association between long-term exercise loading and lumbar spine trabecular bone score (TBS) in different exercise loading groups. J Musculoskelet Neuronal Interact. 2015;15(3):279–85.
165. Shawwa K, Arabi A, et al. Predictors of trabecular bone score in school children. Osteoporos Int. 2015. [Epub ahead of print].
166. Winzenrieth R, Cormier C, et al. Influence of age and gender on spine bone density and TBS microarchitectural texture parameters in infants. Rotterdam, The Netherlands: ICCBH; 2013.
167. Del Rio L, Di Gregorio S, et al. Bone microarchitecture (TBS) and bone mass development during childhood and adolescence in a Spanish population group. Sevilla, Spain: ECCEO-IOF Congress; 2014.
168. Del Rio L, Winzenrieth R, et al. Bone quality and quantity in Duchenne muscular dystrophy patients. Salzburg, Austria: ICCBH; 2015.
169. Del Rio L, Winzenrieth R, et al. Evolution of bone quality and quantity in patients suffering from Duchenne muscular dystrophy. Salzburg, Austria: ICCBH; 2015.
170. Libber J, Winzenrieth R, et al. TBS increases over time in pre-teen girls. Salzburg, Austria: ICCBH; 2015.
171. Roschger P, Grabner BM, et al. Structural development of the mineralized tissue in the human L4 vertebral body. J Struct Biol. 2001;136(2):126–36.
172. Taylor JR, Twomey LT. Sexual dimorphism in human vertebral body shape. J Anat. 1984;138(Pt 2):281–6.
173. Peters JR, Chandrasekaran C, et al. Age- and gender-related changes in pediatric thoracic vertebral morphology. Spine J. 2015;15(5):1000–20.
174. Seeman E. Structural basis of growth-related gain and age-related loss of bone strength. Rheumatology (Oxford). 2008;47 Suppl 4:iv2–8.
175. Roschger P, Paschalis E, et al. Bone mineralization density distribution in health and disease. Bone. 2008;42:456–66.
176. Komarova SV, Safranek L, et al. Mathematical model for bone mineralization. Front Cell Dev Biol. 2015;3:51.
177. Kroger H, Kotaniemi A, et al. Bone densitometry of the spine and femur in children by dual-energy x-ray absorptiometry. Bone Miner. 1992;17:75–85.
178. Katzman DK, Bachrach LK. Clinical and anthropometric correlates of bone mineral acquisition in healthy adolescent girls. J Clin Endocrinol Metab. 1991;73(6):1332–9.

# Appendix A

**Table 1** National and international societies with interest in bone health

**American Dietetic Association Nutrition Resources**
120 Riverside Plaza, Suite 200
Chicago, IL 60606
Tel: (800) 877-1600 (Toll-Free)
Fax: (312) 899-4873
http://www.eatright.org

**American Society for Bone and Mineral Research**
2025M Street NW, Suite 800
Washington, DC 20036
Tel: (202) 367-1161
Fax: (202) 367-2161
E-mail: asbmr@asbmr.org
http://www.asbmr.org

**Best Bones Forever! A Bone Campaign for Girls**
http://bestbonesforever.gov
http://girlshealth.gov

**Bone Biology for Kids**
http://www.depts.washington.edu/bonebio/

**Centers for Disease Control and Prevention**
1600 Clifton Road
Atlanta, GA 30333
Tel: (404) 639-3311
Tel: (404) 639-3534 (public inquiries)
Tel: (800) 311-3435 (public inquiries, Toll-Free)
http://www.cdc.gov

(continued)

© Springer International Publishing Switzerland 2016
E.B. Fung et al. (eds.), *Bone Health Assessment in Pediatrics*,
DOI 10.1007/978-3-319-30412-0

**Table 1** (continued)

**American Bone Health**
1814 Franklin Suite #620
Oakland, CA 94612
Tel: (888) 266-3015
Fax: (510) 208-7174
http://www.americanbonehealth.org

**International Bone and Mineral Society (IBMS)**
330 N. Wabash Suite 1900
Chicago, IL 60611
Tel: (312) 321-5113
Fax: (312) 673-6934
http://www.ibmsonline.org

**International Osteoporosis Foundation (IOF)**
9, rue Juste-Olivier
CH-1260 Nyon
Switzerland
Tel:+41 22 994 0100
Fax:+41 22 994 0101
E-mail: info@osteofound.org
http://www.iofbonehealth.org

**International Society for Clinical Densitometry (ISCD)**
955 South Main Street Building C
Middletown, CT 06457
Tel: (860) 259-1000
Fax: (860) 259-1030
http://www.iscd.org

**Kids and Their Bones: A Guide for Parents**
http://www.niams.nih.gov/hi/topics/osptoporosis/kidbones.htm
A resource developed by the National Institute of Arthritis and Musculoskeletal and Skin Disease

**National Dairy Council**
*In the United Kingdom*
The Dairy Council
Henrietta House
17/18 Henrietta Street
London WC2E 8QH
Tel: 020-735-4030
Fax: 020-7240-9679
E-mail: info@dairycouncil.org.uk
http://www.milk.co.uk

**National Dairy Council**
*In the United States*
National-Dairy Council
10255 W. Higgins Road, Suite 900
Rosemont, IL 60018
Use online directory to locate state or local NDC representative
http://www.nationaldairycouncil.org

(continued)

**Table 1** (continued)

---

**National Institutes of Health, Osteoporosis, and Related Bone Diseases,
National Resource Center**
1 AMS Circle
Bethesda, MD 20892-3676
Tel: (301) 495-4484
Tel: (301) 565-2966 (for hearing impaired)
Tel: (877) 226- 4267 (Toll-Free)
Fax: (301) 718-6366
E-mail: http://www.niams.nih.gov/health_info/bone

**National Organization for Rare Disorders (NORD)**
55 Kenosia Avenue
P.O. Box 1968
Danbury, CT 06813-1968
Tel: (800) 999-6673 (Toll-Free)
Tel: (203) 744-0100
Fax: (203) 798-2291
E-mail: orphan@raredisease.org
http://www.rarediseases.org

**National Osteoporosis Foundation**
1150 17th Street, NW
Suite 850
Washington, DC 20036
Tel: (202) 223-2226
Tel: (800) 231-4222 (Toll-Free)
http://www.nof.org

**National Osteoporosis Society (NOS)**
*United Kingdom*
Camerton
Bath, BA2 0PJ
Tel: 01761 471771
E-mail: info@nos.org.uk
http://www.nos.org.uk

**Northern California Institute for Bone Health, Inc**
50 Vashell Way Suite #400
Orinda, CA 94563
Tel: (510) 625-9100
Fax: (510) 625-9123
http://Betterbones.org

**Nutrition Explorations: Kids**
http://www.superkidsnutrition.com

**Osteogenesis Imperfecta Foundation**
804 West Diamond Avenue, Suite 210
Gaithersburg, MD 20878
Tel: (800) 981-BONE (toll-free)
Tel: (301) 947-0083
Fax: (301) 947-0456
http://www.oif.org

(continued)

**Table 1** (continued)

**Osteoporosis Australia**
Level 2, 255 Broadway
Glebe NSW 2037
Tel: 02 9518 8140
Fax: 02 9518 6306
Toll-free: 1800 242 141 (in Australia)
http://www.osteoporosis.org.au/

**Osteoporosis Canada**
1090 Don Mills Road, Suite 301
Toronto, Ontario M3C 3R6
Tel: (416) 696-2663
Fax: (416) 696-2673
Toll-free (English): 1-800-463-6842 (in Canada only)
Toll-free (French): 1-800-977-1778 (in Canada only)
E-mail: info@osteoporosis.ca
http://www.osteoporosis.ca

**Paget Foundation**
P.O. Box 24432
Brooklyn, NY 11202
Tel: (212) 509-5335
Fax: (212) 509-8492
E-mail: pagetfdn@aol.com
http://www.niams.nih.gov/health_info/bone/Pagets

**Table 2** Contact information for DXA manufacturers

**General Electric Medical Systems**
Lunar iDXA
726 Heartland Trail
Madison, WI 53717
Tel: (800) 535-7339 (Toll-Free)
E-mail: info@gemedicalsystems.com
http://www3.gehealthcare.com

**Hologic, Inc.**
35 Crosby Drive
Bedford, MA 01730-1401
USA
Tel: (800) 343-9729 (toll-free)
Tel: (781) 999-7300
Fax: (781) 280-0669
E-mail: support@hologic.com
http://www.hologic.com

**Norland, CooperSurgical, Inc.**
95 Corporate Drive
Trumbull, CT 06611
USA
Tel: (203) 601-5200
http://www.coopersurgical.com

**Table 3** Useful bone densitometry reference texts

Allgrove J and Shaw N. Eds. *Calcium and Bone Disorders in Children and Adolescents*. Karger. 2009; Vol 16. ISBN-13:978-3805591614

Bonnick SL, ed. *Bone Densitometry in Clinical Practice: Application and Interpretation*, 3rd Ed. Totowa, NJ. Humana Press, 2010. ISBN-13:978-1603274982

Bonnick SL, Lewis LA. *Bone Densitometry for Technologists*. 3rd Ed. New York. Springer, 2013. ISBN-13:978-1461436249

Bronner F, Farach-Carson MC, Roach HI. Eds. *Bone and Development: Topics in Bone Biology*. London, Springer, 2010. ISBN-13:978-1848828216

Glorieux FH, Pettifor JM, Juppner H. Eds. *Pediatric Bone, Biology & Diseases*. 2nd Ed. New York, Elsevier, Academic Press. 2012. ISBN-13:978-0123820402

Holick MF and Nieves JW Eds. *Nutrition and Bone Health* 2nd Ed. Totowa, NJ. Humana Press. 2015. ISBN-13:978-1493920006

Klein G. Ed. *Bone Drugs in Pediatrics: Efficacy and Challenges*. New York, Springer. 2014. ISBN-13:978-1489974358

Martino F, Defilippi C, Caudana R. Eds. *Imaging of Pediatric Bone and Joint Trauma*. New York, Springer. 2011. ISBN-13:978-8847016545

Mencio GA, Swiontkowski MF. Eds. *Green's Skeletal Trauma in Children*. 5th Ed. Philadelphia, Elsevier Sauders. 2015. ISBN-13:978-0323187732

Rosen CJ, Bouillon R, Compston JE, Rosen V. Eds. *Primer on the Metabolic Bone Diseases and Disorders of Mineral Metabolism*. 8th Edition. American Society for Bone Mineral Research. Wiley Blackwell Publishers. 2013. ISBN-13:978-1118453889

**Table 4** Training & certification available for dual energy X-ray absorptiometry: training & education

There are a number of local and regional training opportunities available to technologists, too numerous to highlight here. There are also numerous online educational resources that offer Continuing Medical Education units for radiologic technologists [through the American Society of Radiologic Technologists (AART)] and trained bone densitometry technicians. Most of these are offered for a fee can can be located through internet search engines

*The International Osteoporosis Foundation (IOF)*: furthers patient care and scientific advances in the field of osteoporosis and bone, muscle and joint health by running and supporting a number of the world's leading training courses and educational programs

*International Society for Clinical Densitometry (ISCD)*: Offers a number of educational opportunities in different teaching formats. ISCD is an accredited provider and therefore is able to provide Continuing Medical Education (CME) courses designed to meet the educational needs of physicians and technologists

Most recently the IOF and ISCD have joined efforts to offer a combined 'Osteoporosis Essentials' course:

*Osteoporosis Essentials of Densitometry, Diagnosis and Management (Offered by ISCD + IOF)*: The International Society for Clinical Densitometry (ISCD) and the International Osteoporosis Foundation (IOF) have combined their resources and expertise in order to introduce a single course which is available worldwide. Developed under the auspices of a Joint Entity of IOF and ISCD, this course replaces the Bone Densitometry Course previously offered by each organization. It is offered in partnership with Local Organizing Committees (LOCs). Find details on ISCD & IOF websites

*Pediatric Bone Densitometry Course (Offered by ISCD)*

There are challenges that arise in the interpretation of BMD results from growing and developing children. This course focuses on the assessment of children who may be at risk for a low BMD; a definition of osteoporosis in pediatric patients; diagnosis and management of osteoporosis in the child or adolescent with chronic disease; appropriate reporting of pediatric bone density results. See more at:
http://www.iscd.org/education/cmece-live-courses/pediatric-bone-densitometry-course-peds-bdc/

*Pediatric Bone Health Training Course: (Offered by IOF)*

This course provides an overview of diagnostic issues, endocrine and non-endocrine causes, and osteoporosis treatment in children. The course material is designed for pediatricians, nutritionists, pediatric physical therapists, as well as participants from pharmaceutical industries. To date the one-day course has been held exclusively in Latin America

*Vertebral Fracture Recognition Course (Offered by ISCD)*

This course provides and overview of vertebral fracture imaging, with specific attention to patient positioning, image acquisition and analysis, to optimize the visualization of vertebral fractures, as well as fracture recognition and methods used for their definition and classification. See more at: http://www.iscd.org/education/cmece-live-courses/#sthash.wYm8gVhq.dpuf

*DXA Body Composition Analysis Course (Offered by ISCD)*

To educate healthcare professionals to successfully use DXA body composition analysis in the management of obesity, geriatric sarcopenia and other low muscle mass states, general health and pediatric skeletal disease. See more at:
http://www.iscd.org/education/cmece-live-courses/#sthash.wYm8gVhq.dpuf

(continued)

**Table 4** (continued)

*Certification*

The ISCD Certification encompasses Clinicians and Technologists in Bone Densitometry through one of three certification programs; Certified Clinical Densitometrist (CCD), Certified Bone Densitometry Technologist (CBDT), and Certified Densitometry Technologist (CDT). A practitioner or physician's certification can be verified on the ISCD website using the "Search the Certification Registry Tool" — See more at: http://www.iscd.org/certification/#sthash.8UEUIfs9.dpuf

*Certified Clinical Densitometrist (CCD™®)* is a professional certification in the field of bone densitometry for medical practitioners. It recognizes those who meet specified knowledge requirements measured through a standardized computer-based testing process. Successful candidates can use the CCD™® designation after their names. It is a five year (5) certification. See more at:

http://www.iscd.org/certification/certified-clinical-densitometrist-ccd/#sthash.Jizu99lv.dpuf

*Certified Bone Densitometry Technologist (CBDT™®)* is a professional certification in the field of bone densitometry for technologists who perform bone densitometry scans. The credential signifies that an individual has passed a computer-based examination that has been designed to meet established certification industry standards and best practices in the U.S. (*Offered in the U.S. and Internationally*) - See more at: http://www.iscd.org/certification/certified-bone-densitometry-technologist-cbdt/#sthash.bPaUZ2WB.dpuf

*Certified Densitometry Technologists (CDT™®)* is a professional designation previously awarded to individuals, practicing internationally, who meet specified knowledge requirements measured through a standardized testing process in bone densitometry for performing central DXAs. Internationally this is a renewable five-year certification to those who have already earned the designation. The CDT™® is no longer recognized in the US. - See more at: http://www.iscd.org/certification/certified-densitometry-technologist-cdt/#sthash.E1V87CLe.dpuf

*Radiology Technologists (RT-BD)*

There is also a professional certification for individuals who already hold a radiology technology (RT) license. In 2001 the American Registry of Radiologic Technologists (ARRT) began offering an exam and credentialing for individuals who already held a Radiologic Technologist (RT) license. It is a specialty certification in bone densitometry, those who are certified may use the following initials RT(BD) after their name

*State Licenses in Bone Densitometry:*

Approximately two-thirds of the states in the U.S. have laws covering the practice of radiologic technology. Though similar training to ISCD certification, state licensure is a separate procedure, and performed through the American Registry of Radiologic Technologists (ARRT). ARRT-administered exams are used by 37 states for state licensing purposes. To find out more about AART licensure, please visit:

https://www.arrt.org/certification/bone-densitometry

To find out if your state requires licensure, visit: https://www.arrt.org/State-Licensing/

# Appendix B

**Table 1** Anthropometric techniques: assessment of weight and height

| |
|---|
| *Weight* |
| Equipment: |
| • An electronic or beam balance scale or wheelchair electronic scale: should be calibrated regularly and set to zero between readings |
| Technique: |
| • Children should wear an examination gown or lightweight clothing without shoes or orthopedic apparatuses |
| • Infants should be weighed without clothing or diapers |
| • Children should be weighed to the nearest 0.1 kg; infants, to the nearest 0.01 kg |
| *Stature* |
| (for children without contractures or scoliosis who can stand independently) |
| Equipment: |
| • Digital or electronic stadiometer (calibrated daily) is ideal; otherwise, use a sturdy board with secured tape measure and two stable paddle boards for the head and feet set at 90°. Measurements should be to the nearest 0.1 cm |
| • Head paddle, firmly perpendicular to the backboard (should glide smoothly) |
| • Heel plate, in alignment with the backboard |
| • Solid flooring (not carpeting) |
| Technique: |
| • Stature measurements begin with children >2 yr of age |
| • Child must be able to stand unsupported and should be without significant scoliosis or contractures |
| • Child should be relaxed, with arms at sides |
| • Weight should be evenly placed on both feet |
| • Feet should be against the heel plate and shoulder width apart, or as is comfortable |
| • Heels, buttocks, shoulders, and head should be touching the back of the stadiometer |
| • The head should be held with the Frankfurt plane (an imaginary line from the upper margin of the ear to the lower margin of the eye socket) parallel to the floor |
| • With obesity or kyphosis, standard position may not be possible; positioning of feet and head should align the spine as erect as possible |

(continued)

© Springer International Publishing Switzerland 2016
E.B. Fung et al. (eds.), *Bone Health Assessment in Pediatrics*,
DOI 10.1007/978-3-319-30412-0

**Table 1** (continued)

- Hair clips must be removed from top of head
- Lower paddle gently to top of head; any pressure lowering the paddle will alter child's posture
- Use a foot stool to view reading at eye level, when necessary
- Repeat

*Length*

(for children aged < 2 yr or any child unable to stand independently) Equipment:

- Digital infantometer (calibrated daily) is ideal; otherwise, use a sturdy board with secured tape measure and two stable paddle boards for the head and foot set at 90°. Measurements should be to the nearest 0.1 cm

Technique:

- Requires two people to hold and position the child correctly: one person (the parent can assist) holds the head gently but firmly against the headboard, cupping the cheeks and the back of the head
- Position the head with the Frankfurt plane perpendicular to the board
- The torso should rest flat on the length board, with the midline centered on the board
- Legs should be extended gently but firmly, with the knees flat and the hips even
- With the feet together and flexed at a 90° angle, glide the foot board to the heel
- Best measurements are obtained when the child is relaxed

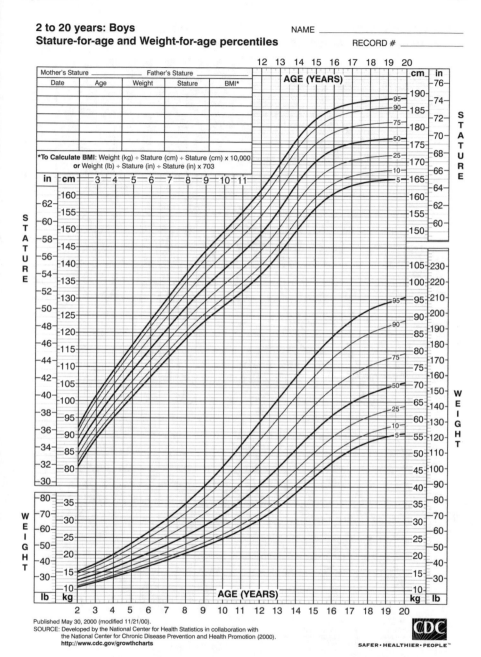

**2 to 20 years: Boys**
**Stature-for-age and Weight-for-age percentiles**

Fig. 1 Centers for Disease Control and Prevention (CDC), Pediatric Growth Chart for Boys aged 2–20 years. Stature-for-age & weight-for-age percentiles. Developed by the National Center for Health Statistics in collaboration with the National Center for Chronic Disease Prevention and Health Promotion (2000)

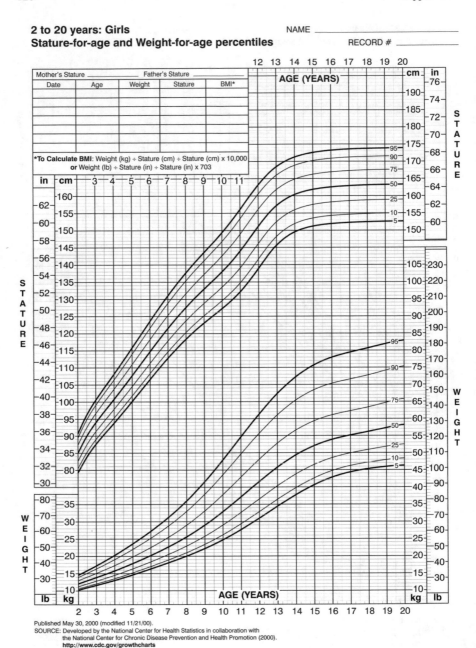

**2 to 20 years: Girls**
**Stature-for-age and Weight-for-age percentiles**

NAME _____

RECORD # _____

Published May 30, 2000 (modified 11/21/00).
SOURCE: Developed by the National Center for Health Statistics in collaboration with
the National Center for Chronic Disease Prevention and Health Promotion (2000).
http://www.cdc.gov/growthcharts

**Fig. 2** Centers for Disease Control and Prevention (CDC), Pediatric Growth Chart for Girls aged 2–20 years. Stature-for-age & weight-for-age percentiles. Developed by the National Center for Health Statistics in collaboration with the National Center for Chronic Disease Prevention and Health Promotion (2000)

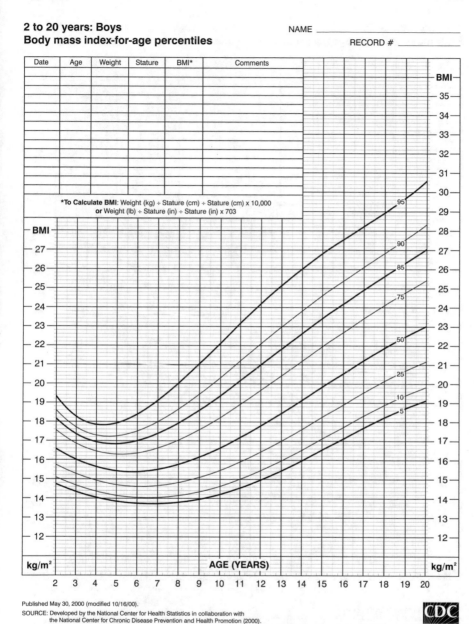

**2 to 20 years: Boys**
**Body mass index-for-age percentiles**

NAME _____

RECORD # _____

**Fig. 3** Centers for Disease Control and Prevention (CDC), Pediatric Growth Chart for Boys aged 2–20 years. Body Mass Index-for-age percentiles. Developed by the National Center for Health Statistics in collaboration with the National Center for Chronic Disease Prevention and Health Promotion (2000)

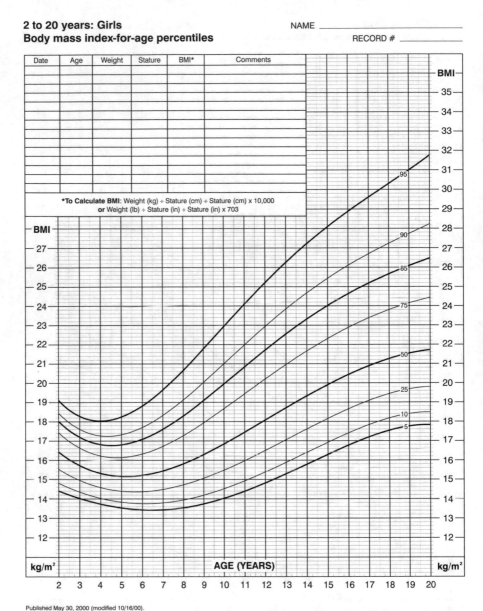

**Fig. 4** Centers for Disease Control and Prevention (CDC), Pediatric Growth Chart for Girls aged 2–20 years. Body Mass Index-for-age percentiles. Developed by the National Center for Health Statistics in collaboration with the National Center for Chronic Disease Prevention and Health Promotion (2000)

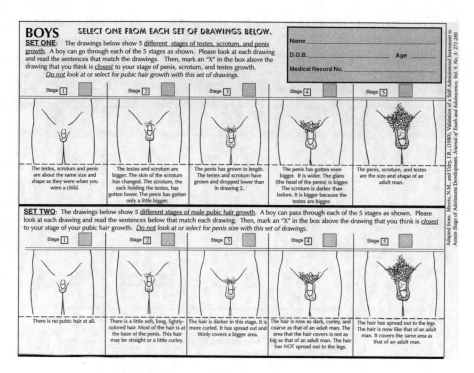

Adapted from: Morris, N.M., and Udry, J.R., (1980), Validation of a Self-Administered Instrument to Assess Stage of Adolescent Development. *Journal of Youth and Adolescence*, Vol. 9, No. 3: 271-280.

**BOYS**   SELECT ONE FROM EACH SET OF DRAWINGS BELOW.

**SET ONE:** The drawings below show 5 different stages of testes, scrotum, and penis growth. A boy can go through each of the 5 stages as shown. Please look at each drawing and read the sentences that match the drawings. Then, mark an "X" in the box above the drawing that you think is *closest* to your stage of penis, scrotum, and testes growth. *Do not look at or select for pubic hair growth with this set of drawings.*

Name _____
D.O.B. _____   Age _____
Medical Record No. _____

Stage 1 — The testes, scrotum and penis are about the same size and shape as they were when you were a child.

Stage 2 — The testes and scrotum are bigger. The skin of the scrotum has changed. The scrotum, the sack holding the testes, has gotten lower. The penis has gotten only a little bigger.

Stage 3 — The penis has grown in length. The testes and scrotum have grown and dropped lower than in drawing 2.

Stage 4 — The penis has gotten even bigger. It is wider. The glans (the head of the penis) is bigger. The scrotum is darker than before. It is bigger because the testes are bigger.

Stage 5 — The penis, scrotum, and testes are the size and shape of an adult man.

**SET TWO:** The drawings below show 5 different stages of male pubic hair growth. A boy can pass through each of the 5 stages as shown. Please look at each drawing and read the sentences below that match each drawing. Then, mark an "X" in the box above the drawing that you think is *closest* to your stage of your pubic hair growth. *Do not look at or select for penis size with this set of drawings.*

Stage 1 — There is no pubic hair at all.

Stage 2 — There is a little soft, long, lightly-colored hair. Most of the hair is at the base of the penis. This hair may be straight or a little curley.

Stage 3 — The hair is darker in this stage. It is more curled. It has spread out and thinly covers a bigger area.

Stage 4 — The hair is now as dark, curley, and coarse as that of an adult man. The area that the hair covers is not as big as that of an adult man. The hair has NOT spread out to the legs.

Stage 5 — The hair has spread out to the legs. The hair is now like that of an adult man. It covers the same area as that of an adult man.

**Fig. 5** Self-administered pubertal assessment form: boys. Adapted from Morris NM and Udry JR. J Youth Adolescence 1980; 9(3) 271–80. With Permission

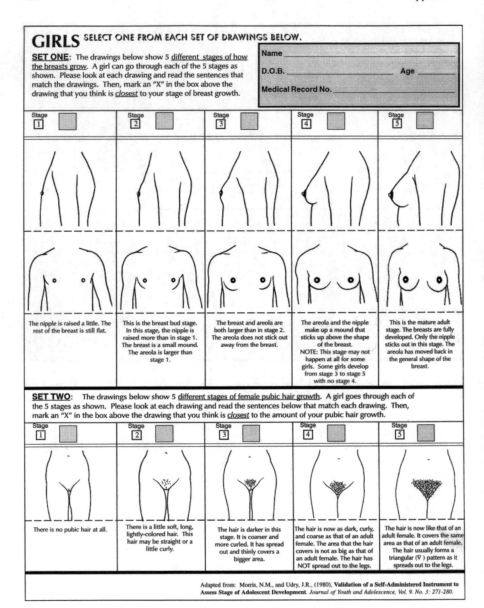

**GIRLS** SELECT ONE FROM EACH SET OF DRAWINGS BELOW.

**SET ONE:** The drawings below show 5 different stages of how the breasts grow. A girl can go through each of the 5 stages as shown. Please look at each drawing and read the sentences that match the drawings. Then, mark an "X" in the box above the drawing that you think is closest to your stage of breast growth.

Name _____
D.O.B. _____ Age _____
Medical Record No. _____

| Stage 1 | Stage 2 | Stage 3 | Stage 4 | Stage 5 |
|---|---|---|---|---|
| The nipple is raised a little. The rest of the breast is still flat. | This is the breast bud stage. In this stage, the nipple is raised more than in stage 1. The breast is a small mound. The areola is larger than stage 1. | The breast and areola are both larger than in stage 2. The areola does not stick out away from the breast. | The areola and the nipple make up a mound that sticks up above the shape of the breast. NOTE: This stage may not happen at all for some girls. Some girls develop from stage 3 to stage 5 with no stage 4. | This is the mature adult stage. The breasts are fully developed. Only the nipple sticks out in this stage. The areola has moved back in the general shape of the breast. |

**SET TWO:** The drawings below show 5 different stages of female pubic hair growth. A girl goes through each of the 5 stages as shown. Please look at each drawing and read the sentences below that match each drawing. Then, mark an "X" in the box above the drawing that you think is closest to the amount of your pubic hair growth.

| Stage 1 | Stage 2 | Stage 3 | Stage 4 | Stage 5 |
|---|---|---|---|---|
| There is no pubic hair at all. | There is a little soft, long, lightly-colored hair. This hair may be straight or a little curly. | The hair is darker in this stage. It is coarser and more curled. It has spread out and thinly covers a bigger area. | The hair is now as dark, curly, and coarse as that of an adult female. The area that the hair covers is not as big as that of an adult female. The hair has NOT spread out to the legs. | The hair is now like that of an adult female. It covers the same area as that of an adult female. The hair usually forms a triangular (∇) pattern as it spreads out to the legs. |

Adapted from: Morris, N.M., and Udry, J.R., (1980), **Validation of a Self-Administered Instrument to Assess Stage of Adolescent Development**. *Journal of Youth and Adolescence, Vol. 9. No. 3: 271-280.*

**Fig. 6** Self-administered pubertal assessment form: girls. Adapted from Morris NM and Udry JR. J Youth Adolescence 1980; 9(3) 271–80. With Permission

# Appendix C

**Table 1** Universal standardized equations

| |
|---|
| **Posteroanterior spine BMD conversions among central DXA devices** |
| Hologic QDR-2000 = (0.906 × Lunar DPX-L) − 0.025 |
| Hologic QDR-2000 = (0.912 × Norland XR-26 ) + 0.088 |
| Lunar DPX-L = (1.074 × Hologic QDR-2000) + 0.054 |
| Lunar DPX-L = (0.995 × Norland XR-26) + 0.135 |
| Norland XR-26 = (0.983 × Lunar DPX-L) − 0.112 |
| Norland XR-26 = (1.068 × Hologic QDR-2000) − 0.07 |
| **sBMD (mg/cm²) conversion formulas for manufacturer-specific** |
| *Spine BMD* |
| SBMD = 1000 (1.0761 × Norland XR-26 BMDspine) |
| SBMD = 1000 (0.9522 × Lunar DPX-L BMDspine) |
| SBMD = 1000 (1.0755 × Hologic QDR-2000 BMDspine) |
| **Standardized BMD (sBMD, mg/cm²) conversion formulas for manufacturer-specific** |
| *Total hip BMD* |
| SBMD = 1000 [(1.012 × Norland XR-26 BMDhip) + 0.006] |
| SBMD = 1000 [(0.979 × Lunar DPX-L BMDhip) − 0.031] |
| SBMD = 1000 [(1.008 × Hologic QDR-2000 BMDhip) + 0.006] |

*Note*: although specific models of the central dual-energy X-ray absoptiometry (DXA) devices are noted in the equations, the formulas may be used to convert bone mineral density (BMD) measured on any model for a given manufacturer to the BMD for a model of the other manufacturer. However, it must be recognized that these formulas were generated from data obtained on *adult patients only*. Also, the errors inherent in these conversions are too great to allow for serial monitoring of BMD to be useful among different manufacturers. All equations are multiplied by 1000 to express the standardized BMD (sBMD) in Data from Genant HK, Grampp S, Gleur CC, Faulkner KG, Jergas M, Engelke K, Hagiwara S, Van Kuijk C. Universal standardization for dual X-ray absorptiometry: Patient and phantom cross-calibration results. J Bone Miner Res 1994;9:1503–1514; and Hanson J. Standardization of femur BMD. J Bone Miner Res 1997;12:1316–1317

© Springer International Publishing Switzerland 2016
E.B. Fung et al. (eds.), *Bone Health Assessment in Pediatrics*,
DOI 10.1007/978-3-319-30412-0

**Table 2** Important calculations and conversions

---

**English to metric:**

Length: 1 in. = 2.54 cm

Weight 1 lb = 0.45 kg

**Metric to English:**

Length: 1 cm = 0.39 in.

Weight: 1 kg = 2.2 lb

**Temperature:**

$°F = (1.8 × °C) + 32$

**Radiation dosages:**

Gray = Gy

Sieverts = Sv

1 mrad = 10 $\mu$Gy

1 mREM = 10 $\mu$Sv

**Z-score=** $\dfrac{\text{(observed − mean*)}}{\text{Standard deviation}}$

The number of standard deviations by which the measured value departs from the *mean value of individuals matched for age and gender

**T-score=** $\dfrac{\text{(observed − mean*)}}{\text{Standard deviation}}$

The number of standard deviations by which the measured value departs from the *mean value of a group of healthy 25- to 35-yr-old individuals

---

**Table 3** Lateral distal femur reference data

# *The Lateral Distal Femur (LDF)*

An Alternative Site for Measuring Bone Mineral Density by DXA

## URL: www.lateraldistalfemur.org

*Purpose:* This site is designed to serve as the resource for information about the Lateral Distal Femur (LDF)

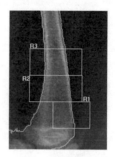

| | DXA Technologists |
| --- | --- |
| *Target* | Pediatricians |
| Audience: | Physicians managing patients with disabilities |
| | Clinicians interpreting DXA |
| | Bone research personnel |

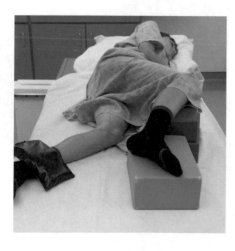

*Overview:* The LDF technique is described on this website, including:

- Origins of the technique
- Application of the LDF and target populations
- Scan acquisition instructions
- Scan analysis instructions
- Normative values
- Interpretation of results
- Examples of analyzed scans
- Selected bibliography
- Links to other bone densitometry resources

www.lateraldistalfemur.org

# Appendix D

## *Forms and Handouts*

As many institutions are shifting from paper forms to the Electronic Medical Record (EMR), few institutions are using traditional referral forms and paper registration forms. For those that do, we have provided a few examples here in the Appendix that may be useful.

For institutions that use EMR, for which the DXA order is placed online, often the ordering physician will be asked to complete basic questions about the referred patient which may include: patient diagnosis, reason for referral, medication and history of fracture, need for interpreter services, and presence of developmental delays, mobility status, and existence of non-removable metal (e.g. spinal rods).

Similarly, for DXA reporting, notes can be dictated or entered directly into the EMR using a series of templates for various different types of patients (pediatric-general; pediatric – motor impairment, with distal femur scan; Pediatric – Short Stature requiring height adjustment). For key elements to be included in the Pediatric DXA report, please refer to Chapter 7.

© Springer International Publishing Switzerland 2016
E.B. Fung et al. (eds.), *Bone Health Assessment in Pediatrics*,
DOI 10.1007/978-3-319-30412-0

***Bone Densitometry Clinic***
***Departmental Referral for DXA Scan***
*< Local address here >*
*Phone: (XXX) XXX-XXXX     Fax: (XXX) XXX-XXXX     Email: XXX@XXX.XXXX*

Ordering Doctor or Provider_____
Clinic Address:_____
Phone:_____     Fax:_____

Patient Name:_____

Date of Birth:___/___/____ Medical Record#:_____

Parent/Guardian Name_____

Primary Diagnosis_____ ICD-10 Code:_____

Reason for Referral:_____

Type of Insurance:_____ Authorization #:_____

Interpreter services required        Yes            No
        If yes, language spoken:_____

Current list of medications:_____

Fracture history      Yes      No
        If yes, briefly list: _____

Bone Age:      Yes      No
        If Yes, result:_____

Comments_____

**Fig. 1** Example referral form

Please complete this questionnaire while waiting for your bone mineral density test.
This document will be reviewed with you. A staff member will measure your height and weight.

Name: _____Date: _____

Date of Birth: _____ Female    Male

*If you answer yes to any of the following 3 questions, please speak to the receptionist immediately*

1.  Is there any chance that you are pregnant?                          ☐ Yes        ☐ No

2.  Have you had a barium enema or barium drink in the last 2 weeks?  ☐ Yes        ☐ No

3.  Have you had a nuclear medicine scan or x-ray dye in the last week? ☐ Yes      ☐ No

*The following information will help us to assess your future risk for fracture.*

4.  Have you ever had a bone density test before?                      ☐ Yes        ☐ No

    If yes, when and where? _____

5.  Have you ever had surgery of the spine or hips?                    ☐ Yes        ☐ No

6.  Have you ever broken any bones?                                    ☐ Yes        ☐ No

    If yes please state:

| Bone Broken | Age Bone Broken | Cause of Broken Bone |
|---|---|---|
|  |  |  |
|  |  |  |
|  |  |  |
|  |  |  |

7.  Have you taken steroid pills (such as prednisone or cortisone)      ☐ Yes        ☐ No

    For more than 3 months in the last 12 months?

    If yes, are you currently taking steroid pills?                    ☐ Yes        ☐ No

    How long have you been taking them?_____

    What is your current dose? _____

    What is the reason you take steroid pills? _____

8.  Have you ever been treated with medications for osteoporosis?      ☐ Yes        ☐ No

    If yes, which medication(s), and for how long? _____

_____

*From the Department of Diagnostic Imaging, The Hospital for Sick Children; Toronto, ON, Canada*

**Fig. 2** Example patient questionnaire

## University of Manchester

**Patient Information**
Name: _____DOB: _____ID:_____
Primary Disease: _____Time since diagnosis: _____
Any other health problems: _____
Height: _____ Weight: _____BMI: _____

**Original Referral**                          **DXA Referral**
Consultant Specialty: _____          Consultant Specialty:_____
Hospital _____              Hospital_____

**Fractures:**

| | | |
|---|---|---|
| Have you ever fractured any bones | ☐ Yes | ☐ No |

If yes, when, which bone, and how?_____

Have you had any persistent back pain in the last 12 months?   ☐ Yes   ☐ No

Has a family member suffered from osteoporosis?   ☐ Yes   ☐ No
    If yes, who?_____

**Mobility and Physical Activity: Mobile patients**
How much physical activity do you do per week?
    ☐ Less than 2 hours (school activity only)
    ☐ 3-5 hours (school + organized activities)
    ☐ More than 5 hours (sports clubs)

Have you had any periods of immobility?   ☐ Yes   ☐ No
    If yes, when and for how long?_____

**Mobility and Physical Activity: Immobile patients**

| How do you usually get around? | Never | Occasionally | Frequently | Always |
|---|---|---|---|---|
| Walk | ☐ | ☐ | ☐ | ☐ |
| Walk with crutches | ☐ | ☐ | ☐ | ☐ |
| Chair | ☐ | ☐ | ☐ | ☐ |
| Bed | ☐ | ☐ | ☐ | ☐ |

Do you use a standing frame?   ☐ Yes   ☐ No
    If yes, how often?_____

Do you have a regular hydrotherapy   ☐ Yes   ☐ No
    If yes, how often?_____

Do you have any other physical activity?   ☐ Yes   ☐ No
    If yes, how often?_____

**Diet**
Do you have any feeding or nutritional problems?   ☐ Yes   ☐ No
    If yes, please give details: _____
If no, how much milk do you drink daily?

| | | | |
|---|---|---|---|
| None | ☐ | ½ to ¾ pint (450 mL) | ☐ |
| 0- ¼ pint (150 mL) | ☐ | ¾ to 1 pint (600 mL) | ☐ |
| ¼-1/2 pint (300 mL) | ☐ | More than 1 pint (600 mL) | ☐ |

**Fig. 3** Children's bone density registration questionnaire

| How often do you eat the following foods? | Occasionally | 1-3 times/wk | Most days |
|---|---|---|---|
| Cheese | ☐ | ☐ | ☐ |
| Yogurt | ☐ | ☐ | ☐ |
| Ice Cream | ☐ | ☐ | ☐ |
| Fromage Frais | ☐ | ☐ | ☐ |
| Milk Chocolate | ☐ | ☐ | ☐ |
| Milk Pudding | ☐ | ☐ | ☐ |

Do you take a calcium supplement?        ☐ Yes      ☐ No

Do you take a vitamin supplement?        ☐ Yes      ☐ No

**Medications**

Do you or have you ever taken oral corticosteroids (e.g. prednisolone?)  ☐ Yes      ☐ No
  If yes, how much and for how long?_____

Do you take any medication for your bones (e.g. pamidronate?)    ☐ Yes      ☐ No
  If yes, for how long?_____

Hve you ever taken hormone replacement therapy (HRT) or the oral contraceptive pill?

                                                          ☐ Yes      ☐ No
  If yes, for how long?_____

Do you take any other medications?                        ☐ Yes      ☐ No
  If yes, which ones, and for how long?_____

**Puberty**

Do you have any signs of puberty?                         ☐ Yes      ☐ No

If yes, please complete the appropriate information below using the pubertal self-assessment tool provided:
  *Girls:*                          *Boys:*
  Age at menarche: _____yr       Age at voice breaking: _____ yr
  Regular     ☐ Yes   ☐ No           Testicular volume: _____
  Pubic hair:           1 2 3 4 5    Pubic hair:    1 2 3 4 5
  Breast development:   1 2 3 4 5

*(Taken from, "A practical guide to bone densitometry in children: National Osteoporosis Society, November, 2004)*

**Fig. 3** (continued)

Patient's Name (Last, First):_____ Today's Date:____/____/_____

Gender:  o Male     o Female                          Date of Birth: ____/____/_____

Ethnicity (*circle the group that best describes your child*):   Asian / Black / Hispanic / White

Referring Doctor: _____ Department:_____
                   (who you would like to receive report)

Have you had this type of examination before?        o Yes    o No

    If yes, where did you have this done?_____

Have you ever been told you have scoliosis or a curvature of the spine?  o Yes    o No

Why have you been referred for a bone density scan? _____

Have you ever had surgery on your hip?        o Yes    o No

If yes, which hip was it performed on?          o Right  o Left   o Both

Do you participate in at least 60 min of physical activity every day?      o Yes    o No

Have you ever broken (fractured) a bone?                       o Yes    o No

    If yes, when was your last fracture? _____

Have you had any exams within the last 7 days where a contrast material was used (e.g. barium, MRI)?

    If so, which exam? _____When was this done?_____

Does your family have a history of osteoporosis?                     o Yes    o No

 If yes, please describe relation to patient (e.g. mother, grandmother, aunt etc.)_____

 If yes, was this a hip fracture?_____ Is this person taking medication for osteoporosis?_____

Have you ever taken corticosteroids (e.g. steroids/prednisone)?      o Yes    o No

Do you currently take any prescribed medications?              o Yes    o No

    If so, please list them here:_____

Do you take **calcium supplements** on a regular basis?     o Yes    o No

    If yes, how much?_____mg   and how frequently? _____

Do you take **vitamin D supplements** on a regular basis?     o Yes    o No

    If yes, how much?_____IU   and how frequently? _____

**For FEMALE patients only:**  Have you begun to menstruate?                 o Yes    o No

                If yes, Do you have a regular menstrual period?        o Yes    o No

          Is there any chance that you may be pregnant?        o Yes    o No

**Calcium Intake:**   For each food listed below, please indicate the number of servings you (the patient) consumes of these calcium rich foods <u>in a typical week</u>. If you consume 1/2 cup of milk on your cereal each morning you can respond:      Milk = 0.5 servings per day **OR**  3.5 servings per week

|  | Serving Size | # servings / week |
|---|---|---|
| Milk any type (including fortified soy milk) alone or in co | 1 cup |  |
| Calcium fortified orange juice | 1 cup |  |
| Yogurt | 1 cup |  |
| Cheese (alone or in sandwiches, casseroles etc) | 1 slice |  |
| Ice Cream, frozen yogurt, pudding or custards | ½ cup |  |
| Macaroni & cheese, quesadillas, tacos/burritos | 1 cup or item |  |
| Pizza (any type) | 1 slice |  |
| Tofu | ½ cup |  |
| Beans (white, navy, pinto, baked) | ½ cup |  |
| Almonds or Pistachios | 1 oz (about 24) |  |
| Cooked green vegetables | ½ cup |  |
| Breakfast Cereal: specify cereal type:_____ | 1 cup |  |

**Fig. 4**  Bone densitometry clinic – children's registration questionnaire

# Index

© Springer International Publishing Switzerland 2016
E.B. Fung et al. (eds.), *Bone Health Assessment in Pediatrics*,
DOI 10.1007/978-3-319-30412-0

Printed in the United States
By Bookmasters